TUBERCULOSIS

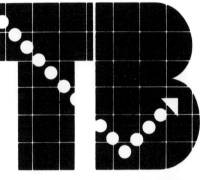

BACK TO THE FUTURE

London School of Hygiene & Tropical Medicine
Third Annual Public Health Forum

TUBERCULOSIS

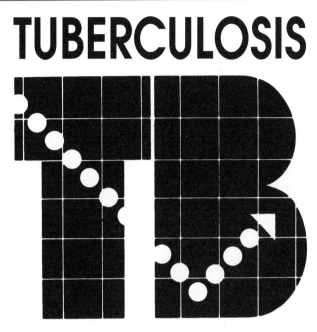

BACK TO THE FUTURE

Edited by
John D.H. Porter and Keith P.W.J. McAdam

Series Editor
Barbara M. Judge

*London School of Hygiene
& Tropical Medicine*

JOHN WILEY & SONS

Chichester · New York · Brisbane · Toronto · Singapore

RA644.T7 L747 1994
London School of Hygiene and
Tropical Medicine Public
Health Forum (3rd : 1993)
Tuberculosis : back to the
future

Jacaranda Wiley Ltd, 33 Park Road, Milton,
Queensland 4064, Australia

John Wiley & Sons (Canada) Ltd, 22 Worcester Road,
Rexdale, Ontario M9W 1L1, Canada

John Wiley & Sons (SEA) Pte Ltd, 37 Jalan Pemimpin #05-04,
Block B, Union Industrial Building, Singapore 2057

Library of Congress Cataloging-in-Publication Data

London School of Hygiene and Tropical Medicine Public Health Forum (3rd : 1993)
    Tuberculosis : back to the future/edited by John D.H. Porter and Keith P.W.J. McAdam.
        p.   cm.
    "London School of Hygiene & Tropical Medicine Third Annual Public Health Forum."
    Forum was held Apr. 18–21, 1993.
    Includes bibliographical references and index.
    ISBN 0–471–94121–2.
    1. Tuberculosis — Congresses. I. Porter, John D.H. II. McAdam, Keither P.W.J. III. Title.
    [DNLM: 1. Tuberculosis — congresses. 2. Developing Countries — congresses. WF 200 L847t
1993].
    RA644. T7L747 1993.
    616.9'95—dc20
    DNLM/DCL
for Library of Congress   93-38817
                                                                                      CIP

British Library Cataloguing in Publication Data

A catalogue record for this book is available from the British Library

ISBN 0 471 94121 2 (cloth)
ISBN 0 471 94346 0 (paper)

Typeset in 10/12 Times by Mackreth Media Services, Hemel Hempstead
Printed and bound in Great Britain by Bookcraft (Bath) Ltd

Contents

Contributors

Barry R. Bloom Weinstock Professor, Department of Microbiology and Immunology, The Albert Einstein College of Medicine, Forchheimer Building, 1300 Morris Park Avenue, Bronx, New York 10461, USA

Reginald C. Boulos Director General, Centres pour le Développement et la Santé, 16 Rue Frères Simmonds, Cité Militaire, PO Box 1666, Port-au-Prince, Haiti

Jaap F. Broekmans Director, Royal Netherlands Tuberculosis Association, PO Box 146, 2501 CC The Hague, The Netherlands

Stewart T. Cole Chef, Unité de Génétique Moléculaire Bactérienne, Institut Pasteur, 28 rue du Dr Roux, 75724 Paris, Cedex 15, France

M. Joseph Colston Head, Laboratory for Leprosy and Mycobacterial Research, MRC National Institute of Medical Research, The Ridgeway, Mill Hill, London NW7 1AA, UK

Sir John Crofton Professor Emeritus of Respiratory Diseases and Tuberculosis, University of Edinburgh, UK

Kevin M. de Cock Department of Clinical Sciences, London School of Hygiene & Tropical Medicine, Keppel Street, London WC1E 7HT, UK, *and* Centers for Disease Control and Prevention, Atlanta, GA 30333, USA

Hazel M. Dockrell Department of Clinical Sciences, London School of Hygiene & Tropical Medicine, Keppel Street, London WC1E 7HT, UK

Alison M. Elliott Fellow in Infectious Diseases, University of Colorado, Health Services Center, 4200 E 9th Avenue, Denver, Colorado, USA

Jerrold J. Ellner Professor of Medicine and Pathology, Case Western Reserve University School of Medicine, 10900 Euclid Avenue, Cleveland, Ohio 44106-4984, USA

Donald A. Enarson Director of Scientific Activities, International Union against Tuberculosis and Lung Disease, 68 boulevard Saint Michel, 75006 Paris, France

Paul E.M. Fine Communicable Disease Epidemiology Unit, Department of Epidemiology and Population Sciences, London School of Hygiene & Tropical Medicine, Keppel Street, London WC1E 7HT, UK

William H. Foege Fellow for Health Policy, The Carter Center Inc, 1 Copenhill, Atlanta, Georgia 3037, USA

Susan Foster Department of Public Health and Policy, London School of Hygiene & Tropical Medicine, Keppel Street, London WC1E 7HT, UK

Erik Glatthaar Head, Department of Community Health, Faculty of Medicine, University of Pretoria, PO Box 667, Pretoria 0001, Republic of South Africa

Peter Godfrey-Faussett ZAMBART Project, Department of Medicine, Lusaka, Zambia and Department of Clinical Sciences, London School of Hygiene & Tropical Medicine, Keppel Street, London WC1E 7HT, UK

Jacques H. Grosset Head, Department of Bacteriology and Virology, Laboratoire Central de Bacteriologie, Groupe Hospitalier Pitie-Salpetrière, 75651 Paris, France

Ralph H. Henderson Assistant Director-General, World Health Organization, CH-1211 Geneva 27, Switzerland

Philip C. Hopewell Chief, Division of Pulmonary and Critical Care Medicine, University of California, San Francisco General Hospital, 1001 Potrero Avenue, San Francisco, California 94110, USA

D.K. Kibuga Head, National Leprosy and Tuberculosis Programme, Ministry of Health, Nairobi, Kenya

Richard O. Laing Drug Use Coordinator, Management Sciences for Health, 165 Allandale Road, Boston, Massachusetts 02130, USA

Keith P.W.J. McAdam Head, Department of Clinical Sciences, London School of Hygiene & Tropical Medicine, Keppel Street, London WC1E 7HT, UK

Denis A. Mitchison Department of Bacteriology, Royal Postgraduate Medical School, University of London, Hammersmith Hospital, Du Cane Road, London W12 0NN

Dale L. Morse Visiting Consultant Epidemiologist, Field Service Unit, PHLS Communicable Disease Surveillance Centre, 61 Colindale Avenue, London

NW9 5EQ, UK. Director, Bureau of Communicable Disease Control and State Epidemiologist for the New York Department of Health, Albany, New York, USA

Christopher J.L. Murray Center for Population and Development Studies, Harvard University, Roger and Ellen Revelle Building, 9 Bow Street, Cambridge, Massachusetts 02138, USA

Alwyn G. Mwinga Department of Medicine, University of Zambia, PO Box 50110, Lusaka, Zambia

Paul Nunn Medical Officer, Operational Research Unit, Tuberculosis Programme, World Health Organization, CH-1211 Geneva 27, Switzerland

Richard J. O'Brien Medical Officer, Tuberculosis Programme, World Health Organization, CH-1211 Geneva 27, Switzerland

Michel Pletschette DG-XII, B-4, STD-Health, Commission of the European Communities, 200 rue de la Loi, B-1040 Brussels, Belgium

John D.H. Porter Department of Clinical Sciences, London School of Hygiene & Tropical Medicine, Keppel Street, London WC1E 7HT, UK

Graham A.W. Rook Department of Medical Microbiology, University College London Medical School, 67–73 Riding House Street, London W1P 7PP, UK

M. Angelica Salomão Chief of Division of Endemic Disease, Ministry of Health, CP 264, Maputo, Mozambique

Peter G. Smith Head, Department of Epidemiology and Population Sciences, London School of Hygiene & Tropical Medicine, Keppel Street, London WC1E 7HT, UK

Dixie E. Snider Jr Associate Director for Science, National Center for Prevention Services, Centers for Disease Control and Prevention, Atlanta, Georgia 30333, USA

John L. Stanford Department of Medical Microbiology, University College London Medical School, 67–73 Riding House Street, London W1P 7PP, UK

Neil G. Stoker Department of Clinical Sciences, London School of Hygiene & Tropical Medicine, Keppel Street, London WC1E 7HT, UK

Richard B. Sykes Deputy Chairman and Chief Executive, Glaxo Holdings plc, Lansdowne House, Berkeley Square, London W1X 6BP, UK

Jan D.A. van Embden Head, Molecular Microbiology Unit, National Institute of Public Health and Environmental Protection, Antonie van Leeuwenhoeklaan 9, PO Box 1, 3720 BA Bilthoven, The Netherlands

Diana E.C. Weil Operational Research Officer, Tuberculosis Programme, World Health Organization, CH-1211, Geneva 27, Switzerland

Douglas B. Young MRC Tuberculosis and Related Infections Unit, Royal Postgraduate Medical School, Hammersmith Hospital, Du Cane Road, London W12 0HS, UK

Foreword

Opening Address to the Forum from
the Rt Hon. the Baroness Chalker of Wallasey,
Minister for Overseas Development

Two years ago the London School held its first Annual Public Health Forum—on malaria. This major communicable disease was once thought to have been conquered. Yet it is back—with a vengeance. Participants considered how best to tackle malaria while we wait for a vaccine. The London School's Malaria Forum paved the way for much international effort: the latest milestone is the WHO's conference on malaria in Amsterdam last autumn. I want to reflect on some of the conclusions of the Malaria Forum. Perhaps this is my way of going 'Back to the Future!'

The Forum agreed that malaria is having a massive debilitating effect on human populations and that the situation has worsened in recent years. It concluded that urgent responses are essential and called for national and local malaria control programmes to make cost effective use of existing tools for controlling the parasite and its vector, or for mitigating the disease. There was also general agreement that present tools are inadequate and that new—and effective—means to combat both parasite and mosquito are sorely needed. The Forum concluded that well-targeted high quality, scientific research is needed to develop these tools. I would not be surprised if the conclusions of this Forum have a similar ring to them.

My Senior Health and Population Adviser, Dr Pene Key, spoke at the Malaria Forum. She said, 'As we consider the scientific solutions, we must take a responsible look at the context in which they are to be delivered. National governments (of developing countries) have to face harsh realities, they have to choose the problems that they will tackle, and select the most cost-effective technologies.' These words apply to many of the serious health problems faced by people of developing countries—HIV disease, high blood pressure, diarrhoea, unsafe motherhood and even mental illness. They apply also to tuberculosis.

The harsh realities have changed little over the last two years. Recurrent public expenditure on health averaging between $2 and $5 per person per year. Ministers of Health tell me that not all the priorities seen as urgent or vital by their health professionals can possibly be met from the public purse. They face public outcry because their health systems are falling apart. As a result of cash shortages they cannot pay adequate salaries to their staff. Nor can they purchase sufficient fuel for their vehicles, maintain health centres or purchase drugs and dressings. We donors sometimes help to meet the recurrent costs of priority activities, but this is only a short-term solution.

ODA is trying to help governments with the long-term and difficult task of restructuring health—and other—sectors. Ministers of health have to take account of the limited budget available for health care. At the same time, developing country Health Ministers have to tackle the priority health needs of their people. They try to concentrate their funds on cost-effective health care. They are expected to maintain tight control of expenditure. Ministers tell me that they have to make very hard choices. I know that these are often unpopular with different vested interests.

Ministers responsible for bilateral aid also have to make hard choices. My officials and I spend hours agreeing the allocation of our precious funds between activities, or between countries, especially if each makes a strong case. Similar difficulties are faced when we divide the diminishing cake between different international programmes that are each designed to tackle a priority health problem. We do not find it easy to choose between competing demands for research when each claims to be finding solutions to a pressing global problem.

Tuberculosis is a world health problem of staggering proportions. Like malaria it has returned to haunt us, and seems to be getting worse. It is a disease of poverty, affecting many millions of people in the world's poorest countries. And it is difficult—and expensive—to control. This Forum is an excellent opportunity for the world's experts on tuberculosis to guide those of us who allocate resources between competing priorities. We want to learn from those involved in the fight against TB. We want to know how the battle progresses. We want Forum participants to tell us how we should deploy our limited resources to best effect.

ODA has come to expect a lot of London School Fora. We expect much from this one, too. I thought I would share some of these expectations with you—not least to know whether our thoughts are on the right track.

We know that the Forum will review the severity of tuberculosis as a global health problem. How does the disability caused by TB compare with that caused by malaria, infections of childhood and non-communicable diseases? The Forum will examine the impact of HIV disease on TB in the world today. We hope that it will explain the way in which HIV will alter the pattern of TB in tomorrow's world and guide us on how we can minimise some of the dire consequences of the HIV/TB interaction that have been predicted in the media during recent months.

We know that TB control will be considered. We have three expectations here. Firstly, we hope that the Forum will undertake a thorough review of existing measures to prevent TB infection and control the disease, examining both their effectiveness and their costs. We would like it to reach conclusions about their utility in different situations. Secondly, we hope that the Forum will look at national and international strategies for TB control in the context of resources—both cash and people—that governments invest in them. Are these strategies feasible and affordable? Thirdly, we hope that the Forum will look at systems for financing and managing TB control strategies. How do we ensure that governments have the people, the institutions and the management systems needed to implement these strategies successfully?

We would like to know what is thought of the control measures available now or, at least, being field tested. Is there a range of promising new tools on the horizon? Should all of us involved in the financing and management of health care reconsider the priority we give to tuberculosis? Should we question the present tendency to integrate TB control into the existing elements of primary health care? We know the Forum will be thinking about research: we would like its views on priority areas for future research in tuberculosis. We hope the Forum will be able to suggest how the limited funds available for research can most efficiently be used.

TB has been described as an 'inseparable but terrible companion of man.' We all have to live with the tubercle bacillus around us. We cannot afford to let it win. The challenge is to find cost-effective means by which we can maintain the upper hand. I expect that the discussions at the Forum will be of enormous significance in the ongoing battle. I hope that this meeting will be a watershed. I wish the Forum well in its vital mission.

Preface

The Third Annual Public Health Forum at the London School of Hygiene and Tropical Medicine was held between April 18–21, 1993 on the topic of 'tuberculosis—back to the future.' Each year the Forum addresses an international public health issue and this year the Forum focused on tuberculosis in developing countries.

The objectives of the Forum were:

- To bring together for constructive interaction scientists working on different aspects of tuberculosis research and public health experts involved in planning and implementing control strategies.
- To describe the global burden of tuberculosis and predict the likely trends over the next decade with special attention to the impact of the HIV epidemic.
- To identify and prioritise major research issues relating to: pathogenesis, diagnosis, clinical management, molecular biology, epidemiology, economics and control of tuberculosis.
- To address specific questions relating to: diagnosis and clinical management, immunology and vaccination, chemoprophylaxis and drug therapy, control strategies and resource allocation.
- To raise international awareness of the challenge facing international public health by the epidemic of tuberculosis accompanying HIV infection.
- and to produce a major publication on the current state of the art of tuberculosis research and control.

The 1980s and 1990s have seen a resurgence of tuberculosis. Changes in the environment lead to changes in the epidemiology of infectious diseases and tuberculosis is an example of how the altered economic and social patterns in the world have lead to a change in the characteristics and distribution of this disease. Tuberculosis is essentially a disease of poverty and deprivation and by joining forces with the human immunodeficiency virus (HIV), another infectious disease which also affects economically deprived populations, it has once again made us all aware of the divisions in the world. We recognise the political conflicts which lead to mass migrations of people encouraging the spread of diseases like tuberculosis, of the widening economic gulf between the north and the south and of the world economic recession which has lead to increased homelessness in industrialised countries and the collapse of health care infrastructures in some developing countries.

When we started to plan the Forum two years ago, we decided that a major objective was to bring together scientists working in all areas of tuberculosis, to provide the opportunity for dialogue between professionals in different scientific disciplines. We felt it was important for immunologists to speak to economists and for molecular biologists to discuss tuberculosis control issues with public health professionals in order to provide everyone attending with an overview of the problem and to help us understand where our particular research interests fit in to an overall strategy of tuberculosis control.

The Forum brought together a distinguished group of invited guests and delegates from 53 different countries. Because the Forum was orientated towards work in developing countries we made sure that as many as possible of these countries were represented. There was a particularly strong contingent from Africa, which reflects the long standing collaborative links that the London School of Hygiene and Tropical Medicine has had with many African countries.

To deal with the changing public health impact of tuberculosis, we need new imaginative ideas and the Forum challenged people with new possibilities and options for tackling their problems, whether they were immunologists, public health practitioners, economists or other health care professionals.

As Max Planck, the father of quantum theory, wrote in his autobiography, 'The pioneer scientist must have a vivid intuitive imagination for new ideas not generated by deduction, but by artistically creative imagination.' We hope that this book will highlight new ideas and strategies to deal with this great public health challenge, discussed at the Forum.

We are grateful to the major sponsors of the Forum, the Overseas Development Administration (ODA), Commission of the European Communities (CEC), the International Union against Tuberculosis and Lung Disease (IUATLD), the World Health Organization (WHO), the UK Department of Health, and the Wellcome Trust. Other organisations, notably the British Council and the Foreign and Commonwealth Office, financed the attendance of overseas delegates. A donation from Glaxo Holdings plc has enabled production of a paperback edition of this book.

The Forum programme was developed by a committee of many people at the School who work on tuberculosis. A smaller Executive Committee bore the brunt of organising this international meeting. Particular thanks go to Alice Dickens who continued the work of Andrea Bonsey as Conference Secretary and was tireless in her contribution to the running of the Forum.

As a result of the Forum and the WHO CARG Meeting which followed it, the World Health Organization declared tuberculosis to be an international public health emergency.

John Porter
Conference Director
Keith McAdam
Conference Chair

OPENING SESSION ADDRESSES

Opening Session Address I

Michel Pletschette

CEC, Brussels, Belgium

It is a great pleasure for me to greet you here at the opening of the Third Public Health Forum on tuberculosis, on behalf of the Commission of European Communities' (CEC) research programme on Life Sciences and Technologies for Developing Countries. I wish to congratulate the organizers for their timely initiative. The CEC is pleased to support this Forum. Life Sciences and Technology for Developing Countries is a research programme initiated some ten years ago and exclusively geared towards health problems in developing countries. The purpose was to mobilize resources to world health problems in developing countries and to develop appropriate research capacities in the developing world and in Europe, through coordination of research and joint research projects, accompanied by meetings and workshops. There are many former and present research contractors of our programme here at this Forum. Just under a fifth of our yearly research budget is dedicated to bacteriology, of which research on mycobacteria represents a key part. This has been so for many years, and the programme is not only related to discovering new information about tuberculosis, but is also trying to promote better use of existing knowledge. Our most recent projects share a molecular biology approach to mycobacterial infections. Roughly half of the projects deal with tuberculosis, and the other half deal with leprosy. Researchers funded by the programme are investigating the molecular basis and the epidemiology of virulent and chemoresistant strains and modern methods of their diagnosis. Other studies focus on the interaction of HIV and *Mycobacterium tuberculosis* infections. Their aim is to determine the individual contribution of reinfection, relapse or reactivation of TB in HIV-infected patients and to characterize the mycobacterial isolates from HIV-positive and HIV-negative patients with regard to differences in species, strain distribution and drug resistance.

The aforementioned projects constitute, together with projects on HIV transmission and co-transmission, the core of the ongoing AIDS research under the CEC's Life Sciences and Technologies for Developing Countries ('STD-3') programme. All the projects comply with the basic philosophy of the programme: the strengthening of the research capacities in developing countries and in Europe

Tuberculosis: Back to the Future. Edited by J.D.H. Porter and K.P.W.J. McAdam
© 1994 John Wiley & Sons Ltd

on development-related health problems with a substantial training component in each project. As the Commission's research programme is asked to focus more and more during the forthcoming years, we will have a very close look naturally at the proceedings of this Forum, from which we expect important input and support, possibly allowing for a better definition of the research issues related to tuberculosis.

Opening Session Address II

Richard B. Sykes

Glaxo Holdings plc, London, UK

Tuberculosis is a disease that many in the West believed to have been eradicated or, at the least, brought under control. But it is clear that tuberculosis has become a major health threat all round the world; it is emerging again within industrialized countries as well as the developing nations. Changes in society (with the emergence of AIDS, the increasing problems of drug addiction and homelessness) and also, perversely, advances in the practice of medicine, particularly in the fields of organ transplantation and cancer therapy, have resulted in an increasing number of immunosuppressed individuals. These individuals are not only open to infection with *Mycobacterium tuberculosis* but their condition also makes them susceptible to reactivation of the organism which has lain dormant within their bodies for years under the control of a once effective immune system.

What must be a particular concern is that we are now seeing the emergence of a variant of the organism responsible which has developed resistance to the currently available antibiotic therapies. These therapies have in the past been successful in the treatment of the TB patient. This resistant organism is now spreading from patients into health care workers looking after them. The spectre of a worldwide tuberculosis epidemic has always been in the background but must now be taken even more seriously. We should accept that the changed mycobacterium poses a very significant threat to world health. If this threat is to be averted, the academic, and health care communities together with the pharmaceutical industry and government must all accept the challenge and work together employing the arsenal of modern science to overcome the disease.

It is 50 years since Selman Waksman and his team discovered streptomycin and thus provided the first pharmaceutical alternative to fresh air, diet and exercise as the basis of tuberculosis treatment. During the years that have followed, other drugs have emerged but our knowledge of their modes of actions remains pitifully small. I think it is interesting to contrast the situation with HIV. AIDS as a disease was not identified until 1981, HIV was isolated in 1983 and its link to AIDS only established in 1984. Yet—to all intents and purposes—we had the HIV life cycle explained biochemically by 1990.

Tuberculosis: Back to the Future. Edited by J.D.H. Porter and K.P.W.J. McAdam
© 1994 John Wiley & Sons Ltd

Why is it that the basic biochemistry of the causative agent of tuberculosis is so sketchy? Simply speaking, it is because the mycobacterium is such a difficult bacterium to work with: it is so highly infectious, it has such a slow rate of growth, and the models for the intracellular form have been so poor. All these factors, and others, have combined to make a formidable barrier to better understanding.

The challenge we are now faced with requires major efforts in two fields. First, effective new drugs are required. The development of resistant mycobacteria is not new in the history of tuberculosis, and we have been faced in the past with the need for new antibiotics to deal with organisms resistant to those previously available. In this regard, we also need to bear in mind that non-tuberculosis mycobacterial species, such as *Mycobacterium avium* complex, are intrinsically more resistant to conventional drugs than TB. Their potential for infection, particularly amongst the immunocompromised, must not be overlooked either.

The problem of discovering new medicines becomes more demanding each time. And TB presents an extremely tough nut to crack for the drug hunters. As well as physical considerations, like its waxy coat that presents a barrier for drugs to cross, there are the basics of its existence in the body—tolerated by the very cells that should be destroying it. Dividing cells as a target for drug discovery are one thing; the semi-dormant, non-dividing mycobacterium hiding inside the macrophage is quite another. Now, however, we have available to us the tools of biochemistry and molecular biology. Using these we can map and sequence the genome of *Mycobacterium*, probe the mechanisms underlying its resistance to antibiotics and point the way to new targets for drug action.

The unique polymers found in the cell walls of mycobacteria clearly provide specific targets and we know that disruption of cell wall synthesis can be an effective way of dealing with infectious bacteria. However, some pretty fundamental work on the enzymes involved needs to be carried out first. Things are moving forward for the drug discoverer, though. Our ability to clone and express mycobacterial genes in other microorganisms opens up TB to researchers who do not have high containment laboratories. In addition, new, genetically-engineered screening methods are 'throwing some light' on the slow growth rate of mycobacteria and hold out the prospect of faster evaluation of drug candidates.

It is unlikely that we can prevent the emergence of yet more resistant forms of the organism in the future, and so an essential second weapon in the war against TB must be the development of more effective, and safe, vaccines to enhance the protective immune response in whole populations. The new knowledge we have gained of the cellular and molecular basis of immunology must be harnessed so that we can determine which of the surface antigens will provide a protective immune response.

The solutions to this world scale problem can be most effectively found by those working in the basic science laboratory and the clinic, the epidemiologists, industry and government coming together in *partnership*. We must appreciate that *people* are our most important resource in making progress in the fight against diseases and other major problems facing mankind. It is vital therefore that our schools work to attract young people into science and ensure that they are encouraged with enthusiasm to pursue careers in science and technology. It is important that our universities are in a position to ensure a supply of well trained scientists and technologists for academia, industry and government. We need to combine our resources, disseminate and share our knowledge, and ensure that the necessary financial provisions are made available. Only then can we really harness the promise of such diverse disciplines as cell biology, biochemistry, molecular biology, immunology and structural and medicinal chemistry to defeat this organism and overcome the serious threat it presents to mankind.

Glaxo is committed to these ideals and we are at present establishing a multidisciplinary and multicentre collaborative research programme extending over the next 5 years. This programme will involve interaction between our own basic scientists and those in leading academic centres in the UK and elsewhere. Glaxo will provide up to £10 million to support the collaborating groups involved in this joint initiative. We and our research partners will have clear objectives before us. We want to understand the biochemistry and molecular biology of the organism; we must also explore the immunological, and other, mechanisms involved in the production of host resistance within the human body. We hope that through such a partnership, we will play our part in defeating this organism and others, thus overcoming the serious threat they present to mankind. We and our partners in research do not expect easy solutions to the problems we are setting out to address but we do believe that with a sense of partnership, with commitment and with enthusiasm, we will achieve our goals.

Opening Session Address III

Donald A. Enarson

International Union against Tuberculosis and Lung Disease, Paris, France

The International Union against Tuberculosis and Lung Disease (IUATLD) had its origins over one hundred years ago during the course of the first international meeting of Internal Medicine, at which it was noted that tuberculosis was the most important problem faced by internists. Plans were then made for an international meeting on tuberculosis at which the first steps were taken to organize a society to undertake periodic scientific meetings to address the problems posed by tuberculosis. The first society was formed in Berlin in 1901. This society was disrupted by the war and the society was reconstituted in its present form in 1920 at the Sorbonne in Paris. Its role was noted at that time to be to develop the means, methods and modes of implementation for the fight against tuberculosis and to provide assistance to governments in order to carry it out. The society was constituted as an international association of national associations organized to combat tuberculosis and consisting of the voluntary, non-professional sector and the academic and professional community. The Union has been involved since that time in the development of all major aspects of the fight against tuberculosis including sanatorium treatment, tuberculin surveys, X-ray screening examinations, mass vaccination, and the development, evaluation and use of antibiotics for the treatment and prevention of tuberculosis.

In recent years, under the leadership of the Director of Scientific Activities, Dr Karel Styblo, and with the collaboration of development cooperation agencies and voluntary associations, the Union has developed a 'model' for national tuberculosis programmes in developing countries. This has been shown to achieve the targets required for an epidemiological impact in the control of transmission of tuberculosis infection and has been evaluated by the Health Sectors Priority Review of the World Bank as among the most cost-effective of any health intervention in developing countries. This achievement forms the basis of the strategy of the Tuberculosis Unit of the World Health Organization in its global programme against tuberculosis. Within the context of these activities, and for a very small amount of money provided by donors in Norway, Switzerland and The Netherlands, the Union-assisted national tuberculosis programmes diagnosed and

Tuberculosis: Back to the Future. Edited by J.D.H. Porter and K.P.W.J. McAdam
© 1994 John Wiley & Sons Ltd

treated more than 65 000 cases of active tuberculosis (around one case out of every ten occurring in the region). It has been possible within these programmes to achieve a documented cure of more than 70% of all pulmonary cases diagnosed smear positive.

The involvement of members from the United Kingdom in the work of the IUATLD goes back to its very beginning. Prominent among those who have contributed to the work of the IUATLD during the past few decades are Professor Sir John Crofton who remains a key adviser on tuberculosis control and on the anti-tobacco campaign, Professor Wallace Fox who was chairman of the Executive Committee and Professor Stewart Kilpatrick, chairman of the scientific committees for a number of years.

The fight against tuberculosis must continue. What is needed for this fight? Although we do need more science and more technology, we certainly need more commitment among all those concerned to see the end of the tubercle bacillus, definitely more collaboration (particularly between those involved in basic research and those involved in implementing programmes), and absolutely more generosity from individuals and from organizations to ensure that this 'white plague' has an end.

The Union heartily welcomes the initiative of the London School of Hygiene and Tropical Medicine in this Forum. Tuberculosis today is estimated to be the most common cause of death in the world from a single agent, affecting the segment of the population in the productive years of life. It is our firm belief that tuberculosis can be effectively treated and eventually eliminated. It cannot be done without mobilizing every party concerned with this problem. We strongly appeal to the London School of Hygiene & Tropical Medicine, the Government of the United Kingdom and to all those present to do as was done in 1920 when the Union was constituted, create a group whose aim remains the control and eventual elimination of this scourge from our society.

PLENARY SESSION
ADDRESSES

1
Tuberculosis: the world situation. History of the disease and efforts to combat it

Dixie E. Snider

Centers for Disease Control and Prevention, Atlanta, GA, USA

Introduction

Tuberculosis (TB) is a major health problem in the world. This chapter will review the history of this disease and efforts to combat it. Emphasis will be placed on improvements in diagnosis, treatment and prevention during the past hundred years. Historical trends in the epidemiology of the disease will be briefly reviewed and current estimates of the magnitude and impact of TB will be presented. Strategies for, and obstacles to, control will also be discussed.

Basic facts about tuberculosis

Tuberculosis is a bacterial disease caused mainly by *Mycobacterium tuberculosis* and *Mycobacterium bovis* (Bass *et al.*, 1990). When clinical specimens containing these organisms (e.g. sputum) are examined under the microscope after staining with certain dyes, the organisms are acid-fast, i.e. they retain the dye even after being washed with acid alcohol.

M. bovis infections are uncommon in most countries today. In the past, this infection was often transmitted through the oral route by drinking milk from infected cows.

Virtually all new infections with *M. tuberculosis* are acquired via airborne transmission (Bass *et al.*, 1990). The sources of infections are persons with tuberculosis of the lung or larynx who are coughing. Coughing produces tiny infectious droplets, 1–5 μm in size, known as droplet nuclei. In indoor environments, these droplet nuclei can remain suspended in the air for long periods of time unless they are removed by ventilation, filtration or ultraviolet irradiation.

Tuberculosis: Back to the Future. Edited by J.D.H. Porter and K.P.W.J. McAdam
Published 1994 John Wiley & Sons Ltd

A susceptible individual breathing air contaminated with these droplet nuclei is at risk of becoming infected. The magnitude of this risk is primarily dependent upon the concentration of droplet nuclei in the air and the duration of time the individual breathes this contaminated air. Virtually all transmission occurs in enclosed environments.

Once an individual is infected with *M. tuberculosis*, he or she remains infected for many years, perhaps for life (Bass *et al.*, 1990). A few infected persons develop clinically apparent disease within a few weeks after infection. Most, however, are asymptomatic; the only evidence of the infection may be a positive reaction to TB skin test. However, infected persons can develop clinical disease at any time. Infected persons are particularly likely to develop disease if they come under physical or emotional stress or if they become immunocompromised as occurs with HIV infection. Disease can affect virtually any tissue or organ but most commonly affects the lungs.

Historical background

Tuberculosis is an ancient disease. Tuberculosis was present in Egypt from early dynastic times, perhaps as early as 3700 BC (Morse *et al.*, 1964). Manchester (1984) has reviewed evidence that suggests that human tuberculosis may have evolved during the Neolithic period (seventh and sixth millennia BC) at which time population increases and cattle domestication occurred in Europe and the eastern Mediterranean.

Certainly, tuberculosis was well recognized by the time of Hippocrates (*c.* 460–377 BC) who gave an excellent clinical description of the disease (Hippocrates, 1939). In India, the medical luminary Susruta (*c.* 500 AD) mentioned the disease in his writings (Pierry and Roshem, 1931).

In the New World, tuberculosis appears to have antedated the arrival of Columbus and other European settlers (Buickstra, 1931). Just how and when the disease reached the New World is unknown. Significantly, tuberculosis-like lesions in the Americas are largely confined to the remains found in sedentary agriculturally-based communities and rare among groups of hunters and gatherers who presumably were less exposed to crowding (Buickstra, 1931; Perzigian and Widmer, 1979). As Manchester (1984) has aptly summarized, ' . . . tuberculosis, being a population density-dependent disease, owes its . . . increase to urbanization or at least to the development of aggregate population groups.'

The study of tuberculosis did not really begin until the period of the Renaissance when Girolamo Fracastoro (1483–1553), regarded by some as the first epidemiologist, recognized the contagious nature of tuberculosis (Lowell *et al.*, 1969). The Dutch physician, Franciscus Sylvius (1614–1672) deduced from autopsies that tuberculosis was characterized by the formation of nodules, which he named 'tubercles' (Lowell *et al.*, 1969). Jean-Antoine Villemin (1827–1892), a French army surgeon, performed several experiments and reported to the French Academy of

Medicine in 1865 that tuberculosis was transmissible (Lowell *et al.*, 1969).

Pasteur performed experiments as early as 1862 which suggested that tuberculosis was transmitted via the airborne route (Conant, 1957), but this remained somewhat controversial until the 1930s when the elegant studies of William Wells at the Harvard School of Public Health conclusively proved airborne transmission via droplet nuclei (Wells, 1934).

It was, of course, Robert Koch's report of the isolation of *M. tuberculosis* in 1882 before the Berlin Phthisiological Society (Koch, 1882) that convinced the medical community and the world of the communicable nature of tuberculosis and brought about concerted efforts to combat the disease.

The development of an acid-fast stain by Ehrlich (1885) and the discovery of X-rays by Roentgen in 1895 made possible early and more accurate diagnosis of the disease (Burke, 1955).

Burden of disease prior to 1950

For several reasons, it is not possible to obtain accurate data on the prevalence and incidence of tuberculosis prior to recent times. Until late in the 19th century, many wasting diseases of the chest—cancer, silicosis, lung abscesses—were confused with tuberculosis. Furthermore, many extrapulmonary forms of the disease were not recognized as being caused by the tubercle bacillus. Even if clinical diagnosis had been accurate, most areas did not have good disease surveillance systems until the 20th century. When such systems did come into existence, many physicians refused to report cases. The public viewed tuberculosis as a stigma and patients did not wish others to know of their disease for fear of ostracism, loss of a job, and decreased eligibility for marriage (Dubos and Dubos, 1952).

Despite these limitations, recorded deaths from tuberculosis are useful indicators of the burden of the disease during the 17th to 19th centuries. Rene and Jean Dubos state that, in England and Wales, pulmonary tuberculosis was rare in the country districts around 1650 but caused some 20% of all deaths in urban areas (Dubos and Dubos, 1952). TB mortality then decreased and accounted for only 13% of deaths in 1715 but began to increase again around 1730, reaching a peak toward the end of the 18th century (Dubos and Dubos, 1952).

In Salem, Massachusetts, during the 5 year period 1768–73, pulmonary tuberculosis accounted for 18% of deaths; for the period 1799–1808, the proportion rose to 25%. During the first half of the 19th century, most cities in the eastern United States reported case rates in excess of 400 per 100 000 population and 15 to 30% of all deaths were attributed to TB. Death rates from TB in the United States probably peaked around the middle of the 19th century (Lowell *et al.*, 1969).

Grzybowski (1991) has recently pointed out that epidemic waves of tuberculosis have affected different populations at different times. In western Europe and in the white population of North America, the epidemic probably achieved its height in

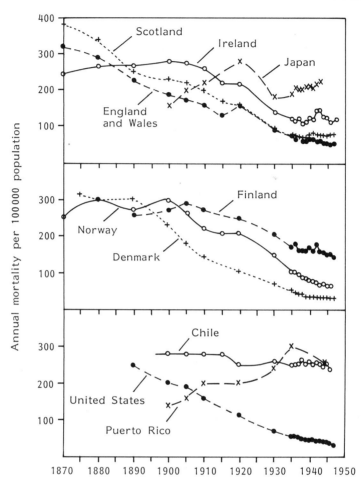

Figure 1.1 Deaths per 100 000 population per year in selected countries, 1870–1950 (from Dubos and Dubos, 1952)

the late 18th or early 19th century. The peak was delayed by several decades in eastern Europe. The large countries of Asia experienced the height of the epidemic in the late 19th or early 20th century. These varying patterns are illustrated in Figure 1.1. The epidemic in sub-Saharan Africa may be at its peak now.

The impact of the deprivations and disruptions of World War I and World War II in selected countries is shown in Figure 1.2. The decline in the death rate from tuberculosis in industrialized countries clearly occurred prior to the introduction of effective chemotherapy (Dubos and Dubos, 1952). This decline has been attributed to a progressive improvement in the standard of living. However, Wilson (1990) has recently called attention to the evidence, first espoused by Sir Arthur

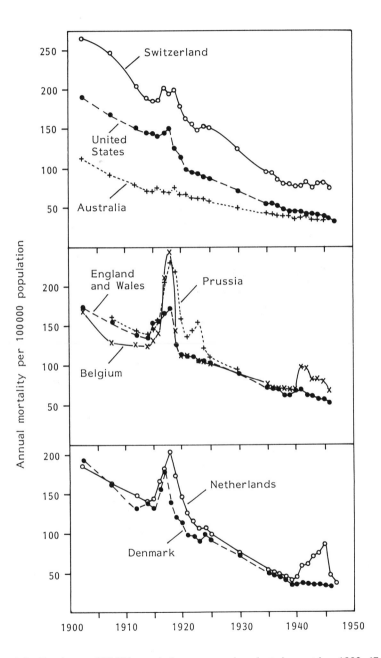

Figure 1.2 Deaths per 100 000 population per year in selected countries, 1902–47 (from Dubos and Dubos, 1952)

Newsholme (1924), that the decline of tuberculosis was the result of a reduction in exposure to infection brought about by the segregation of persons with infectious TB in England and Poor Law infirmaries. In fact, Newsholme's data showed no relationship between a decline in tuberculosis and standard of living.

Combating tuberculosis

Prior to the development of effective chemotherapy in the 1950s, a variety of remedies had been used to treat tuberculosis but none showed significant efficacy.

Koch's early effort to develop an effective immunotherapy, i.e. by the injection of tuberculin, was an embarrassing failure (Koch, 1890), although it did lead to the development of the tuberculin skin test. The intradermal skin test method developed by Mantoux (Mantoux, 1910) is still the preferred method for identifying persons infected with *M. tuberculosis*.

Koch's failure did not, however, dampen enthusiasm for controlling the disease. A few years before Koch's discovery of the tubercle bacillus, bed rest had been advocated as a treatment of tuberculosis and the sanatorium movement began in both Europe and the United States (Burke, 1955).

Two men, Sir Robert W. Philip in Edinburgh and Dr Hermann M. Biggs in New York, were prime movers in establishing organized systems for the control of tuberculosis (Lowell et al., 1969). The first tuberculosis dispensary in the world was opened by Sir Robert W. Philip in Edinburgh in 1887. Two years later, Dr Biggs created a plan for administrative control of tuberculosis in New York City which involved reporting of cases to health authorities, official inspection of cattle, public education, and disinfection of rooms which had been occupied by patients with pulmonary tuberculosis.

Early in the 20th century the major effort to control tuberculosis in the United States came not from government or from official health agencies but from local voluntary organizations of physicians and lay persons (Lowell et al., 1969). In 1904, the National Association for the Study and Prevention of Tuberculosis (now the American Lung Association) was formed to educate the public and stimulate programmes for the control of tuberculosis. The organization was highly successful in promoting and maintaining public interest in tuberculosis through hundreds of local and state affiliates, and, over the next several decades, each state and most large cities had organized tuberculosis control programmes. Voluntary movements also sprang up in Europe and other areas and in 1920, the International Union Against Tuberculosis was formed (Rouillon, 1991).

National programmes for eradication of tuberculosis in cattle were instituted in many countries in the early 20th century. This involved tuberculin skin testing to identify infected cattle and slaughter of those cattle found to be infected. Pasteurization of milk also contributed to the control of bovine tuberculosis (Lowell et al., 1969).

Treatment

As mentioned above, by the early 20th century, treatment of patients with tuberculosis usually involved bed rest. A dry climate and fresh air were considered important by many clinicians and many of the sanatoria were located in rural areas at higher elevations. Nutritional therapies, fresh air, sunlight, mental tranquillity and optimism were also promoted by many (Dubos and Dubos, 1952).

Surgery

The most dramatic of the therapies to emerge in the late 19th and early 20th centuries were surgical therapies (Gaensler, 1982). Forlanini began using artificial pneumothorax in 1892 (Forlanini, 1906). Subsequently, other surgical techniques were developed including pneumolysis, pneumoperitoneum, artificial phrenic paralysis, extrapleural pneumothorax and plombage, thoracoplasty, subcostal extraperiosteal plombage and pulmonary resection. Although the contribution of these techniques to tuberculosis control efforts remains unclear, they did provide the basis for the development of modern thoracic surgery techniques (Gaensler, 1982).

Chemotherapy

Following Koch's discovery of the tubercle bacillus, an intense interest in chemotherapy of the disease developed. None of the drugs studied in animals and in man showed great promise, however, until the discovery of streptomycin by Waksmann and coworkers in 1944 (Schatz *et al.*, 1944). Trials by the British Medical Research Council (MRC), the United States Public Health Service (USPHS), and the US Veterans Administration–Armed Forces Cooperative Trials Group confirmed its efficacy, but drug resistance emerged as a serious drawback. Therefore, in an effort to prevent resistance, in 1948 the MRC undertook a successful trial of combined streptomycin–PAS therapy (Medical Research Council, 1950). By 1952, isoniazid had become an important part of the initial treatment regimen. It was not until the early 1960s that a MRC trial settled the optimal duration of treatment—2 years (Medical Research Council, 1962). A number of trials conducted during the 1950s and 1960s also demonstrated that treatment could be effectively given on an outpatient basis and that hospitalization and bed rest were unnecessary (D'Esopo, 1982).

Another major advance in chemotherapy in the 1960s was the discovery that therapy could be just as effective when given intermittently (two or three times weekly) as when given daily (Tuberculosis Chemotherapy Centre, Madras, 1963; Sbarbaro and Johnson, 1968; Doyle *et al.*, 1970; Stradling and Poole, 1970). Supervision of intermittently administered therapy is much easier and less costly than supervision of daily therapy.

The next major advance was the development of so-called short-course chemotherapy—usually understood to mean treatment regimens of 9 months or less—in the 1970s (D'Esopo, 1982). Short-course regimens with high cure rates became possible only after the introduction of rifampicin. With the introduction of this drug, the chemotherapeutic armamentarium for TB included two bacterial drugs—rifampicin and isoniazid—and it was subsequently shown that high cure rates could be obtained by giving both these drugs for only 9 months (Fox and Mitchison, 1975). The development of successful 6 month treatment regimens occurred when pyrazinamide (PZA) was added. This drug was first introduced in 1952 but not widely used because of hepatotoxicity. However, by using lower dosages and limiting the duration of treatment with PZA, the MRC Tuberculosis Unit, under the leadership of Professor Wallace Fox, was able to achieve results as good as, or better than, the best regimens of longer duration (Fox, 1981).

Scores of short-course chemotherapy regimens have now been studied (Girling, 1989). Several principles of short-course chemotherapy are worth emphasizing. First, all regimens of 9 months' duration must contain both isoniazid and rifampicin, at least during the first 2 months. Second, all regimens of 6 months' duration must contain isoniazid, rifampicin and pyrazinamide, at least during the first 2 months. Third, there is great flexibility in the rhythm of administration; drugs can be given daily throughout, daily initially and then intermittently, or intermittently from the beginning. The development of short-course chemotherapy was a critical factor enabling the development of effective strategies for global TB control (see below).

Prevention

Vaccination

Efforts to prevent tuberculosis by inducing resistance to infection began early in this century. An attenuated strain of *Mycobacterium bovis* was produced by Calmette and Guerin after 231 passages through media containing glycerin and oxbile (Luelmo, 1982). This BCG vaccine was safely administered to a child in 1921 and its use spread quickly across Europe. It was first administered by mouth but later given by the intradermal route. A disaster in Lubeck, Germany in 1930, in which 72 children died as a result of vaccination with a BCG contaminated with a virulent strain, generated years of controversy concerning the safety of the vaccine. However, subsequent clinical observations, uncontrolled studies and clinical trials established the safety of BCG for immunocompetent individuals (Luelmo, 1982).

Numerous controlled studies of BCG have been conducted. The results have shown a wide variation in protective efficacy, ranging from 0 to 80% (Luelmo, 1982). Several hypotheses have been proposed to explain these disparate results including variations in the potency and/or immunogenicity of the vaccine strain, pre-existing protection as a result of infection with environmental non-tuberculosis mycobacteria, and biases in study design. The contribution of each of these factors remains unclear. There is an emerging consensus, however, that BCG vaccination does not prevent infection, and that, when it is protective, BCG reduces the risk of extrapulmonary forms of disease, e.g. miliary disease and meningitis, more than pulmonary forms. Styblo and Meijer (1976) have shown that BCG vaccination does little to reduce the number of infectious TB cases; thus, it is less important than good case finding and treatment programmes for improving the tuberculosis situation. However, BCG vaccination is of potential benefit in reducing TB mortality among children and, as such, is an important component of the WHO Expanded Programme on Immunization.

Preventive therapy (chemoprophylaxis)

The development of tuberculosis is a two-stage process; first, an infection must become established, and second, that infection must progress to clinical disease. Among all persons who become infected with *M. tuberculosis*, approximately 10% will eventually progress to clinical disease (Bass *et al.*, 1990). The latent period between infection and active disease varies from weeks to months.

With the development of chemotherapy for tuberculosis, it became possible to consider treatment of infected persons to prevent the development of disease. Chemoprophylaxis trials had their genesis in the observations by Lincoln that isoniazid could prevent complications, e.g. meningitis, in recently infected children with clinical manifestations of disease (Lincoln, 1954). Subsequently, at least 14 placebo-controlled trials involving more than 100 000 subjects were conducted. The USPHS trials demonstrated that 1 year of isoniazid chemoprophylaxis reduced the incidence of clinical disease by 55–83% (Ferebee, 1970; International Union Against Tuberculosis, 1982). The primary determinant of effectiveness was patient compliance. Among highly compliant individuals, the effectiveness of isoniazid was greater than 90% (International Union Against Tuberculosis, 1982).

In addition to non-compliance, other major problems with isoniazid chemoprophylaxis have been (i) the occurrence of hepatoxicity, which can be fatal, in approximately 1% of subjects who take the drug (Kopanoff *et al.*, 1978), and (ii) uncertainties regarding the risks and benefits and cost-effectiveness in various populations (Snider, 1988). Nevertheless, isoniazid preventive therapy for high risk individuals, e.g. HIV-infected persons and recent close contacts of infectious cases, has become an integral part of tuberculosis control programmes in the United States (Centers for Disease Control, 1990). Preventive therapy may also be indicated in developing countries for children in the household of infectious cases and for HIV-infected persons.

What is the present magnitude and nature of the global TB problem?

At the very beginning, we must acknowledge that we do not know the precise answer to this question. Surveillance systems in many countries are too incomplete to provide meaningful information on the incidence of, or mortality from, tuberculosis. WHO has divided countries into four groups in terms of the current level and past trends of the annual risk of infection and health resource availability (Kochi, 1991) (Table 1.1). In industrialized countries (group I), tuberculosis has been declining very rapidly. Nevertheless, tuberculosis remains one of the most common notifiable infectious diseases and, in many industrialized countries, the declining trend has slowed down, and, in some countries it has reversed (see below). In some middle-income developing countries (group II), tuberculosis has declined relatively rapidly. In other middle-income developing countries (group III), the decline has been slow and tuberculosis remains a major problem. In most low-income developing countries (group IV), there has been almost no observable decline in tuberculosis. The absolute number of cases in many of these countries is increasing due to population growth, especially in the 15–59 year age group, and with the impact of HIV infection (see below).

Two recent papers have used several epidemiological parameters to estimate indirectly the global burden of TB (Kochi, 1991; Murray et al., 1990) (Tables 1.2 and 1.3). The parameters used include the incidence of sputum smear-positive pulmonary tuberculosis, the proportion of all cases that are smear-positive, the annual risk of infection with *M. tuberculosis* (calculated from tuberculin skin test surveys), and case-fatality rates for smear-positive and other tuberculosis (Styblo, 1980). The necessity of using these indirect methods creates some degree of uncertainty about the magnitude of the global TB problem.

Infection

Kochi (1991) has estimated that about one-third of the world's population (1.7 billion people) are infected with *M. tuberculosis*. The great majority of the world's population, and thus the majority of infected persons, reside in developing

Table 1.1   The epidemiological pattern of tuberculosis

Areas of the world	Annual risk of infection		Health resource availability
	Current level (%)	Annual decline trend (%)	
I Industrialized	0.1–0.01	>10	Excellent
II Middle-income in Latin America, West Asia, and North Africa	0.5–1.5	5–10	Good
III Middle-income in East and South-east Asia	1.0–2.5	<5	Good
IV Sub-Saharan Africa and Indian subcontinent	1.0–2.5	0–3	Poor

From Kochi (1991) *Tubercle*, *72*, 1–6. With permission of Churchill Livingstone.

Table 1.2 Estimated new tuberculosis cases and deaths occurring in 1990 by region

Region	New cases	Deaths
Africa	1 400 000	660 000
Americas[a]	560 000	220 000
Eastern Mediterranean	594 000	160 000
South-east Asia	2 480 000	940 000
Western Pacific[b]	2 560 000	890 000
Europe and other industrialized countries[c]	410 000	40 000
Total	8 004 000	2 910 000

Adapted from Kochi (1991) *Tubercle, 72*, 1–6. With permission of Churchill Livingstone.
[a]Excluding USA and Canada.
[b]Excluding Japan, Australia and New Zealand.
[c]Including USA, Canada, Japan, Australia and New Zealand.

Table 1.3 Estimated new tuberculosis cases and deaths in developing countries, 1990

Region	New cases[a]	Deaths[a]
Sub-Saharan Africa	1 156 000	528 000
North Africa and Western Asia	323 000	99 000
Remainder of Asia	5 102 000	1 709 000
South America	356 000	125 000
Central America and Caribbean	185 000	88 000
Total	7 122 000	2 549 000

Adapted from Murray *et al*. (1990) with permission of the International Union against Tuberculosis and Lung Disease.
[a]Best (midpoint estimates).

countries. In industrialized countries, 80% of infected individuals are aged 50 years or more while, in developing countries, 75% of infected persons are less than 50 years old.

Disease

Murray *et al*. (1990) estimated that the number of new cases of all forms of tuberculosis in developing countries in 1990 was 7.1 million; their estimates ranged from 3.5 million to 10.7 million depending upon the assumptions they used. The midpoint of 7.1 million compares favourably with Kochi's estimate of 7.6 million new cases of tuberculosis in developing countries (Kochi, 1991). Kochi reported there were an additional 400 000 new cases in industrialized countries, bringing the number of new cases occurring annually to 8 million. Thus, 95% of the TB cases are estimated to occur in developing countries and only 5% in industrialized countries. In both studies, the largest estimated number of cases (about 5 million) occurred in Asia. However, the highest estimated case rate was in Africa. Murray *et al*. (1990) estimated a case rate of 229 per 100 000 population in sub-Saharan

Africa; Kochi (1991) estimated a case rate of 272 cases per 100 000 population in WHO's African Region.

Deaths

Murray *et al.* (1990) estimated that there were 2.5 million deaths from all forms of tuberculosis in developing countries in 1990; the low estimate was 1.1 million and the high estimate was 4 million. Kochi (1991) estimated that, worldwide, tuberculosis caused 2.9 million deaths in 1990, all but 40 000 in developing countries. By either estimate, tuberculosis appears to be the largest cause of death from a single pathogen in the world. In both studies, the largest number of deaths (1.7–1.8 million) was estimated to occur in Asia.

According to a 1989 WHO report, 1.3 million cases and 450 000 deaths from tuberculosis in developing countries occur in children under the age of 15 years (World Health Organization, 1989). However, the greatest number of cases and deaths is concentrated in the economically most productive age group of the population (15–59 years); 70–80% of the tuberculosis cases in developing countries fall in this age group (Kochi, 1991). Murray *et al.* (1990) estimate that tuberculosis accounts for 7% of all deaths and 26% of potentially avoidable deaths in the world.

Current status of control efforts

To assess the current status of tuberculosis control efforts in developing countries, WHO held a workshop in Massachusetts in 1989 (World Health Organization, 1990). Presentations at this workshop revealed that the majority of countries do not have a mechanism to monitor treatment outcomes routinely on a national basis, i.e. the percentage of patients who are cured. Partial information on the outcome of treatment based on *ad hoc* surveys in a limited number of treatment centres indicated that, in many developing countries, less than half of the tuberculosis patients who started treatment were cured or completed their course of chemotherapy. Grzybowski (1991) has pointed out that such poor chemotherapy programmes may slow down the natural decline of tuberculosis and may even worsen the situation by keeping infectious cases alive to continue to transmit infection. Another result of poor programmes is an increase in the prevalence of drug resistance.

WHO also estimates that less than half of the existing tuberculosis patients in developing countries, excluding China, are covered by the treatment services (Kochi, 1991).

Strategies for control

Despite the gloomy statistics regarding the large number of deaths from tuberculosis and the low cure rates in conventional tuberculosis control programmes, there is reason to believe that the situation can be improved by implementing the tuberculosis control strategies now being advocated by the WHO (Kochi, 1991). These strategies were developed primarily through the work of the Mutual Assistance Programme of the IUATLD under the leadership of Dr Karel Styblo (Rouillon, 1991). The first successful project was begun in Tanzania in 1982, but later projects were begun in other countries including Malawi, Mozambique and Nicaragua. Using the principles and strategies developed by Dr Styblo, these countries have been able to achieve cure rates of about 80%. The key factors of success in these projects include (Enarson, 1991):

1. The political commitment on the part of the government to TB control.
2. The use of a relatively cheap short-course regimen, namely 2 months of daily isoniazid, rifampicin, pyrazinamide and streptomycin (administered under strict supervision) followed by 6 months of self-administered isoniazid and thiacetazone.
3. A secure supply of high quality drugs and other materials.
4. A network of microscopy centres with quality control.
5. Proper recording and reporting of cases and treatment outcomes.
6. Proper training and supervision of staff.

Murray *et al.* (1991) have carefully examined the cost-effectiveness of this strategy and have found that chemotherapy for smear-positive tuberculosis is cheaper than other cost-effective health interventions such as immunization against measles and oral rehydration therapy.

These findings have prompted the WHO to reinvigorate and expand its TB programme and to develop new strategies for global TB control based on these principles (Kochi, 1991). WHO has established the objectives of detecting at least 70% of smear-positive cases in the world, and curing at least 85% of those detected, by the year 2000. In addition, the above findings have encouraged the World Bank and several large countries, including China, to embark on efforts to reorient the TB control programmes in these countries to conform to the new WHO strategy. The early results of the project in China are very encouraging (R. Bumgarner, personal communication).

Potential obstacles to global TB control

The obstacles to global TB control are numerous and include the HIV pandemic, drug resistance and a lack of application of resources to TB control.

The impact of HIV infection

WHO estimates that about 4.4 million people are dually infected with the tubercle bacillus and HIV in the world (A. Kochi, personal communication). HIV infection is the highest risk factor so far identified which increases the chance of latent infection with tubercle bacilli progressing to active tuberculosis (Selwyn *et al.*, 1989). The risk of active TB in dually infected persons is estimated to be 7–10% per year. At present, less than 5% of TB cases throughout the world are estimated to be associated with HIV infection; the majority of these cases are concentrated in sub-Saharan African countries. In many of these countries, surveys have shown that 20–67% of patients with tuberculosis have HIV infection (De Cock, *et al.*, 1992). The HIV epidemic has caused dramatic increases in tuberculosis, with some countries experiencing a doubling of reported tuberculosis cases in the past 5–7 years (Narain *et al.*, 1992) (Figure 1.3), and further dramatic increases are projected by the year 2000 (Table 1.4) (Schulzer *et al.*, 1992). Similar increases in Asia in the future are a major concern.

The dramatic increase in TB cases in Africa has had a devastating effect. There have been greater demands for diagnostic services, antituberculosis drugs, hospital beds and other supplies and services in countries where they are already in short supply. HIV-infected persons with tuberculosis have a higher frequency of non-reactivity to the tuberculin test, a higher frequency of unusual or atypical chest radiographic findings and a higher frequency of extrapulmonary tuberculosis, all of which make TB more difficult to diagnose in HIV-infected persons (Barnes *et al.*, 1991). Also, since HIV-infected persons have a higher frequency of adverse reactions to drugs, particularly to thiacetazone (Nunn *et al.*, 1991), patient management is more difficult. A higher mortality rate among HIV-related tuberculosis patients may decrease the credibility of the programme in the eyes of the public and policy-makers.

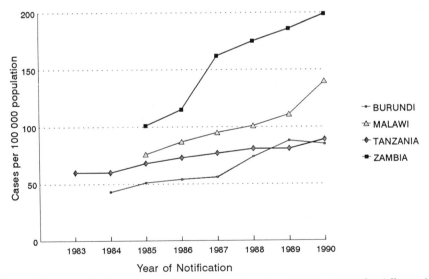

Figure 1.3 Annual tuberculosis notification rates in selected African countries (all cases), 1983–90 (from Narain *et al.*, 1992 *Tubercle and Lung Disease*, *73*, 311–321. Reproduced by permission of Churchill Livingstone.

Table 1.4 Future TB problem in sub-Saharan Africa—four scenarios for the year 2000

Scenario	ARI[a] (%)	TB infection: prevalence[b] (%)	HIV infection: prevalence[b] (%)	% increase in smear-positive TB
1	1	45	2	60
2	2	60	2	52
3	2	60	10	280
4	2	60	20	888

From Schulzer *et al.* (1992) *Tubercle and Lung Disease*, *73*, 52–58. With permission of Churchill Livingstone.
[a]Annual risk of TB infection.
[b]Prevalence in 1989.

Drug resistance

In the years since the development of effective treatment regimens 4 decades ago, tuberculosis control efforts have only occasionally been hampered by the emergence of drug-resistant strains, a problem that has plagued treatment of many other bacterial infections. However, during the past few years, several large outbreaks of multidrug-resistant tuberculosis (tuberculosis caused by organisms resistant to at least isoniazid and rifampicin) have occurred in the United States (Centers for Disease Control, 1991). These outbreaks have primarily involved HIV-infected persons, have caused many deaths, and have resulted in the infection of many health care workers and other persons with multidrug-resistant organisms.

Limited surveillance data from the United States indicate that the incidence of multidrug-resistant disease has increased in the past few years (Centers for Disease Control, unpublished data). Data from other countries are extremely limited, but there is evidence that resistance to isoniazid and rifampicin has also increased in Argentina and Thailand in recent years (B. Vareldzis, personal communication).

The occurrence of multidrug-resistant tuberculosis has potentially disastrous implications for the control of TB in both industrialized and developing countries and underscores the need to prevent the emergence of drug-resistant disease by implementing the basic WHO strategy in all countries.

Lack of money for drugs

Many developing countries do not have the hard currency necessary to purchase drugs, especially those drugs, such as rifampicin and pyrazinamide, that are essential for short-course regimens. External assistance may be needed in some circumstances, although Chaulet (1992) has pointed out that national financial resources could be found in most developing countries if there were a rational and coherent national drugs policy aimed at guaranteeing the availability of essential drugs.

Lack of awareness, political will, and coverage of the population with tuberculosis services

As noted above, WHO estimates that less than half of the existing tuberculosis patients have access to care. There is still a lack of awareness among government officials and other policy-makers about the magnitude of the TB problem, the availability of effective interventions, and the cost-effectiveness of these interventions. Strong advocacy will be needed to change the status quo.

Increases in tuberculosis in industrialized countries

From 1985 to 1991, the United States experienced an 18% increase in cases (Centers for Disease Control, unpublished data). This increase can, in part, be attributed both to TB occurring in HIV-infected persons and to immigration from higher prevalence countries.

Seven of 14 western European countries (Austria, Denmark, Ireland, Italy, The Netherlands, Norway and Switzerland) have also recently experienced increases in reported cases (M. Raviglione, personal communication). The major factor responsible for these increases appears to be immigration from high prevalence countries.

Conclusion

Tuberculosis remains a major world health problem but effective interventions are available to combat the disease. Most of these interventions appear to be very cost-effective relative to other health interventions. Although improvements in the technology for TB control would be useful, the greatest need is for more widespread application of existing technologies in developing countries.

References

Barnes PF, Bloch AB, Davidson PT, Snider DE (1991) Tuberculosis in patients with human immunodeficiency virus infection. *New England Journal of Medicine, 324,* 1644–1650

Bass JB, Farer LS, Hopewell PC, Jacobs RF, Snider DE (1990) Diagnostic standards and classification of tuberculosis. *American Review of Repiratory Disease, 142,* 725–735

Buikstra JE (ed.) (1981) *Prehistoric Tuberculosis in the Americas.* Northwestern University Archeological Program, Evanston, Illinois

Burke RM (1955) *An Historical Chronology of Tuberculosis,* 2nd edition. Charles C Thomas, Springfield, Illinois

Centers for Disease Control, Advisory Committee for the Elimination of Tuberculosis (1990) The use of preventive therapy for tuberculosis infection in the United States and screening for tuberculosis and tuberculous infection in high-risk populations. *Morbidity and Mortality Weekly Report, 39* (RR-8), 1–12

Centers for Disease Control (1991) Nosocomial transmission of multidrug-resistant tuberculosis among HIV-infected persons—Florida and New York, 1988–1991. *Morbidity and Mortality Weekly Report, 40,* 585–591

Chaulet P (1992) The supply of antituberculosis drugs and national drug policies. *Tubercle and Lung Disease, 73*, 295–304

Conant TB (1957) *Harvard Case Histories in Experimental Science*, Vol 2. Harvard University Press, Cambridge Massachusetts. p. 509

DeCock KM, Soro B, Coulibaly IM, Lucas SB (1992) Tuberculosis and HIV infection in sub-Saharan Africa. *Journal of the American Medical Association, 268*, 1581–1587

D'Esopo ND (1982) Clinical trials in pulmonary tuberculosis. *American Review of Respiratory Disease, 125* (3:2), 85–93

Doyle JA, Lambertini A, Dolmann A (1970) Intermittent chemotherapy with three drugs in the treatment of pulmonary tuberculosis. *Tubercle, 51*, 397–402

Dubos R and Dubos J (1952) *The White Plague: Tuberculosis, Man, and Society.* Little Brown, Boston

Enarson DA (1991) Principles of IUATLD collaborative tuberculosis programmes. *Bulletin of the International Union Against Tuberculosis and Lung Disease, 66*, 195–200

Ehrlich P (1885) *Das Sauerstoff-Bedürfniss des Organismus. Eine farbenanalytische Studie.* A Hirschwald, Berlin

Ferebee SH (1970) Controlled chemoprophylaxis trials in tuberculosis. A general review. *Advances in Tuberculosis Research, 17*, 28–106

Forlanini C (1906) Zur Behandlung der Lungenschwindsucht durch künstlich erzengten Pneumothorax. *Deutsche Medizinische Wochenschrift, 32*, 1401–1406

Fox W (1981) Whither short-course chemotherapy? *British Journal of Diseases of the Chest, 75*, 331–357

Fox W, Mitchison DA (1975) Short-course chemotherapy for pulmonary tuberculosis. *American Review of Respiratory Disease, 111*, 325–353

Gaensler EA (1982) The surgery for pulmonary tuberculosis. *American Review of Respiratory Disease, 125* (3:2), 73–84

Girling DJ (1989) The chemotherapy of tuberculosis. In Ratledge C, Stanford J and Grange JM (eds), *Biology of Mycobacteria*. Academic Press, London

Grzybowski S (1991) Tuberculosis in the third world. *Thorax, 46*, 689–691

Hippocrates (1939) *The Genuine Works of Hippocrates* translated by Francis Adams. Williams and Wilkins, Baltimore. pp. 101–133

International Union Against Tuberculosis Committee on Prophylaxis (1982) The efficacy of varying durations of isoniazid preventive therapy for tuberculosis: Five years of follow-up in the IUAT trial. *Bulletin of the World Health Organization, 60*, 555–564

Koch R (1882) Die aetiologie der tuberkulose. *Berliner Klinische Wochenschrift, 19,* 221–230

Koch R (1890) Uber Bacteriologische forschung. *Wiener Medizinische Blätter, 8*, 531–535

Kochi A (1991) The global tuberculosis situation and the new control strategy of the World Health Organization. *Tubercle, 72*, 1–6

Kopanoff DE, Snider DE, Caras GJ (1978) Isoniazid related hepatitis. *American Review of Respiratory Disease, 117*, 991–1001

Lincoln EM (1954) Effect of antimicrobial therapy on prognosis of primary tuberculosis in childhood. *American Review of Tuberculosis, 69*, 682–689

Lowell AM, Edwards LB, Palmer CE (1969) *Tuberculosis. Vital and Health Statistics Monographs, American Public Health Association.* Harvard University Press, Cambridge, Massachusetts

Luelmo F (1982) BCG vaccination. *American Review of Respiratory Disease, 125* (3:2), 70–72

Manchester K (1984) Tuberculosis and leprosy in antiquity: an interpretation. *Medical History, 28*, 162–173

Mantoux C (1910) L'intradermo-reaction à la tuberculine et son interprétation clinique.

Journal de Medecine Internationale, 18, 10–13

Medical Research Council (1950) Treatment of pulmonary tuberculosis with streptomycin and para-amino-salicylic acid. A Medical Research Council Investigation. *British Medical Journal, ii*, 1073–1085

Medical Research Council Tuberculosis Chemotherapy Trials Committee (1962) Long-term chemotherapy in the treatment of chronic pulmonary tuberculosis with cavitation. *Tubercle, 43*, 201–267

Morse D, Brothwell DR, Ucko PJ (1964) Tuberculosis in ancient Egypt. *American Review of Respiratory Disease, 90*, 524–541

Murray CJ, Styblo K, Rouillon A (1990) Tuberculosis in developing countries: burden, intervention, and cost. *Bulletin of the International Union Against Tuberculosis and Lung Disease, 65*, 6–24

Murray CJL, DeJonghe E, Chum HJ, Nyangulu DS, Salomao A, Styblo K (1991) Cost effectiveness of chemotherapy for pulmonary tuverculosis three sub-Saharan African countries. *Lancet, 338*, 1305–1308

Narain JP, Raviglione MC, Kochi A (1992) HIV-associated tuberculosis in developing countries: epidemiology and strategies for prevention. *Tubercle and Lung Disease, 73*(6), 311–321

Newsholme A (1924) *The Elements of Vital Statistics in Their Bearing on Social and Public Health Problems.* D Appleton and Co, New York

Nunn P, Kibuga D, Gathua S *et al.* (1991) Cutaneous hypersensitivity reactions due to thiacetazone in HIV-1 seropositive patients treated for tuberculosis. *Lancet, 337*, 627–630

Perzigian AJ, Widmer L (1979) Evidence for tuberculosis in a prehistoric population. *Journal of the American Medical Association, 241*, 2643–2646

Piery M, Roshem J (1931) *Historie de la Tuberculose.* G Doin, Paris. pp. 5–7

Rouillon A (1991) The mutual assistance programme of the IUATLD. Development, contribution and significance. *Bulletin of the International Union Against Tuberculosis and Lung Disease, 66*, 159–172

Sbarbaro JA, Johnson S (1968) Tuberculous chemotherapy for recalcitrant outpatients administered directly twice weekly. *American Review of Respiratory Disease, 97*, 895–903

Schatz A, Bugie E, Waksman SA (1944) Streptomycin, a substance exhibiting antibiotic activity against gram-positive and gram-negative bacteria. *Proceedings of the Society for Experimental Biology and Medicine, 55*, 66–69

Schulzer M, Fitzgerald JM, Enarson DA, Grzybowski S (1992) An estimate of the future size of the tuberculosis problem in sub-Saharan Africa resulting from HIV infection. *Tubercle and Lung Disease, 73*, 52–58

Selwyn PA, Hartel D, Lewis IA *et al.* (1989) A prospective study of the risk of tuberculosis among intravenous drug abusers with human immunodeficiency virus infection. *New England Journal of Medicine, 320*, 545–550

Snider DE (1988) Decision analysis for isoniazid preventivè therapy: take it or leave it? *American Review of Respiratory Disease, 137*, 2–4

Stradling P, Poole GW (1970) Twice-weekly streptomycin plus isoniazid for tuberculosis. *Tubercle, 51*, 44–47

Styblo K (1980) Recent advances in epidemiological research in tuberculosis. *Advances in Tuberculosis Research, 20*, 1–63

Styblo K, Meijer J (1976) Impact of BCG vaccination programmes in children and young adults on the tuberculosis problem. *Tubercle, 57*, 17–43

Tuberculosis Chemotherapy Centre, Madras (1963) Intermittent treatment of pulmonary tuberculosis. A concurrent comparison of twice-weekly isoniazid plus streptomycin and daily isoniazid plus p-aminosalicylic acid in domiciliary treatment. *Lancet, i*, 1078–1080

Wells WF (1934) On airborne infection II. Droplets and droplet nuclei. *American Journal of Hygiene, 20,* 611–618

Wilson LG (1990) The historical decline of tuberculosis in Europe and America: its causes and significance. *Journal of the History of Medicine and Allied Sciences, 45,* 366–396

World Health Organization (1989) Childhood tuberculosis and BCG vaccine. *EPI Update,* August

World Health Organization (1990) Summary report on the WHO workshop 'Case studies for evaluation of tuberculosis control in various primary health care settings.' WHO/TUB Unit Publication, Sturbridge, Massachusetts, USA

Discussion

Peter G. Smith, London School of Hygiene & Tropical Medicine, UK

Historically, tuberculosis was perceived as a public health problem in developed countries of importance perhaps comparable to the position occupied by cancer in those countries today. Enormous amounts of resources, both human and monetary, were devoted to attempts to control the disease and a very high degree of success was achieved, although, as McKeown (1979) has highlighted, most of the decline in mortality from the disease preceded the development of effective therapy or widespread use of BCG vaccination, and was almost certainly due largely to general improvements in living standards and housing conditions. Dr Snider appeared to call this epidemiologically popular wisdom into some question by quoting the work of Wilson (1990) and Newsholme (1924), questioning the extent to which the decline in tuberculosis was related only to improved standards of living. However, even in the poorest communities it is the poorest of the poor who seem to be at most risk of the disease, and the consistency of the association of tuberculosis with poverty and deprivation is very striking.

In some respects, the effective tools that we have against tuberculosis today were developed at the tail end of the epidemic in developed countries. That they were available, or at least existed, must have influenced thinking about the disease in the early 1970s when new initiatives were taken towards the control of the major tropical diseases. Tuberculosis was not classed as one of the great neglected diseases in the Rockefeller programme of that name and did not feature as one of the six diseases in WHO's Tropical Disease Research Programme, despite the fact that it is almost certainly the most important preventable cause of death afflicting adults in developing countries. Perhaps it was foreseen that with the development of effective short-course chemotherapy and the availability of a vaccine that appeared to have high efficacy, at least in some places, the necessary tools were available for disease control and all that was required was their appropriate application.

If this indeed was the then thinking, it can be seen, with the wisdom of hindsight, to have been more than a little optimistic. Certainly in the 1980s tuberculosis must be classed as one of the truly greatly neglected diseases. During this decade the situation became more bleak for many developing countries. Firstly, the pace of development showed a marked decline, socio-economic circumstances ceased to improve, or got worse, and this in itself may have led to a deterioration in the tuberculosis situation, but also led to a decline in medical services such that the powerful chemotherapy that had been developed was not effectively delivered to those in need. Secondly, the results of the South India BCG trial became available, the first really large-scale trial of BCG in a developing country, and showed no evidence of a protective effect, opening to question the impact on tuberculosis of one of the most successful medical interventions of the 1980s, the expanded programme of immunization, which now gets BCG to most infants in developing countries. But the worst news of all came most recently, and that was of the interaction between HIV and tuberculosis, bringing about a turnaround in the tuberculosis decline in the United States, where only a few years ago, elimination had become the goal. More seriously, increases in rates of tuberculosis were also seen in the small number of countries in Africa where Dr Styblo and his colleagues in International Union against Tuberculosis and Lung Disease had worked with national disease control programmes to implement widespread short-course chemotherapy programmes. As the HIV epidemic takes hold in India and other Asian countries, with already massive tuberculosis problems, the future looks bleak indeed.

In contrasting the burdens of premature mortality in developing and industrialized countries and the resources devoted to research on specific disease problems, the Commission on Health Research for Development (1990) drew attention to the fact that while 93% of potential years of life lost because of premature mortality (from all causes of death) occurred in developing countries, 95% of global medical research expenditure was devoted to the disease problems of industrialized countries. The re-emergence of tuberculosis as a public health problem in at least some industrialized countries may go some small way towards encouraging some redress of this imbalance in research expenditure, at least as far as tuberculosis is concerned.

One of the debates that I am sure we will have at this meeting, and which for many disease problems is a frequent source of discussion, is around the issue of whether we need more research or whether we already know enough about the disease and have sufficiently powerful interventions available to be able to control tuberculosis effectively. All that is required, some may argue, is operations research to find the most cost-effective ways of delivering and applying the tools we already have. I do not wish to preempt that debate but, given this opportunity, I cannot resist the temptation to air some personal biases. To me it is clear that we need both operations and biomedical research, especially since HIV has appeared on the scene. We have a vaccine that works well in some places, does not work in others, and in most places we do not know whether it works or not. We have powerful chemotherapy available, but even 'short' courses last 6 months or more, and there must be scope for developing yet shorter regimens, using new drugs, especially in view of the spectre of multidrug-resistant disease beginning to emerge. Furthermore, most of our knowledge of the epidemiology of tuberculosis is based on studies in now developed countries and there is uncertainty as to how transferable this model of disease is to developing countries, most especially because of the way in which HIV infection forces us to rethink traditional models of the disease. I have no doubt that we need a two pronged attack. On the one hand to apply the tools we now have in the most cost-effective manner, and, on the other hand, to conduct both basic and applied research to develop better tools and better strategies for disease control.

References

Commission on Health Research for Development (1990) *Health Research: Essential Link to Equity in Development.* Oxford University Press, New York

McKeown T (1979) *The Role of Medicine.* Basil Blackwell, Oxford

Newsholme A (1924) *The Elements of Vital Statistics in their Bearing on Social and Public Health Problems.* D Appleton and Co, New York

Wilson LG (1990) The historical decline of tuberculosis in Europe and America: its cause and significance. *Journal of the History of Medicine and Allied Sciences, 45,* 366–396

2
Impact of Interaction with HIV

Kevin M. De Cock

London School of Hygiene & Tropical Medicine, UK and Centers for Disease Control and Prevention, Atlanta, GA, USA

Introduction: evidence for the association between HIV infection and tuberculosis

Five lines of evidence suggest that infection with human immunodeficiency virus (HIV) is a risk factor for the development of tuberculosis. These are clinical observations, epidemiological data on trends in tuberculosis case rates, HIV seroprevalence rates in patients with tuberculosis, and the results of observational and intervention studies among persons with HIV and tuberculous infections.

Although most studies have concerned HIV type 1 (HIV-1), persons with HIV type 2 (HIV-2) are also at increased risk for tuberculosis (De Cock *et al.*, 1991a). Unless otherwise specified, studies quoted refer to persons infected with HIV-1. Although the rate of development of immune deficiency may be slower in persons infected with HIV-2 than in those with HIV-1, disease manifestations are similar. General statements referring to HIV infection, therefore, should be considered to apply to infection with either virus.

Clinical observations

Clinical reports in the early 1980s documented high rates of tuberculosis in patients with AIDS from Haiti (Pitchenik *et al.*, 1983; Pape *et al.*, 1983) and Central Africa (Piot *et al.*, 1984; Van de Perre *et al.*, 1984). This was in marked contrast to the early clinical descriptions of AIDS in the United States, affecting predominantly white homosexual men, in whom tuberculosis was rare.

Results of autopsy studies in Abidjan, Côte d'Ivoire, showed that 35% of deaths among HIV-positive patients were due to tuberculosis (Lucas *et al.*, 1992), and that tuberculosis was the commonest overall cause of death as well as the most frequent cause of pulmonary pathology in patients with HIV disease (Abouya *et al.*, 1992).

Tuberculosis: Back to the Future. Edited by J.D.H. Porter and K.P.W.J. McAdam
© 1994 John Wiley & Sons Ltd

Trends in tuberculosis

The number of tuberculosis cases reported annually in the United States declined steadily until 1984, when surveillance data showed a reduction in the rate of decline, and subsequently an increase in cases (Snider, 1992). Reported cases declined in whites and Native Americans, but increased among blacks, Hispanics, Asians and Pacific Islanders. Rates increased among both men and women.

Although different factors, including immigration, have played a role in this increase in tuberculosis, the groups with the greatest increases, blacks and Hispanics aged 25–44 years, are also the groups with the highest rates of HIV infection and AIDS. Geographic overlap exists, the greatest increases in tuberculosis having occurred in areas where rates of HIV/AIDS are highest. In recent time, therefore, AIDS and tuberculosis have shared the basic characteristics of descriptive epidemiology of time, place, and person.

Increases in tuberculosis cases coincident with the AIDS epidemic have also been reported from countries in East, Central and West Africa. In Abidjan, annual tuberculosis cases increased by 37% between 1985 and 1991, corresponding to an increase in case rates from 149/100 000 to 159/100 000 (Richards *et al.*, 1992).

HIV seroprevalence in patients with tuberculosis

Increased HIV seroprevalence in tuberculosis patients was first reported from Kinshasa, Zaire, in 1986. Since then, numerous studies have been published from industrialized and developing countries documenting higher rates of HIV infection in patients with tuberculosis than in healthy comparison groups. A recent review (De Cock *et al.*, 1992) described HIV seroprevalence rates of 20–67% among tuberculosis cases in different sub-Saharan African countries, the highest rates in TB patients being found where rates are highest in the general population (Table 2.1). In the United States, the seroprevalence in patients attending tuberculosis clinics ranged from 0 to 46.3% (Onorato *et al.*, 1992).

Cohort studies

In a classic prospective cohort study among injecting drug users in New York, NY, Selwyn and colleagues (1989) showed that persons with HIV infection and a previously positive tuberculin skin test had an incidence of tuberculosis of 7.9 cases per 100 person years; in contrast, no cases occurred in HIV-negative persons with a positive tuberculin skin test. A retrospective cohort study among women of childbearing age in Kinshasa, Zaire, showed that after a median follow-up of 32 months HIV-positive women had a 26-fold greater risk of developing tuberculosis than seronegative women (Braun *et al.*, 1991).

Intervention studies

Prospective studies of the use of tuberculosis chemoprophylaxis among HIV-positive persons have shown that this intervention can reduce the incidence of tuberculosis,

Table 2.1 Prevalence of HIV infection in patients with tuberculosis in selected African countries

Countries	HIV seroprevalence
Burkina Faso Guinea Bissau Kenya Swaziland Zaire	20–29%
Central African Republic Côte d'Ivoire Zimbabwe	30–49%
Burundi Malawi Uganda Zambia	>50%

Modified from De Cock *et al.*, © 1992 American Medical Association from *JAMA*, *268*, 1581–1587.

demonstrating the increased risk and a potential way of modifying it. In a controlled trial in Zambia, HIV-infected persons with Walter Reed Stages III and IV disease who did not receive isoniazid prophylaxis had an incidence of 11.3/100 person years, 4.3 times higher than those who did receive it (Wadhawan *et al.*, 1992).

Magnitude and public health impact

About one-third of the world's population is infected with *Mycobacterium tuberculosis*, over half these infected persons living in South-east Asia, China, and the Western Pacific countries (Sudre *et al.*, 1992). Because Africa's population is small compared to that of Asia, it accounts for less than 10% of the global total of persons with tuberculous infection, although sub-Saharan Africa has the highest annual risk of tuberculous infection (1.5–2.5% per year). The estimated number of cases of tuberculosis worldwide in 1990 was approximately 8 million, with 2.6–2.9 million deaths (Sudre *et al.*, 1992). Tuberculosis is the cause of more adult deaths than any other infectious disease (Murray *et al.*, 1990).

The impact of HIV on rates of tuberculosis will be greatest where the two infections most frequently occur together, which currently is in sub-Saharan Africa. Of the approximately 3 million people worldwide infected with *M. tuberculosis* and HIV, almost 80% reside in Africa. Approximately 305 000 excess cases of tuberculosis attributable to HIV were estimated to have occurred globally in 1990, 230 000 of them in Africa (Sudre *et al.*, 1992). While these HIV-associated cases represent only about 4% of the world's total cases, for Africa this has resulted in a 20% increase in case rates. Estimates of the excess mortality due to HIV-associated tuberculosis are that in 1990 there were 120 000–150 000 excess deaths, of which 100 000–120 000 occurred in Africa.

Projections for the future based on data on disease progression and the prevalence of HIV and tuberculous infections in sub-Saharan Africa are sobering. For example, in Kampala, Uganda, where the prevalence of HIV infection in young adults currently exceeds 30%, the annual incidence of tuberculosis by the end of the century may be 2%, representing an excess burden of tuberculosis of about 800% over what should have occurred in the absence of HIV (Schulzer et al., 1992). In African cities with adult HIV seroprevalence rates of about 10%, the excess tuberculosis incidence may be approximately 300%. As the HIV epidemic spreads in Asia, an increasing proportion of the world's HIV-associated cases of tuberculosis will be from that continent.

Natural history and interaction of HIV infection and tuberculosis

HIV infection

The natural history of HIV infection is one of progressive decline in immune function, best characterized by loss of CD4+ T lymphocytes, with the eventual appearance of one or more opportunistic diseases that are included under the surveillance case definition for AIDS. Data from prospective cohort studies show that after 11 years of HIV infection, 54% of patients have AIDS (Rutherford et al., 1990); the majority of patients not meeting the case definition for AIDS after this time nevertheless have immune deficiency, and are highly likely to progress to full disease. Although understanding of the natural history of HIV infection is still incomplete, and antiviral drugs can modify the course of disease, the available evidence suggests that most or all HIV-infected persons will ultimately become ill with immune deficiency.

Tuberculosis

Exposure to tubercle bacilli usually results from contact with a person with sputum smear-positive tuberculosis (Murray et al., 1990). Infection is controlled by cell-mediated immunity, but is generally not eliminated (Hopewell, 1992). The lifetime risk of developing tuberculosis is about 10%, half of the cases occurring within 5 years of infection, and the other half at a more remote time (Murray, 1989). Early disease is especially likely in children.

Interaction of HIV and tuberculosis

Three mechanisms appear relevant for the development of HIV-associated tuberculosis: reactivation, progression from recent infection, and reinfection. A subject of great interest currently is the effect of tuberculosis on the natural history of HIV infection.

Reactivation. The work of Selwyn *et al.* (1989) quoted earlier demonstrated a 24-fold increased risk of developing tuberculosis in HIV-positive patients who had a previously documented positive tuberculin skin test compared with HIV-positive patients with a negative skin test. This has been interpreted to suggest that much tuberculosis associated with HIV infection represents reactivation disease. In developing countries with high annual rates of infection with *M. tuberculosis*, where the majority of adults will have been infected, this is likely to be the commonest mechanism of disease development in HIV-positive persons.

Progression from recent infection. Persons with HIV infection who are exposed to *M. tuberculosis* are at risk of infection and rapid progression to disease. This has been observed in nosocomial outbreaks of tuberculosis (Di Perri *et al.*, 1989; Daley *et al.*, 1992) including multidrug-resistant disease (Edlin *et al.*, 1992) among patients with profound immunodeficiency who were exposed in health care settings. Outbreaks of tuberculosis under such conditions have been characterized by attack rates of 30–40% among those exposed, with disease occurring as little as one month after infection.

Reinfection. Conventional thinking is that immunocompetent patients infected with *M. tuberculosis* are resistant to subsequent infection. Analysis of tuberculous organisms isolated from patients with AIDS using the technique of restriction fragment length polymorphism (RFLP) suggests that reinfection can occur (Hopewell, 1992; Godfrey-Faussett and Stoker, 1992). This raises the possibility that apparent cases of relapse after therapy for tuberculosis in HIV-infected patients may in fact represent reinfections, and has important implications for nosocomial transmission in areas where both infections are frequent.

Effect of tuberculosis on HIV infection. A high death rate in HIV-infected patients with tuberculosis is recognized (Colebunders *et al.*, 1989; Small *et al.*, 1991), although death is apparently rarely due to tuberculosis itself (Nunn *et al.*, 1992). Tuberculosis results in immune activation affecting T cells and macrophages, witnessed by increased serum levels of different cytokines (Wallis *et al.*, 1993). Increased levels of beta-2-microglobulin have also been documented early in HIV-associated tuberculosis, which otherwise is a marker of progression to AIDS. Although firm evidence is limited, tuberculosis has been suggested to lead to immune activation, increased virus expression, and more rapid progression to AIDS.

Clinical features, diagnosis and therapy

Clinical presentation

The clinical presentation of HIV-associated tuberculosis is heavily influenced by the degree of underlying immunodeficiency (Barnes *et al.*, 1991; Hopewell, 1992;

Table 2.2   CD4+ T lymphocyte counts in newly diagnosed outpatients with tuberculosis
(Abidjan, 1992–93)

CD4+ T lymphocyte count	HIV-positive EPTB (%)	HIV-positive PTB (%)	HIV-negative (%)
<200/mm³	51	41	1
200–499/mm³	36	39	16
500+/mm³	13	20	83
Total	100	100	100
Median CD4/mm³	197	262	824

EPTB = extrapulmonary tuberculosis; PTB = pulmonary tuberculosis.

De Cock *et al.*, 1992). In HIV-infected patients with AIDS and tuberculosis in the United States, tuberculosis preceded other AIDS-defining illnesses in about one-half of cases, by periods of up to 2 years. Table 2.2 shows the range of CD4+ T lymphocyte counts found in newly diagnosed outpatients with tuberculosis in Abidjan. Although the range is wide, the median count at presentation in HIV-positive patients is higher than that found in other severe opportunistic infections, in keeping with clinical observations that tuberculosis is an early event in the course of immune deficiency.

In the earlier stages of HIV disease, the pathology of tuberculosis is similar to that seen in patients without HIV infection. As the CD4+ T lymphocyte count falls, the clinicopathological nature changes and tuberculous disease becomes increasingly atypical and disseminated. Histologically, the appearances of caseating giant cell and epithelioid granulomas with scanty tubercle bacilli ('paucibacillary tuberculosis') become less common. In advanced immunodeficiency, the macrophage reaction is diminished, granulomas are rare, and tubercle bacilli are abundant ('multibacillary tuberculosis').

In early HIV disease, the clinical features of tuberculosis resemble those seen in HIV-negative persons. Pulmonary tuberculosis is most frequent, and is often sputum smear-positive. Localized extrapulmonary tuberculosis, especially lymph node disease, occurs in some HIV-positive persons. In late-stage immunodeficiency, disseminated tuberculosis associated with severe wasting and with the features of multibacillary disease is characteristic.

Overall, HIV-positive patients are more likely to have extrapulmonary tuberculosis than HIV-negative patients. Other major clinical differences are a greater frequency of other manifestations of HIV disease such as wasting, oral candidiasis, generalized lymphadenopathy and pruiginous dermatosis.

Diagnosis

Diagnosis of tuberculosis in HIV-positive persons is rendered more difficult by an increased frequency of false negative tuberculin skin tests (Huebner *et al.*, 1992), of sputum smear-negative (pulmonary or extrapulmonary) disease (Elliott *et al.*, 1990), and of atypical radiological manifestations (Pitchenik and Rubinson, 1985; Elliott *et al.*, 1990).

Tuberculin skin tests are of limited diagnostic value in countries where the annual risk of infection is high and where BCG is widely used. The rate of tuberculin skin test positivity in HIV-infected patients with active tuberculosis is related to immune function; this explains the wide range reported, from approximately one-third to three-quarters (Barnes *et al.*, 1991; Hopewell, 1992). For HIV-infected persons, 5 mm induration is recommended as a cut-off for considering a tuberculin skin test positive (American Thoracic Society/CDC, 1990). HIV-infected persons with negative tuberculin skin tests should have anergy testing with two other antigens (*Candida*, mumps or tetanus toxoid).

There have been conflicting reports of the sensitivity of sputum smears in diagnosing pulmonary tuberculosis in HIV-infected persons. In Zambia (Elliott *et al.*, 1990) patients with culture-positive pulmonary tuberculosis were less likely to have a positive sputum smear if they were HIV-infected (63% versus 82% in HIV-positives and HIV-negatives, respectively). In other reports the sensitivity of sputum smears has been similar in HIV-positive and HIV-negative persons. The underlying immune status is again likely to be important, since cavitation is more frequent in patients with preserved immune function. With an increased frequency of extrapulmonary and disseminated disease, the overall sensitivity of sputum smear examination for diagnosing tuberculosis in HIV-infected persons is likely to be reduced.

Early observations placed great emphasis on differences in the radiological appearances in HIV-positive persons (Pitchenik and Rubinson, 1985; Elliott *et al.*, 1990). Compared with HIV-negative patients, HIV-infected patients are less likely to have cavitary lesions, more often have involvement of parts of the lung other than the upper zones, and have an increased frequency of pleural effusions and intrathoracic adenopathy. As the CD4+ T lymphocyte count falls, cavitation becomes less common (Abouya *et al.*, unpublished).

A major problem is diagnosis of tuberculosis in HIV-infected persons with negative sputum smears and atypical or non-diagnostic features on chest X-ray. Fine needle extrathoracic lymph node aspiration with Ziehl–Neelsen staining yields evidence of acid-fast bacilli in a substantial proportion of cases (Lucas, 1991) even with pleural or pericardial tuberculosis (Pithie and Chicksen, 1992). The problem of diagnosis of disseminated tuberculosis, which is often found at autopsy in African patients with 'slim disease' (Lucas *et al.*, unpublished), is especially difficult. Fine needle aspiration of lymph nodes and perhaps liver merits investigation. Use of the polymerase chain reaction (PCR) for the diagnosis of tuberculosis is of research interest currently, but the applicability of this to the problems in developing countries is uncertain.

Therapy

Differences between HIV-positive and HIV-negative patients in their response to therapy are increased rates of side effects from drugs, increased mortality in the HIV-infected, and perhaps increased relapse rates (Barnes *et al.*, 1991; Hopewell *et al.*, 1992; De Cock *et al.*, 1992). In patients treated with modern rifampicin-containing regimens, response to treatment is usually satisfactory, and microbiological response occurs as in HIV-negative patients (Small *et al.*, 1991). However, a significantly increased risk of death has been demonstrated in the HIV-infected, both in industrialized as well as in developing countries. In San Francisco, median survival in HIV-positive patients treated for tuberculosis was 16 months after diagnosis, and 6% of the deaths were considered attributable to tuberculosis (Small *et al.*, 1991). In Nairobi, Kenya, the probability of death after 6 months' therapy for HIV-positive and HIV-negative patients was, respectively, 21% and 6% (Nunn *et al.*, 1992). Death rates of the same order of magnitude have been documented among HIV-positive persons in Abidjan (Kassim *et al.*, 1992).

Definitive autopsy studies to document the causes of the increased mortality in HIV-infected persons with tuberculosis have not been performed. In Nairobi, most of the increased mortality after the first month of treatment was not considered due to tuberculosis itself, but to other HIV-associated complications, especially non-tuberculous bacterial septicaemia (Nunn *et al.*, 1992). In San Francisco, tuberculosis was considered responsible for death in 6% of treated patients; three-quarters of the tuberculosis-attributable deaths occurred in the first month of treatment (Small *et al.*, 1991).

As with treatment for some other opportunistic infections, a greater frequency of adverse side effects from antituberculous medication has been documented in HIV-positive patients. In the report from San Francisco, 18% of patients had their therapy changed because of adverse effects (Small *et al.*, 1991). Reactions consisted of rashes, hepatitis, gastrointestinal disturbance and anaphylaxis. Side effects were attributed, in descending order of frequency, to rifampicin, pyrazinamide, isoniazid and ethambutol. In developing countries that use thiacetazone-containing regimens, this drug is likely to be the most frequently responsible for side effects. Thiacetazone toxicity may occur in up to one-third of HIV-positive patients receiving it, with cutaneous hypersensitivity reactions the most common and frequently fatal (Nunn *et al.*, 1991). These severe side effects are mostly seen early on in the course of treatment, and are generally found in the more immunosuppressed patients.

Following therapy, a relapse rate of 3.6 per 100 person-years was documented in HIV-infected patients in San Francisco, probably not different from that seen in HIV-negative persons in that city (Small *et al.*, 1991). Increased rates of relapse have been reported, however, from Kinshasa (Perriens *et al.*, 1991) and Nairobi (Hawken *et al.*, 1992), where rifampicin-containing regimens were not being used. Since the underlying immune deficiency causing reactivation of tuberculosis persists after therapy, it would be surprising if relapse was not more frequent in HIV-positive persons in due course. Increased mortality may be one reason why relapse is not being seen more often.

Multidrug-resistant tuberculosis

The emergence of multidrug-resistant tuberculosis (MDR-TB) in association with HIV infection must rank as one of the most important events in public health in recent years. Since 1990, the Centers for Disease Control and Prevention (CDC) have participated in or learnt of about a dozen outbreaks or clusters of MDR-TB in the United States, involving hospital patients, health care workers, prison inmates, prison guards, and clients in a substance-abuse treatment facility (Centers for Disease Control, 1991a; 1991b; 1992a; Edlin et al., 1992; Fischl et al., 1992). Of the approximately 300 persons affected, about 230 have died. These outbreaks have been concentrated in New York State, including New York City, and Florida, but MDR-TB in HIV-positive persons and their contacts has also been reported in Michigan (Centers for Disease Control, 1991a) as well as in France (Bader, 1992) and Italy (Monno et al., 1991).

The outbreaks described have some common features. They involved HIV-positive patients confined in restricted environments such as prisons or hospitals. Diagnosis of tuberculosis and availability of drug sensitivity patterns were frequently delayed, giving ample opportunity for dissemination of infection. Facilities were often inadequate to isolate infectious patients. Molecular characterization of strains by RFLP demonstrated identical strains affecting persons in outbreaks, and provided evidence for nosocomial transmission. The time between exposure and illness in HIV-infected persons was often short, illustrating the high attack rate and reduced incubation period for tuberculosis in persons with advanced immunodeficiency. Mortality has exceeded 80% in some of the outbreaks. Most strains isolated have been resistant to rifampicin and isoniazid, while some have been resistant to as many as seven or more drugs.

Management of patients with MDR-TB is imperfect. Drug susceptibility of the relevant strain should govern the choice of therapy, with known data on patterns of resistance in the community determining the choice of therapy if susceptibility tests are not available. Maximal drug levels should be aimed for, and surgery may need to complement medical therapy to remove localized concentrations of drug-resistant bacilli. Addition of individual drugs to a failing regimen is likely to be ineffective and lead to further drug resistance. Fluoroquinolones such as ofloxacin and sparfloxacin are being investigated for their potential role in treatment.

CDC have published a National Action Plan to combat MDR-TB (Centers for Disease Control, 1992b). Important elements include specific recommendations to limit nosocomial transmission, conduct surveillance to determine patterns of drug susceptibility, widen the capacity for rapid determination of drug susceptibility, and place increased emphasis on directly observed therapy. However, many experts have pointed out how the epidemic of tuberculosis, resistant and sensitive to drugs, reflects fundamental problems with the provision of medical care to those most at risk for HIV infection and tuberculosis (Brudney and Dobkin, 1991; Bloom and Murray, 1992).

Implications for programmes and policy

Tuberculosis control programmes

Tuberculosis control programmes in countries with high rates of HIV infection will be severely if not impossibly stretched by the increased case load secondary to the HIV epidemic. This will tax resources for diagnosis and therapy. Patients presenting with tuberculosis will often have other medical complaints needing attention, for which investigational and therapeutic facilities may not be available. Use of antituberculous drugs will increase outside of the direct supervision of the tuberculosis control programme, when hospitalized patients need treatment. This may lead to reduced therapeutic discipline, inconsistent treatment criteria, and poor compliance, all risk factors for the development of drug resistance. Finally, but very importantly, morale of staff may suffer because of an increased case load combined with a high mortality rate, and public confidence in the programme may decline.

Policy

Five important issues of policy are coordination between tuberculosis and AIDS control programmes, HIV testing and counselling, use of BCG, chemoprophylaxis, and surveillance.

Co-ordination. In developing countries with high rates of HIV infection, AIDS and tuberculosis are often indistinguishable, since tuberculosis is the dominant opportunistic infection causing death in HIV-infected persons. Control programmes for the two diseases clearly need to coordinate their activities in almost all areas, including health education, clinical management, epidemiological surveillance, and policy on issues such as chemoprophylaxis. This coordination has unfortunately often been lacking.

HIV testing and counselling. In many countries in Africa, one-third to one-half of tuberculosis patients are HIV-infected. Their management is currently not different in most countries from that for HIV-negative patients, but that may not always be so. In addition, such patients require counselling about their condition and ways of avoiding transmission of HIV to others. This raises issues of policy concerning voluntary HIV testing and counselling of patients with tuberculosis, and the resources required for this.

BCG. This is currently given to infants at birth in developing countries under the Expanded Programme on Immunization (Citron, 1993). In HIV-infected adults given BCG there is a risk of dissemination. While there is no evidence that vaccinated infants of HIV-positive mothers have suffered disseminated BCG disease, neither are there definitive studies to show that dissemination cannot occur in HIV-infected children. A reasonable policy is to continue to give BCG at birth to all infants, but to avoid its use later in life in areas where HIV infection is common.

Chemoprophylaxis. In persons without HIV infection who are infected with *M. tuberculosis* chemoprophylaxis (usually with isoniazid alone) reduces the incidence of tuberculosis by up to about 90% (Porter and McAdam, 1992). The extremely high incidence of tuberculosis in HIV-positive persons led to recommendations for use of chemoprophylaxis for all those infected with *M. tuberculosis* and HIV (Centers for Disease Control, 1990), despite the lack of data from prospective clinical trials to establish the efficacy of such an intervention. Preliminary data from Zambia have shown that treatment with isoniazid reduces the incidence of tuberculosis in persons infected with HIV (Wadhawan *et al.*, 1992), although increased long-term survival has not been demonstrated thus far.

Unresolved issues include which drug or combination of drugs is optimal, the long-term effect on drug resistance, whom to target, and what screening to perform prior to initiating therapy. Feasibility and cost will be major questions to consider in developing countries whose tuberculosis control programmes are not succeeding in treating all HIV-negative, smear-positive cases of tuberculosis. Chemoprophylaxis for tuberculosis in HIV-infected persons is one of the most critical research and policy questions to be addressed today.

Surveillance. As of January 1993, CDC is using an expanded case definition for AIDS surveillance that considers all persons to have AIDS who meet the 1987 revised case definition, or who are HIV-positive and have tuberculosis, recurrent pneumonia, invasive carcinoma of the cervix, or a CD4+ T lymphocyte count below 200 μl (Centers for Disease Control, 1993). Inclusion of tuberculosis as an AIDS-defining illness in HIV infection under the expanded CDC case definition has broad implications for the rest of the world, especially developing countries with high rates of both infections. Further discussion is needed to make international AIDS surveillance case definitions more uniform.

International surveillance for tuberculosis is weak, and has not taken account of HIV infection. Systematic serosurveillance in tuberculosis patients, allowing estimates of tuberculosis cases attributable to HIV, would be of value.

Future research

The most important questions are how currently available technology can be used to improve case detection and management, and how HIV-infected persons can best be prevented from developing tuberculosis. These questions need to be addressed not only in terms of efficacy but also feasibility. Issues of clinical management that require addressing are optimal duration of treatment for HIV-infected patients with tuberculosis, the need for maintenance therapy, and the causes of increased mortality in HIV-positive patients with tuberculosis and ways of modifying this. Research is required to establish the degree to which MDR-TB occurs internationally, and to develop better drugs. Development and evaluation of depot preparations, for MDR-TB as well as non-resistant strains, deserves attention.

Priorities for epidemiological research include development and evaluation of projections of the tuberculosis case load, assessment of the extent to which HIV infection increases the overall burden of tuberculosis, and investigation of the effect of the HIV epidemic on paediatric tuberculosis. Whether or not tuberculosis affects the natural history of HIV infection needs study since data confirming this hypothesis would argue for increased emphasis on chemoprophylaxis.

Many fundamental needs in tuberculosis research are independent of but highlighted by the HIV epidemic. Few of the advances of the molecular era have until now been applied to this disease. Development of tools such as RFLP permit molecular epidemiological studies of patterns of transmission and outbreaks, and, potentially, distinction between reinfection and relapse. Better understanding of tuberculosis immunology, molecular biology, and pathogenesis will be required for long-term goals of improved diagnostics and vaccines.

Finally, to bring the science of tuberculosis into the 21st century will take manpower and resources not currently applied to it (Bloom and Murray, 1992). A modern cadre of well-funded researchers and public health professionals is required who are prepared to devote their careers to this disease. Paradoxically, the AIDS epidemic has contributed more than any other phenomenon to the recent global increase in tuberculosis, but also has brought scientific and political attention to what has been an extraordinarily neglected disease. Scientific and public health leadership are required to seize the opportunities now available.

Acknowledgements

Some of the Abidjan work quoted was funded in part by the Global Programme on AIDS, WHO; and the Rockefeller Foundation. I thank the Ministry of Health of Côte d'Ivoire; staff of Projet RETRO-CI, Abidjan; colleagues in the Division of HIV/AIDS, NCID, CDC; and Drs I.-M. Coulibaly, D. Coulibaly and S.B. Lucas.

References

American Thoracic Society/Centers for Disease Control (1990) Diagnostic standards and classification of tuberculosis, *American Review of Respiratory Disease, 142*, 725–735
Abouya YL, Beaumel A, Lucas S *et al.* (1992) *Pneumocystis carinii* pneumonia. An uncommon cause of death in African patients with acquired immunodeficiency syndrome. *American Review of Respiratory Disease, 145*, 617–620

Bader JM (1992) France: nosocomial multidrug-resistant TB. *Lancet, 340,* 1533

Barnes PF, Bloch AB, Davidson PT, Snider DE (1991) Tuberculosis in patients with human immunodeficiency virus infection. *New England Journal of Medicine, 324,* 1644–1650

Bloom BR, Murray CJL (1992) Tuberculosis: commentary on a reemergent killer. *Science, 257,* 1055–1064

Braun MM, Badi N, Ryder R *et al.* (1991) A retrospective cohort study of the risk of tuberculosis among women of childbearing age with HIV infection in Zaire. *American Review of Repiratory Disease, 143,* 501–504

Brudney K, Dobkin J (1991) Resurgent tuberculosis in New York City. Human immunodeficiency virus, homelessness, and the decline of tuberculosis control programs. *American Review of Respiratory Disease, 144,* 745–749

Centers for Disease Control. Advisory Committee for Elimination of Tuberculosis (1990) Screening for tuberculosis and tuberculous infection in high risk populations [and] the use of preventive therapy for tuberculous infection in the United States. *Morbidity and Mortality Weekly Report, 39,* RR8, 1–12

Centers for Disease Control (1991a) Transmission of multidrug-resistant tuberculosis from an HIV-positive client in a residential substance-abuse treatment facility—Michigan. *Morbidity and Mortality Weekly Report, 40,* 129–131

Centers for Disease Control (1991b) Nosocomial transmission of multidrug-resistant tuberculosis among HIV-infected persons—Florida and New York, 1988–1991. *Morbidity and Mortality Weekly Report, 40,* 585–591

Centers for Disease Control (1992a) Transmission of multidrug-resistant tuberculosis among immunocompromised persons in a correctional system—New York, 1991. *Morbidity and Mortality Weekly Report, 41,* 507–509

Centers for Disease Control (1992b) National action plan to combat multidrug-resistant tuberculosis. *Morbidity and Mortality Weekly Report, 41,* RR-11, 1–48

Centers for Disease Control (1993) 1993 revised classification system for HIV infection and expanded surveillance case definition for AIDS among adolescents and adults. *Morbidity and Mortality Weekly Report, 41,* No R17, 1–19

Citron KM (1993) BCG vaccination against tuberculosis: international perspectives. *British Medical Journal, 306,* 222–223

Colebunders RL, Ryder RW, Nzilambi N *et al.* (1989) HIV infection in patients with tuberculosis in Kinshasa, Zaïre. *American Review of Respiratory Disease, 139,* 1082–1085

Daley CL, Small PM, Schecter GF *et al.* (1992) An outbreak of tuberculosis with accelerated progression among persons infected with the human immunodeficiency virus. An analysis using restriction-fragment-length polymorphisms. *New England Journal of Medicine, 326,* 231–235

De Cock KM, Gnaore E, Adjorlolo G *et al.* (1991) Risk of tuberculosis in patients with HIV-I and HIV-II infections in Abidjan, Ivory Coast. *British Medical Journal, 302,* 496–499

De Cock KM, Soro B, Coulibaly IM, Lucas SB (1992) Tuberculosis and HIV infection in sub-Saharan Africa. *Journal of the American Medical Association, 268,* 1581–1587

Di Perri G, Cruciani M, Danzi MC *et al.* (1989) Nosocomial epidemic of active tuberculosis among HIV-infected patients. *Lancet, ii,* 1502–1504

Edlin BR, Tokars JI, Grieco MH *et al.* (1992) An outbreak of multidrug-resistant tuberculosis among hospitalized patients with the acquired immunodeficiency syndrome. *New England Journal of Medicine, 326,* 1514–1521

Elliott AM, Luo N, Tembo G *et al.* (1990) Impact of tuberculosis in Zambia: a cross sectional study. *British Medical Journal, 301,* 412–415

Fischl MA, Uttamchandani RB, Daikos GL *et al.* (1992) An outbreak of tuberculosis caused by multiple-drug-resistant tubercle bacilli among patients with HIV infection. *Annals of Internal Medicine, 117,* 177–183

Godfrey-Faussett P, Stoker NG (1992) Aspects of tuberculosis in Africa: 3. Genetic "fingerprinting" for clues to the pathogenesis of tuberculosis. *Transactions of the Royal Society of Tropical Medicine and Hygiene, 86*, 472–475

Hawken M, Nunn P, Gathua S *et al.* (1992) HIV-I infection and recurrence of tuberculosis, Nairobi, Kenya. VIII International Conference on AIDS/III STD World Congress, Amsterdam, The Netherlands, 19–24 July 1992, Volume 1, Abstract TuB 0538

Hopewell PC (1992) Impact of human immunodeficiency virus infection on the epidemiology, clinical features, management, and control of tuberculosis. *Clinical Infectious Diseases, 15*, 540–547

Huebner RE, Villarino ME, Snider DE (1992) Tuberculin skin testing and the HIV epidemic. *Journal of the American Medical Association, 267*, 409–410

Kassim S, Sassan-Morokro M, Doorly R *et al.* (1992) Prospective study of pulmonary tuberculosis and HIV-1 and HIV-2 infections, Abidjan, Côte d'Ivoire. VIII International Conference on AIDS/III STD World Congress, Amsterdam, The Netherlands, 19–24 July 1992. Volume 2, Abstract PoB 3086

Lucas SB (1991) Tuberculosis, lymphadenopathy, and HIV. *Lancet, 337*, 428

Lucas S, Hounnou A, Beaumel A *et al.* (1992) The pathology of adult HIV infection in Abidjan, Côte d'Ivoire. VIII International Conference on AIDS/III STD World Congress, Amsterdam, The Netherlands, 19–24 July 1992. Volume 2, Abstract PoB 3751

Monno L, Angarano G, Carbonara S *et al.* (1991) Emergence of drug-resistant *Mycobacterium tuberculosis* in HIV-infected patients. *Lancet, 337*, 852

Murray CJL, Styblo K, Rouillon A (1990) Tuberculosis in developing countries: burden, intervention and cost. *Bulletin of the International Union Against Tuberculosis and Lung Disease, 65*, 6–24

Murray JF (1989) The white plague: down and out, or up and coming? *American Review of Respiratory Disease, 140*, 1788–1795

Nunn P, Brindle R, Carpenter L *et al.* (1992) Cohort study of human immunodeficiency virus infection in patients with tuberculosis in Nairobi, Kenya: analysis of early (6-month) mortality. *American Review of Respiratory Disease, 146*, 849–854

Onorato IM, McCray E, and the Field Services Branch (1992) Prevalence of human immunodeficiency virus infection among patients attending tuberculosis clinics in the United States. *Journal of Infectious Diseases, 165*, 87–92

Pape JW, Liautaud B, Thomas F *et al.* (1983) Characteristics of the acquired immunodeficiency syndrome (AIDS) in Haiti. *New England Journal of Medicine, 309*, 945–950

Perriens JH, Colebunders RL, Karahunga C *et al.* (1991) Increased mortality and tuberculosis treatment failure rate among human immunodeficiency virus (HIV) seropositive compared with HIV seronegative patients with pulmonary tuberculosis treated with "standard" chemotherapy in Kinshasa, Zaire. *American Review of Respiratory Disease, 144*, 750–755

Piot P, Quinn TC, Taelman H *et al.* (1984) Acquired immunodeficiency syndrome in a heterosexual population in Zaire. *Lancet, ii*, 65–69

Pitchenik AE, Rubinson HA (1985) The radiographic appearance of tuberculosis in patients with the acquired immune deficiency syndrome (AIDS) and pre-AIDS. *American Review of Respiratory Disease, 131*, 393–396

Pitchenik AE, Fischl MA, Dickinson GM *et al.* (1983) Opportunistic infections and Kaposi's sarcoma among Haitians: evidence of a new acquired immunodeficiency state. *Annals of Internal Medicine, 98*, 277–284

Pithie AD, Chicksen B (1992) Fine-needle extrathoracic lymph-node aspiration in HIV-associated sputum-negative tuberculosis. *Lancet, 340*, 1504–1505

Porter JDH, McAdam KPWJ (1992) Aspects of tuberculosis in Africa. 1. Tuberculosis in

Africa in the AIDS era—the role of chemoprophylaxis. *Transactions of the Royal Society of Tropical Medicine and Hygiene, 86*, 467–469

Richards SB, Nieburg P, Coulibaly IM, Coulibaly D, Doorly R, De Cock KM (1992) Changes in the epidemiology of tuberculosis (TB) since the advent of human immunodeficiency virus (HIV)–Abidjan, Côte d'Ivoire. VII International Conference on AIDS in Africa, Yaoundé, Abstract TO001

Rutherford GW, Lifson AR, Hessol NA *et al.* (1990) Course of HIV-1 infection in a cohort of homosexual and bisexual men: an 11 year follow up study. *British Medical Journal, 301*, 1183–1188

Schulzer M, Fitzgerald JM, Enarson DA, Grzybowski S (1992) An estimate of the future size of the tuberculosis problem in sub-Saharan Africa resulting from HIV infection. *Tubercle and Lung Disease, 73*, 52–58

Selwyn PA, Hartel D, Lewis VA *et al.* (1989) A prospective study of the risk of tuberculosis among intravenous drug users with human immunodeficiency virus infection. *New England Journal of Medicine, 320*, 545–550

Small PM, Schecter GF, Goodman PC, Sande MA, Chaisson RE, Hopewell PC (1991) Treatment of tuberculosis in patients with advanced human immunodeficiency virus infection. *New England Journal of Medicine, 324*, 289–294

Snider D (1992) The impact of tuberculosis on women, children and minorities in the United States. *World Congress on Tuberculosis,* Bethesda. (Abstract C1)

Sudre P, Dam GT, Kochi A (1992) La tuberculose aujourd'hui dans le monde. *Bulletin of the World Health Organization, 70*, 297–308

Van de Perre P, Rouvroy D, Lepage P *et al.* (1984) Acquired immunodeficiency syndrome in Rwanda. *Lancet, ii*, 62–65

Wadhawan D, Hira S, Mwansa N, Perine P (1992) Preventive tuberculosis chemotherapy with isoniazid among persons infected with HIV-1. VIII International Conference on AIDS/III STD World Congress, Amsterdam, The Netherlands, 19–24 July 1992. Volume 1, Abstract TuB 0536

Wallis RS, Vjecha M, Amir-Tahmasseb M *et al.* (1993) Influence of tuberculosis on human immunodeficiency virus (HIV-1): enhanced cytokine expression and elevated beta-2 microglobulin in HIV-1-associated tuberculosis. *Journal of Infectious Diseases, 167*, 43–48

Discussion

Paul Nunn

World Health Organization, Geneva, Switzerland

Nobody who has entered a TB ward in Africa in recent years can doubt the seriousness of the interaction of HIV and tuberculosis. But the interaction is complex, with many implications and Dr De Cock has dissected them with skill and clarity, exposing the issues for patients and physicians in both the developing and the developed world. If there is one perspective that could be added it is that of the national TB control programme (NTP) in a developing country, and it is from this viewpoint that I will base most of my remarks.

First, how big is the problem on a global scale? Using only one of many possible ways of estimating the magnitude of the impact of HIV on TB it appears unlikely that HIV-associated tuberculosis will greatly exceed 11% of all cases of tuberculosis by the year 2000. Although this figure may appear small, it represents a total of some 1.14 million cases per year by the year 2000, and in addition, it can only rise with time. It is reasonable, if depressing, to assume that any HIV vaccine or treatment would only slowly become available to the developing world. We must begin to plan for this disaster now, and especially in Asia, where two-thirds of the world's TB-infected population live, and where many countries do not yet have effective TB control programmes. Before HIV reaches its peak, effective TB control must be introduced. Emphasis should be placed on the cities, which will probably bear the brunt of the HIV-associated TB epidemic, in contrast to the current rural predominance of TB in many developing countries.

Dr De Cock implies that reactivation of latent tuberculosis infection will be more important in the development of TB in dually infected people than newly acquired infection. However, it may not be so. The risk of infection with *Mycobacterium tuberculosis* may be higher in HIV-infected people. Susceptibility may be greater, and in addition, both diseases are poverty related and may cluster. Thus, local infection rates may be much higher than average in areas where HIV infection is also high, including hospital wards and outpatient clinics. Further, any protection afforded by previous tuberculous infection is likely to be diminished by HIV. It is thus too early to exclude newly acquired infections as a significant source of HIV-associated TB.

In the area of diagnosis, although it appears that sputum smear microscopy is less sensitive in HIV-associated TB, it is not clear how this impacts on programmes. Even in the presence of HIV, diagnosis based on sputum smear alone may be sufficient for control of TB transmission. The hard fact remains that it is the smear-positive cases that are important to diagnose from the public health viewpoint. For the individual patient, health workers must know that a negative smear must be repeated if symptoms persist. While the smear-negative patient may be the smear-positive case of the future, and therefore important to detect not only for his/her own sake but also for public health reasons, HIV-infected smear-negative patients have a shorter lifespan than HIV-negative patients with TB and thus a smaller probability of developing into chronic tuberculosis cases.

The main practical problem in diagnosis is quite different: in Malawi, for example, while the number of smear-positive cases has almost doubled since 1985, the number of smear-negative cases has more than quadrupled. The enormous case load that has resulted is threatening to break the TB programme. The major problem facing TB control programmes in sub-Saharan Africa now is how to cope with this situation. In other words, how can we discriminate between those with HIV disease alone and those with genuine smear-negative TB? What are the most appropriate treatment and supervision strategies for tuberculosis when HIV prevalence is high?

On the outcome of treatment, mortality from both TB and other causes is all too common among patients with HIV-associated TB. In Nairobi, HIV-positive patients with TB were nearly four times more likely to die from TB than HIV-negative patients (rate ratio 3.8 (95%, confidence intervals (CI) 1.3–11) unpublished data) within 13 months of diagnosis. Most of these deaths were in the first month of treatment. However, they were even more likely to die from other causes (rate ratio 14 (4.4–42)), and these are, in descending order of frequency, non-tuberculous bacterial infections, intracranial lesions and toxic epidermal necrolysis. NTPs therefore need to diagnose patients earlier, and be able to diagnose and treat non-tuberculous infections.

Does TB accelerate mortality from HIV infection by activating the immune system and thereby increasing HIV replication? If it is true that a raised beta-2-microglobulin represents immune system activation (Wallis *et al.*, 1993), then it appears that HIV-positive patients with TB have more activated systems than HIV-negative patients: 48/64 (75%) compared to 51/124 (41%) with a beta-2-microglobulin level $\geqslant 5.5$ mg/dl at diagnosis in one study (Nunn *et al.*, 1992). However, while raised beta-2-microglobulin was a significant risk factor for death among HIV-negative patients, it was not for the HIV-positive group (RR 12.2 (1.5–100) compared to 1.0 (0.3–3.2)).

From the programme standpoint the main problem with therapy in developing countries is thiacetazone toxicity. Twenty-eight per cent of the world's population live in areas where thiacetazone is part of the recommended antituberculosis regimen. This is even higher in Africa (65%), the eastern Mediterranean (45%), and South-east Asia (68%). While WHO has recommended that thiacetazone be avoided in patients known or suspected to be HIV positive (WHO, 1992), this does not, of itself, provide NTPs with the necessary information to determine the most appropriate policy. The possibilities are to replace thiacetazone completely with rifampicin or ethambutol, to replace it only in those positive on HIV testing, or to train health workers to recognize and treat cutaneous hypersensitivity reactions before they become life-threatening. The choice will depend, amongst other things, on the prevalence of HIV infection among TB patients, the financial resources available, and the logistic, social and political consequences of HIV tests for TB patients.

There is no doubt that the near obsession of health care workers in the USA with multidrug-resistant strains of tuberculosis (MDR-TB) in HIV-positive patients reflects a major problem. It is not yet clear if it is also a major problem in developing countries (Braun *et al.*, 1992; Githui *et al.*, 1992). But it should be emphasized that it is not clear because there are almost no data. What information there is suggests there is no room whatsoever for complacency. MDR-TB is certainly present in the developing world (Jain, 1992).

With regard to the five policy issues addressed by Dr De Cock, while co-ordination between AIDS and TB control programmes may be desirable, the priority must be for TB control programmes to achieve far higher cure rates for TB.

BCG and chemoprophylaxis, on present evidence, are likely to have little role in the containment of HIV-associated TB among the general public.

More fundamental questions have yet to be answered. They include: how can adequate, sustainable funding for NTPs in developing countries be achieved? How can expansion of NTPs to cope with greatly increased case loads, and the treatment of non-tuberculous opportunistic infections be realized? What measures should be taken to enable NTPs in Asia to prepare for the coming epidemic of HIV-associated TB? How can highly infectious smear-positive cases be separated from highly susceptible HIV-positive individuals in hospitals and clinics? How can diagnostic precision be improved in HIV-associated TB? What is the most cost-effective thiacetazone-free treatment regimen for HIV-associated TB? What is the most cost-effective method of surveillance of HIV and drug resistance among TB patients?

References

Braun M, Kilburn J, Smithwick R et al. (1992) HIV infection and primary resistance to antituberculosis drugs in Abidjan, Côte d'Ivoire. AIDS, 6, 1327–1330

Githui W, Nunn P, Juma E et al. (1992) Cohort study of HIV positive and HIV negative tuberculosis, Nairobi, Kenya: comparison of bacteriological results. Tubercle and Lung Disease, 73, 203–209

Jain NK (1992) Drug resistance in India: a tragedy in the making. Indian Journal of Tuberculosis, 39, 145–148

Nunn P, Brindle R, Carpenter L et al. (1992) Cohort study of human immunodeficiency virus infection in patients with tuberculosis, Nairobi, Kenya. American Review of Respiratory Disease, 146, 849–854

Wallis R, Vjecha M, Amir-Tahmasseb M et al (1993) Influence of tuberculosis on human immunodeficiency virus, HIV-1: enhanced cytokine expression and elevated beta-2 microglobulin in HIV-1 associated tuberculosis. Journal of Infectious Diseases, 167, 43–48

World Health Organization (1992) Severe hypersensitivity reactions among HIV-seropositive patients with tuberculosis treated with thioacetazone. Weekly Epidemiological Record, 67, 1–3

3
Immunities in and to tuberculosis: implications for pathogenesis and vaccination

Paul E.M. Fine

London School of Hygiene & Tropical Medicine, UK

Introduction

Immunology has played an important role in the history of tuberculosis research and control. After discovering *Mycobacterium tuberculosis* in 1882, Robert Koch went on to experiment with therapeutic vaccines before the turn of the century; Von Pirquet introduced tuberculin as a test for infection in 1907; and Calmette and Guerin derived BCG (the oldest prophylactic vaccine still in use today) in the first two decades of this century, employing it first in humans in 1921. The tuberculin skin test has long served as the paradigm for a delayed-type hypersensitivity reaction; and tuberculin reagents, as improved by Seibert in 1934, were employed by the World Health Organization during the 1950s and 1960s in the largest immunological surveys ever carried out. More people alive today have received BCG than have received any other vaccine.

Despite this long and global immunological experience, we are in deep immunological trouble over tuberculosis today. Though tuberculosis was the major infectious killer in Europe and North America during the last century, it was thought only 20 years ago that BCG vaccine—in conjunction with effective drugs and socio-economic improvements—were solving the problem. Infection rates declined steadily in wealthier countries, and the creation of the Expanded Programme on Immunization in 1974 ensured routine BCG vaccination in poorer countries. Reflecting this optimism, it was not thought necessary to include tuberculosis among the six diseases of WHO's Tropical Disease Research (TDR) programme, the major agencies funding medical research showed little interest in the disease, and few scientists entered a field in which the key problems appeared to have been solved. This was pride before a fall. In 1979 it was revealed that BCG

Tuberculosis: Back to the Future. Edited by J.D.H. Porter and K.P.W.J. McAdam
© 1994 John Wiley & Sons Ltd

vaccines had failed to provide any protection against tuberculosis in a very large trial in South India (Tuberculosis Prevention Trial, Madras, 1980). Then came the appearance during the 1980s of HIV, a pandemic virus targeted selectively at the cellular basis of immunity to tuberculosis. Before the decade was out, strains of *M. tuberculosis* appeared which were resistant to most of the available antibiotics, the downward trend of tuberculosis was reversed in countries which had confidently predicted its elimination, and the disease was again recognized to be among the top public health problems in the world.

The only fortunate aspect of these events has been the return of scientific attention to this important disease. Much of the ensuing research activity has been immunological, and has revealed mechanisms of almost bewildering complexity. It is the task of this report to summarize briefly this complexity in the context of the overall goal of tuberculosis control, and to comment on appropriate directions for the future. As immuno-diagnostic methods are covered elsewhere in this volume, emphasis will here be placed upon the implications of immunology for tuberculosis pathogenesis and for the nature of protective responses which might be relevant for therapeutic or prophylactic vaccines.

Patterns of infection and disease

There are striking patterns which are typical of tuberculosis in human populations, and which are probably immunologically mediated. These are summarized in this section (and in Figure 3.1) to provide a broad context within which to consider more detailed immunological data and investigations.

Primary infection

It is thought that infection generally occurs by respiration of a very small number of bacilli into the alveoli (Comstock, 1982). High dose exposures, and exposure by ingestion, also occur but less frequently. Most individuals develop some degree of delayed-type hypersensitivity (DTH) to tuberculin within 6–8 weeks of infection with *M. tuberculosis* (or related bacteria). The quality, magnitude and duration of this response, which provides our best measure of infection status, vary with method of assessment and between populations.

Age and infection

The prevalence of tuberculin 'positivity' (however defined) rises with age at a rate reflecting the intensity of exposure in the community (Figure 3.1a,b). This strong age dependence must be taken into consideration when comparing tuberculin sensitivity levels between populations. Regardless of what criterion is used for tuberculin positivity, its prevalence never reaches 100%, even in highly endemic communities (Roelsgaard *et al.*, 1964; Tuberculosis Prevention Trial, 1980;

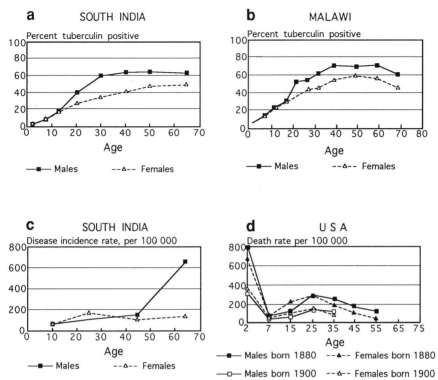

Figure 3.1   Typical patterns of infection (a, b) and disease (c, d) by age and sex, illustrated with data from different populations. Figures 3.1a and 3.1b show the prevalence of tuberculin positivity in South India (>10 mm to RT23, 1 IU) and Malawi (>5 mm to RT23, 2 IU), each showing similarity in prevalence among male and female children but a male excess among adults. Figure 3.1c shows the incidence of clinical tuberculosis in the same South Indian population portrayed in 3.1a. Figure 3.1d shows data on tuberculosis mortality in Massachusetts, USA, from before the antibiotic era, plotted by birth cohort. Note the excess of disease among young adult females and older males in c and d. Data: 3.1a and 3.1c from National Tuberculosis Institute, Bangalore (1974); 3.1b from Fine *et al.* (in preparation); 3.1d from Frost (1939)

Sutherland *et al.*, 1983). This indicates that some individuals escape infection, or that the test is not 100% sensitive, and/or that some individuals lose infection with age. The prevalence of tuberculin positivity generally declines in older adults (over age 50), reflecting either selective mortality of tuberculin positives, or else 'ageing' of the immune system and declining sensitivity of the test as an indicator of infection, or a combination of reversions to negativity and reduced exposure.

Sex and infection

Prevalence of tuberculin positivity is generally similar between males and females up to adolescence, after which the prevalence of tuberculin positivity is higher among males (Roelsgaard *et al.*, 1964; Tuberculosis Prevention Trial, 1980; Sutherland *et al.*, 1983) (Figures 3.1a,b). This has often been interpreted as reflecting greater exposure among adult males, but may equally reflect a sex difference in predisposition to DTH-type responsiveness. If the latter, then the sensitivity and/or specificity of DTH tuberculin tests are different between the sexes.

Age and 'primary' disease

There is evidence that the risk of progressive disease soon after primary infection is a function of the age at which infection occurs, being high among young children (less than 5 years old), then low (less than 5%) between ages 5 and 12, rising again to 10–20% in young adults. The high disease risks among the very young may reflect high dose challenge within home environments, but why young adults should also be at high risk of primary disease is not known (Frost, 1939; Comstock *et al.*, 1974) (Figure 3.1d).

Age and post-primary disease

Most tuberculosis in older adults appears many years after primary infection. This may either arise through endogenous reactivation of a latent focus of infection or it may reflect reinfection of the individual. The proportion of disease attributable to the two mechanisms varies between populations dependent upon the risk of infection in the community. If transmission rates are very low then almost all the disease in older individuals must be due to endogenous reactivation (Sutherland, 1976).

Sex and disease risk

In many populations, the risk of clinical tuberculosis in young adults is higher among females (sometimes attributed to the physiological stresses of reproductive activity) but among older adults it is much higher among males (Figure 3.1c,d). The female excess in disease in young adults contrasts paradoxically with the male excess in tuberculin positivity in this age group, indicating important gender differences in propensity to manifest DTH and/or susceptibility to disease (National Tuberculosis Institute, Bangalore, 1974; Sutherland *et al.*, 1982).

Age and clinical type

That meningitic disease is more common among children and genitourinary disease more common among adults is well established. There is good evidence that the proportion of pulmonary cases increases with age, though observed numbers may be influenced by difficulties in diagnosing pulmonary disease in children.

Ethnic/racial/geographic differences

Even taking into account variations in diagnosis and reporting between populations, there is good evidence for important differences in clinical tuberculosis between populations. Glandular disease is more common among Asians and genitourinary disease is more common in Europeans. Many authors have noted that pulmonary disease is more severe among Eskimos and blacks than among Caucasians (Comstock, 1982). Some of these differences may reflect differences in route or dose of exposure, but some probably reflect genetic differences between human populations (Stead 1992).

BCG and protection against tuberculosis

Studies of BCG have found widely differing protection in different populations. Though the reasons for these differences are not entirely clear, it is nonetheless true that at least some BCG vaccines, in at least some populations, can and do provide 'good' (in the order of 80%) protection at least against some forms of clinical tuberculosis. Unfortunately, the opposite is also true (Fine, 1989). The need to explain this paradox, and to answer its corollary of defining the nature of and prerequisites for effective vaccination against tuberculosis, is the great challenge posed by the public health community to immunologists with the courage to study this disease.

Basic mechanisms of infection and the immune response

M. tuberculosis is a facultative intracellular parasite which requires aerobic conditions for growth, and has a predilection for invading phagocytic monocytes. This invasion triggers a complex series of events involving many aspects of the immune system. These are summarized in Figure 3.2 and described below.

1. Infection generally occurs as small numbers of bacilli reach terminal alveoli of the lung, typically in the mid or lower lobes. They are then ingested by alveolar macrophages within which they are carried to the local (hilar) lymph nodes. Some replication of the bacilli may occur in the macrophages, but some of the bacilli are destroyed and broken up within phago-lysosomes. Certain proteins or polypeptides are released from the phago-lysosomes and are transported to the surface of the macrophages, where they are 'presented' in association with MHC (major histocompatibility complex) molecules determined by the HLA alleles of the host cell. It is these combinations of parasite antigen plus host HLA determinant which are recognized by circulating thymus-derived (T) lymphocytes.
2. If a T lymphocyte recognizes the presented antigen—because its combining site is complementary to the presented MHC–parasite antigen combination— various peptide mediators (cytokines) are released, in particular the

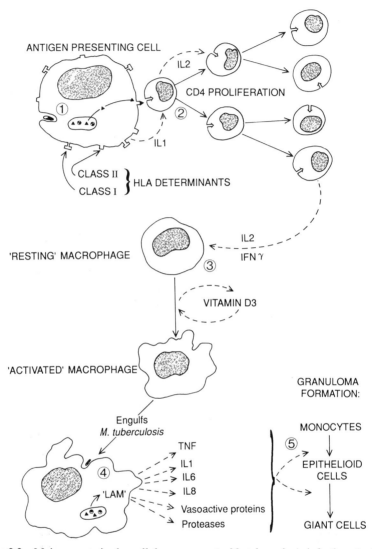

Figure 3.2 Major events in the cellular response to *M. tuberculosis* infection. 1: Antigen presenting cell (macrophage) ingests a tubercle bacillus and breaks it up within a phago-lysosome. Some of the antigens are expressed on the cell's surface in conjunction with molecules determined by the MHC (HLA) system. 2: A CD4 thymus-derived lymphocyte recognizes a combined *M. tuberculosis*–Class II antigen structure, and is induced to proliferate under influence of interleukins IL1 and IL2. 3: Activated CD4 lymphocytes secrete IL2 and γIFN, which in turn activate a resting macrophage. This is further encouraged by vitamin D3 metabolites. 4: Activated macrophage engulfs *M. tuberculosis*. Release of lipo-arabino-mannan ('LAM') from the bacterial cell wall encourages production of various cytokines. 5: These cytokines, in particular TNF, encourage conversion of monocytes into epithelioid cells and Langhans giant cells, forming a granuloma

'interleukin' IL1 by the macrophage, and IL2 by the T cell. These in turn induce the T cell to proliferate into a clone of cells with its particular specificity.

What happens next depends upon the type of lymphocyte which has been activated: whether it is 'TH1' or 'TH2,' and whether it is 'CD4' or 'CD8.' The choice of CD4 versus CD8 cells depends upon whether the antigen had been presented in association with an HLA DR, DP or DQ (= 'Class II') or an HLA A, B or C (= 'Class I') derived antigen on the surface of the macrophage, respectively; the mechanism of selection between TH1 and TH2 type cells is less clear, but may be dose-dependent, with low dose challenges favouring TH1 responses (Bretscher, 1992).

3. It is generally believed that the TH1–CD4 type cells play the most important role in the subsequent pathogenesis and immune response in tuberculosis. These cells secrete cytokines, most importantly IL2 and γIFN (gamma interferon), which can in turn 'activate' macrophages to ingest and digest mycobacteria and to secrete other cytokines such as IL8 (which may serve to attract T cells and neutrophils), IL6 and TNF (tumour necrosis factor) which activate the acute phase inflammatory response.

There is much evidence that TNF plays a particularly important role in the response to tubercle infection. Its production by infected macrophages is induced by the presence of a cell wall constituent of *M. tuberculosis* called 'LAM' (lipo-arabino-mannan) (Rook, 1990). It assists in granuloma formation, by attracting monocytes and encouraging their transformation into epithelioid and giant cells, whose clusters are so characteristic of the pathology of tuberculosis (Kindler *et al.*, 1989). It is also one of the factors responsible for cell death, as occurs in the centre of granulomata. Granuloma formation thus performs a protective role by physically containing the tubercle bacilli, and also by providing an anaerobic environment in which the bacilli cannot thrive.

Though it has been assumed that mycobacteria within macrophages are killed by reactive oxygen metabolites (e.g. hydrogen peroxide or nitric oxide) within phago-lysosomes, this has not actually been demonstrated *in vitro* for human macrophages, and thus the precise mechanism for killing *M. tuberculosis* in man is unknown.

There is some recent evidence that CD4 type cells may also, under certain conditions, cause lysis of macrophages containing *M. tuberculosis* (Kumararatne *et al.*, 1990).

4. In addition to the CD4-dependent processes, there is evidence that T cells of the CD8 series, which recognize antigens presented by macrophages in conjunction with Class I HLA-A, B or C determinants, are also involved in the response to tubercle infection (Kaufmann, 1988). These cells can be directly cytotoxic, and have the ability to recognize and to kill infected macrophages. *M. tuberculosis* may be destroyed with lysis of their host cells, or may be released into the extracellular environment and then engulfed by other activated macrophages.

5. Though antibodies are not thought to play a major role in protective immunity against tuberculosis, TH2 and B cells are involved in the overall response, and antibodies are produced to several proteins of the tubercle bacillus (Jackett *et al.*, 1988). The functions of these antibodies are unknown.

Such an abbreviated description overlooks many well-described cellular interactions which are now known to be involved in the response to *M. tuberculosis* infection. A large literature has appeared over the past decade reflecting efforts to unravel these complicated proceedings. One approach has been to define the antigens and epitopes of *M. tuberculosis*, in particular those which are presented on the surface of macrophages and which are recognized by host lymphocytes. This work has produced a catalogue of antigens and epitopes, identifying many that are shared with other mycobacterial species and some that are similar to an ubiquitous family of proteins (the 'heat-shock-proteins' = 'stress proteins') which are found in most species and types of living cells (Kaufmann and Young, 1992; Young *et al.*, 1992). A prime motivation of this research has been the hope of finding antigens or epitopes which are 'protective,' i.e. are associated with protective immune responses and which might therefore be appropriate as vaccines (Collins, 1991).

Another perspective has been that of identifying the various cell types and cytokine mediators involved in the response to infection with the tubercle bacillus, using a variety of animal and *in vitro* systems (Orme, 1991; Kaufmann, 1993). The availability of monoclonal antibodies specific for individual T lymphocyte subsets and cytokines, and of genetically manipulated mice, has allowed recognition, measurement and specific removal of successive steps in the immune network. We thus know that the response to tubercle infection involves at least: TH1/CD4, TH1/CD8,TH2/CD4, α/β, γ/δ, natural killer and B lymphocytes; neutrophils, macrophages, epithelioid and Langhans giant cells; interleukins 1, 2, 4, 6 and 8; γIFN, TNF, vitamin D3 derivatives, acute-phase proteins and various antibodies, including agalactosyl IgG. Other components which might be involved include platelet activating factor, endothelium-leucocyte adhesion molecules, granulocyte/macrophage colony stimulating factor, intercellular adhesion molecule, etc. (Rook, 1990). The problems of unravelling the interactions between so many factors are formidable.

Immune responses and pathology

The large majority of individuals infected with *M. tuberculosis* suffer no recognizable ill effects. Their bacilli are successfully ingested by macrophages and (apparently) contained within granulomata inside the lungs or regional lymph nodes, where they may remain viable for many years. The fact that this occurs is prima facie evidence that humans are capable of mounting an effective protective immune response against the tubercle bacillus.

In some individuals, however, for one or another reason, the primary infection is not effectively contained, and goes on to cause substantial tissue damage and clinical disease. The process may be initiated by haematogenous spread of bacilli from the initial lung site to some other organ of the body, where protective mechanisms are less efficient. This is most likely to occur in young individuals, some weeks or months after primary infection (Wallgren, 1948; Stead and Bates, 1971). Alternatively, the granulomatous defence mechanism in the lung or hilar nodes may be unable to contain local proliferation of the bacilli, thereby initiating a process of local pulmonary disease. The pathology is sometimes interpreted as a malfunction of the immune response, involving an 'excessive' cellular hypersensitivity reaction to antigens of the tubercle bacillus, leading to inflammation, release of large amounts of TNF, death of infected macrophages and other cells, release of tubercle bacilli and their ingestion by new activated macrophages and to the accumulation of necrotic (or 'caseous') debris within the growing granuloma. Though patients can be extremely ill with these various forms of 'primary' disease (called primary because they are thought to arise directly, within months or a very few years, from a primary infection) they are generally not infectious to others.

Infectious pulmonary disease, upon which the tubercle bacillus is dependent for transmission to new susceptibles, has a more complicated origin. This usually arises many years after primary infection (though it may arise as a consequence of primary infection in young adults), either by breakdown of a localized lesion within the lung, or by aerosol reinfection of an individual whose resistance has weakened. Either mechanism implies a waning or suppression of the immune capabilities which serve to contain the infection in the large majority of individuals at the time of first infection. This may be brought about as a consequence of age (this vague notion covers a multiplicity of immunological changes), malignant disease, immunosuppressive treatment, malnutrition, alcoholism or other insults associated with deterioration of cell-mediated immune capabilities. The host still attempts to contain the bacilli within macrophages and granulomata, but under these conditions the lesion enlarges until ultimately it breaks open into the lungs, discharging the debris and forming open cavities with abundant oxygen in which *M. tuberculosis* can proliferate freely. Such is the origin of the 'open' pulmonary case whose sputum consists of purulent material and large numbers of bacilli (up to 10^8 per day) direct from the cavity (Rees and Meade, 1974).

Tuberculosis associated with HIV infection and AIDS is thought to be due mainly to reactivation of latent infection and is associated with a declining CD4 count (Selwyn *et al.*, 1989; Barnes *et al.*, 1991). It is less likely to be pulmonary and sputum-positive, perhaps because the HIV-determined suppression reduces hypersensitivity responses in the tissues (Elliott *et al.*, 1990).

The cough and haemoptysis of pulmonary tuberculosis are readily understood in terms of lung lesions. The characteristic fever may reflect a variety of pyrogens associated with the inflammatory process, and also the specific pyrogenic activity of certain cytokines, in particular IL1, IL6 and TNF. Just why the fevers should typically occur at night ('night sweats') is less clear, but may reflect the imposition of the body's circadian rhythms upon the physiological disruption associated with the disease process. The loss of weight associated with tuberculosis reflects generalized tissue breakdown. This may be attributable in part to the large amounts of TNF produced by infected macrophages, as the effect is well enough described for TNF to be known also as 'cachectin.'

Pathogenesis of the delayed-type hypersensitivity response

Discussions of the pathogenesis of tuberculosis include frequent mention of hypersensitivity. The most familiar such response is the delayed-type hypersensitivity 'tuberculin' reaction which can be palpated 48–72 hours after intradermal injection of soluble antigens of the tubercle bacillus (Beck, 1988). The response begins in a non-specific manner, as dermal and immigrant macrophages engulf and process the foreign antigens. If the injected individual had previously met these antigens, specific T cells (CD4 and CD8) will be available to recognize the presented antigens. Antigen recognition by and activation of these T cells leads to their proliferation and to cytokine production which in turn acts on local blood vessels, allowing tissue fluid with large numbers of monocytes and lymphocytes to leak into the site. Such reactions generally disappear within a few days, except in individuals with active clinical disease, in whom (because of certain combinations of cells or cytokines?) the local reaction may be sufficiently severe to progress to local necrosis.

Vaccines and the manipulation of immunity

The story of vaccination against tuberculosis is largely the story of BCG (Ten Dam, 1984; Fine, 1989). These vaccines are all derivatives of an uncloned strain of *M. bovis*, originally isolated from a cow and passaged 231 times over 13 years in a medium containing oxbile before first being used in humans. Despite a long history of controversy, first over their safety and more recently over their efficacy, these vaccines have been used very widely since the 1950s in most countries of the world. Only the USA and The Netherlands have not used them on a national scale. Their efficacy has been evaluated in a dozen large controlled trials, and in numerous observational studies, the results of which show efficacies ranging from approximately nil to approximately 80% (Figure 3.3). Scrutiny of these studies suggests that protection has been generally high against tuberculous meningitis but has ranged widely with reference to pulmonary disease. Despite efforts of many apologists and critics, no clear pattern or explanation has emerged for these disparate results. The major explanations are as follows:

1. *Artefact*: Some authors have in the past suggested that the observed variation was attributable to inadequacies of and differences between the designs of the

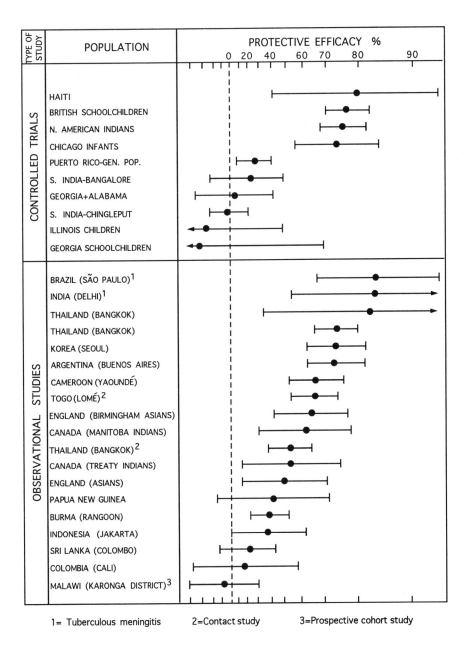

1= Tuberculous meningitis   2=Contact study   3=Prospective cohort study

Figure 3.3 Efficacy of BCG as determined in controlled trials and observational studies in various populations. Lines reflect 95% confidence intervals. For primary references, see Fine (1989), Smith (1993)

various studies (Clemens *et al.*, 1983). Few observers would accept this explanation today, and there is a general consensus that the great variation in estimates of protection reflects real biological variation.

2. *Differences between vaccines*: It is recognized that BCG strains differ between manufacturers, and possible that these differences could have immunological implications (Osborn, 1983; Comstock, 1988). On the other hand, similar sorts of vaccines have shown very different protection in different trials (e.g. Danish vaccine in the UK MRC trial and the Chingleput trial), and different vaccines have shown similar protection in some trials (e.g. Paris and Danish vaccines in Chingleput, BCG and vole bacillus in the UK MRC trial), making it unlikely that vaccine differences can provide all the explanation.

3. *Differences in environmental mycobacteria*: It is known that exposure to an infection with a variety of widespread environmental mycobacteria can induce skin test sensitivity to tuberculin and some degree of protection against tuberculosis. It has thus been proposed that immunity to these mycobacteria could mask protection imparted by BCG (Palmer and Long, 1966). A more recent suggestion is that responses to various mycobacteria may act either synergistically or antagonistically with BCG (Stanford *et al.*, 1981). There is animal evidence for masking of the protective effect of BCG by prior infection with environmental mycobacteria, but no evidence for direct antagonism.

4. *Differences in pathogenesis*: The failure of BCG to protect against pulmonary disease in the Chingleput trial led to the hypothesis that BCG may protect against primary disease, and against haematogenous spread of bacilli as occurs in extrapulmonary disease or in endogenous reactivation (Fok *et al.*, 1976; Wiegeshaus and Smith, 1989), but that it may not protect against disease attributable to exogenous reinfection (Ten Dam and Pio, 1982; Smith *et al.*, 1988).

5. *Genetic differences between human host populations*: The identification of an autosomal dominant gene ('*bcg*') which regulates T-cell independent antimycobacterial function in mice, and which may have a homologue on chromosome 2 in man, raises the possibility of genetic control of the response to BCG vaccination and subsequent natural exposure (Skamene, 1989). However, epidemiological studies indicate that BCG protects Asians living in Britain better than it does Asians in Asia, and thus genetics is unlikely to provide the entire answer (Rodrigues *et al.*, 1991).

Various other explanations have been raised in the literature, but have failed to provide convincing evidence. These include geographic differences in strains of *M. tuberculosis*, nutrition and sunlight exposure (Palmer, 1952; Ten Dam, 1984; Fine, 1989). No consensus has been reached among these competing explanations. It is possible that several of them contribute to the observed variation in protection.

Despite the large-scale use of BCG over several decades, measurement of its impact has proved as difficult as estimation of its efficacy. This is in part because countries with good records, which might have allowed impact evaluation, were experiencing an extraordinary, longstanding and rapid decline of tuberculosis (approximately 10% per annum) even prior to the introduction of BCG (Styblo and Meijer, 1976). Furthermore, the large-scale introduction of BCG coincided with the introduction of effective antibiotics during the 1950s, and these should also have led to reductions in infection transmission and in disease incidence. A third issue is the fact that BCG is given to young individuals, whereas tuberculosis is predominantly a disease of older adults; and thus many years are required for any vaccine-derived protection to reach the important elder population.

We thus have the extraordinary situation of a global vaccination programme of uncertain overall impact, maintained in part by the momentum of history and in part by the hopeful belief that even if it is not always highly effective, it is at least, on balance, preventing the rarer serious forms of tuberculosis, and, to a lesser and variable extent, some cases of pulmonary disease, without causing too much harm.

This issue of BCG's safety has arisen repeatedly and is now of concern because of the increased prevalence of HIV infection and AIDS. Very few cases of HIV-associated BCG disease have been reported, however, and thus recommendations for its use continue except for the proviso that it not be given to individuals with overt AIDS (World Health Organization, 1987).

There are as yet no data on whether or to what extent HIV infection and AIDS may influence protection by BCG vaccines.

Improving upon BCG

Efforts to improve upon the obvious inadequacies of BCG vaccines have taken three approaches. The first, which considers itself the 'rational approach' and which has attracted most attention over the past decade, has concentrated upon detailed dissection of the antigens of *M. tuberculosis* and of the immune response to these antigens, with the long range goal of constructing a new vaccine based on this knowledge. Some advocates of this approach emphasize the need to identify 'protective antigens' (though not all would agree that such antigens exist as such) and others have emphasized the need for subtle modulation of the immune response (though we have as yet little idea where to begin with this) (Collins, 1991; Orme, 1991; Rook, 1991; Kaufmann, 1992). As of today, we are still far from the development, let alone evaluation, of a 'rationally' constructed vaccine.

A second approach has been to select another known mycobacterium and to try it out as a therapeutic vaccine. *M. vaccae* was chosen because it grows easily and because it induces a non-necrotic type hypersensitivity (Stanford *et al.*, 1990). Anecdotal reports have appeared indicating that immunotherapy based on one or more injections of killed *M. vaccae* may reduce the severity of clinical tuberculosis (Onyebujoh and Rook, 1991; Etemadi *et al.*, 1992). Proper clinical therapeutic trials are soon to begin.

A third approach has consisted of efforts to improve upon the way in which current BCG vaccines are used. One suggestion has been to reduce the dose of BCG vaccine, on the premise that it would thereby be more likely to induce a beneficial TH1 cell dependent response (Bretscher, 1992). Experiments are currently underway in animals to explore these dose implications. Another is to capitalize upon the adjuvant and delivery qualities of BCG, but to increase its immunogenicity by the addition of genes for appropriate 'protective antigens' (see above) using molecular genetic techniques (Bloom, 1986; Jacobs *et al.*, 1989). Finally there are efforts to evaluate multiple doses of BCG, as repeated BCG vaccination is policy in many countries but has never formally been evaluated. A large leprosy and tuberculosis vaccine trial currently underway in Malawi will provide the first controlled trial of one versus two BCG vaccinations (Fine and Pönnighaus, 1988).

Regardless of the design of any new antituberculosis vaccine, the experience of BCG vaccination is relevant. Given that BCG is used widely in most populations at high risk of tuberculosis, any new vaccines will have to contend with BCG's influences, whatever they may be. Beyond that practical consideration, the recognition that BCG vaccines can provide good protection in one population, but not in another, will haunt any effort to evaluate and to extrapolate the effects of new vaccine products (Fine, 1989).

Immunological correlates of protection—the key

Both the immunology and the vaccinology of tuberculosis are bogged down in jungles of complex data. Scientists in each discipline attempt to explain these data with flowcharts of increasing complexity, but both groups are lost—at least in so far as neither is able to explain adequately how either an unvaccinated or a vaccinated individual resists infection with the tubercle bacillus. For both groups the key to the puzzle lies in the concept—or reality—of (immunological) correlates of protective immunity.

The critical necessity for a measurable immunological correlate of protective immunity is evident from the observation that a BCG vaccine can work against pulmonary disease in some populations (e.g. the United Kingdom) but very poorly if at all in others (e.g. South India). If this observation is accepted as fact, it means that *epidemiological—and thus also some immunological—results relating to vaccines can not necessarily be extrapolated from one population to another*. It thus strikes at the fundamental need for generalizable results in science and public health.

Many people believe that induction of a 'positive' tuberculin skin test as a consequence of a (BCG) vaccine indicates that protective immunity has been induced. This misconception is in part semantic, as to some basic scientists any production of antibodies or cell sensitivity may be described as a form of 'immunity,' whereas the epidemiological community prefers to apply this term to changes associated with protection against disease. Beyond this, there has been an important tradition in immunology which has argued that delayed-type hypersensitivity is associated with protection. Thus no less a figure than Mackaness wrote 'The immunizing conditions required for inducing resistance to the tubercle bacillus are substantially the same as those needed to induce delayed type hypersensitivity . . . The capability of BCG to provide a background of hypersensitivity that is the sine qua non of acquired resistance gives us good cause to foster its use' (Mackaness, 1971). This view was institutionalized by organizations such as UNICEF and became an important rationale underlying the global use of BCG during the 1950s–1970s (Tuberculosis Program PHS/USA, 1955; WHO Tuberculosis Research Office, 1955). It lives on in national policies, for example in recommendations to repeat a BCG vaccination to individuals who have failed to become tuberculin positive, in regulations for potency testing vaccines on the basis of DTH production, and in the opinions of many nurses and doctors involved in vaccine delivery.

There is a contrary view. Many immunologists have argued that the DTH response associated with tuberculosis does more harm than good, that it is part of the mechanism leading to tissue destruction in the disease, and that an ideal vaccine should not induce skin test positivity at all. Evidence for this view is supported by animal experiments first carried out during the 1930s which showed that desensitized guinea pigs which could no longer mount a DTH response to tuberculin could still resist the infection. More recent experiments have shown that it is possible to transfer selectively either DTH or protective immunity to tuberculosis in mice with separate cell fractions (Orme and Collins, 1984). Such results have led to the view that DTH and protective immunity are separate and dissociable phenomena (Youmans, 1979; Dannenberg, 1989).

It is important to appreciate that skin test assessment of DTH is the *only* immunological parameter which has been studied epidemiologically as a potential correlate of immunity, and that the epidemiological evidence does *not* support a simple relationship between DTH and protective immunity. Three sorts of studies and data are available on this point. First, follow-up of individuals in the UK MRC BCG trial, which showed a high overall protection by BCG, revealed no relationship between the degree of tuberculin sensitivity induced by vaccination and the subsequent risk of disease (Table 3.1) (Hart *et al.*, 1967). Second, a combined analysis of all the trials of BCG against tuberculosis found no relationship between the proportion of vaccinees who became tuberculin positive after vaccination, and the proportion of vaccinees protected against tuberculosis in each of the trials (Comstock, 1988). Third, follow-up studies of large numbers of individuals with prior tuberculin tests show a J shaped relationship with subsequent tuberculosis risk (Palmer, 1957) (Figure 3.4). This suggests that low or moderate levels of tuberculin sensitivity, which may be attributable to non-specific responses to infection with environmental mycobacteria, may be associated with reduced risk, whereas the absence, or higher levels, of sensitivity are associated with increased risk. Among the important implications of such data is the recognition that skin tests should not just be treated as negative or positive (as they usually are)—at least

Table 3.1 Incidence of tuberculosis among BCG vaccinated participants in the British MRC trial, over the first 10 years after vaccination, broken down by degree of BCG-attributable tuberculin conversion. All vaccinated individuals were tuberculin negative (0–4 mm to both 3 and 100 TU) at recruitment. The table shows incidence numbers and risks by post-vaccination tuberculin status, among 7332 vaccinees who were retested within 12 months after vaccination, and 6266 vaccinees who were not retested. There is no evidence for higher risks of disease among those who failed to convert to tuberculin positivity. Note that 1155/7332 (16%) of vaccinees apparently failed to become tuberculin positive after vaccination (from Hart *et al.*, 1967, *Tubercle*, 48, 201–210, by kind permission of Churchill Livingstone)

Results of first tuberculin test following vaccination (in order of diminishing sensitivity)		Number of BCG vaccinated participants	Cases of tuberculosis	
3 TU (mm induration)	100 TU (mm induration)		No.	Incidence risk (%)
15 mm or more	—	1 320	3	0.23
10–14 mm	—	2 669	12	0.45
5–9 mm	—	2 188	14	0.64
0–4 mm	5 or more mm	1 044	2	
0–4 mm	not tested	94	1	0.26
0–4 mm	0–4 mm	17	0	
All tested within 1 year of vaccination		7 332	32	0.44
Not tested within 1 year of vaccination		6 266	17	0.27
Total		13 598	49	0.36

three categories may be necessary to capture their full implications. There are data indicating that BCG-induced tuberculin sensitivity is more durable in some populations (e.g. Danish schoolchildren) than in others (e.g. Egyptians, or South Indian villagers) (Palmer, 1952; Horwitz and Bunch-Christensen, 1972; Tuberculosis Prevention Trial, Madras, 1980). The reasons for this differential, and its implications for vaccine-derived protection, are unclear.

The need to identify correlates of protective immunity has often been discussed. Among the strategies which have been proposed for their demonstration are animal model challenge experiments and comparisons of healthy infected (i.e. healthy tuberculin positive) individuals with clinically ill patients (Kaufmann and Young, 1992). Neither of these methods is ideal. Many authors have pointed out that mice and guinea pigs are not natural hosts of *M. tuberculosis*, and that these species deal with tubercle infection in ways different to man. No animal model to date has proved able to predict the efficacy of BCG in humans (Wiegeshaus and Smith,

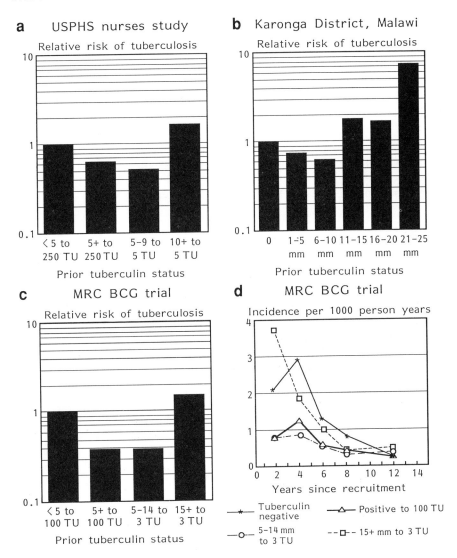

Figure 3.4 Relationship between prior tuberculin status and subsequent risk of tuberculosis, in different populations. US nurses study data (3.4a) based on 7 years' follow-up after dual testing with 5 or 250 TU PPD-S (from Palmer, 1957). Malawi data (3.4b) presented as age–sex standardized relative risks based on 10 years' follow-up after testing with RT23, 2 TU (Fine *et al.*, in preparation). British MRC trial data (3.4c,d) based on 15 years' follow-up after dual testing with 3 and 100 TU (Medical Research Council, 1972). The incidence peaks 4 years after start of follow-up in the MRC trial data reflect primary disease among recently infected young adults, but the declining risk with time also reflect the rapid decline in *M. tuberculosis* transmission in the population. Note that in all these populations the individuals with low or moderate initial tuberculin sensitivity were at lowest risk of disease

1989); and, given the observed geographic variation in efficacy, it is unclear how any animal model could do so. Mice and guinea pigs are not humans. The comparison of healthy infected versus diseased individuals raises other problems (Vordermeier et al., 1992). The presence or absence of certain cells or mediators in diseased individuals may reflect a consequence of the disease, not the reason for their having contracted disease. Furthermore, given the long incubation period of tuberculosis, just because an infected individual is healthy today does not mean that he or she is not one of the unfortunate minority who will suffer disease in future. This suggests that there may be no effective short-cut to the recognition of correlates of protection and that the only convincing way to identify those responses which are protective is by longitudinal studies of groups of people whose prior immunological status has been carefully characterized.

Conclusions

Much has been learned over the past decade concerning the immunological mechanisms involved in the response to *M. tuberculosis* infection. We now know of the involvement of many antigens, cell types, antibodies and mediators of which we were totally unaware only a few years ago. The unconventional term 'immunities' was used in the title of this paper to call attention to this wide variety of immunological processes now known to be associated with tuberculosis. Some of these are probably beneficial, some are probably deleterious, and some may be irrelevant as far as the host's well-being is concerned.

The challenge of sorting out the implications of these immunological phenomena raises many problems. In the background is the need to understand the basic age and sex pattern of natural tuberculosis. The striking patterns in Figure 3.1 may have counterparts in cellular mechanisms—in which case laboratory workers may need to pay particular attention to the demographic details of their material. Another problem is the need to move from qualitative flow-chart descriptions as expressed in diagrams such as Figure 3.2 to consider the quantitative implications of these complex processes. It is likely that the optimal response for the host individual reflects a balance of many factors, and that this balance is maintained by various threshold and feedback mechanisms. Understanding the quantitative relationships will require attention to doses and numbers of cells, and may benefit from mathematical models to explore the inevitable non-linear relationships. A third problem is the need to confirm the mechanism whereby *M. tuberculosis* are killed in human hosts. This may yet be possible through experiments on human cells. A fourth and most critical challenge is the need to identify the cell types or processes associated with low and with high risks of disease. This will require epidemiology.

Despite the continued use of BCG on a vast scale, there has been less progress in the last decade in understanding the practical consequences of this intervention than there has been in basic immunology. The large trial in South India came to an end, but its detailed results have yet to be published. A major advance in BCG vaccine research came with the application of observational case control and contact study methods to evaluate the effectiveness of BCG in various countries, and these have produced a range of efficacy estimates similar to those observed in the controlled trials (Smith, 1982, 1993). Available data show relatively consistent protection by BCG against tuberculous meningitis, but the conditions appropriate for protection against the vastly more frequent pulmonary disease remain unknown.

The need for improved vaccines against tuberculosis is obvious and great. Research towards that goal is compromised severely in the absence of clear evidence as to what constitutes a beneficial immunological response against *M. tuberculosis*. In this sense the needs of immunologists and vaccinologists, and indeed of tuberculosis control in general in the face of increasing drug resistance and HIV, focus upon the identification of immunological correlates of low and high long-term risk of disease among infected, uninfected, vaccinated and unvaccinated individuals. Such tests or assays should distinguish those processes which are pathogenic from those which are protective, a distinction which would accelerate greatly the development, identification, evaluation and extrapolation of improved vaccines against tuberculosis. It is likely that the only way to obtain such information is by appropriate longitudinal studies of individuals of known prior immunological profile (or whose cells and sera have been stored in such a way as to permit retrospective assessment of relevant immunological status). Such studies should be of high priority for the future of immunology, pathology and vaccine-related tuberculosis research.

Acknowledgements

I thank many colleagues, most recently Hazel Dockrell, Sebastian Lucas, Graham Rook and Douglas Young, for having tried to initiate me into the mysteries of cell-mediated immunity—but take full responsibility for any errors of interpretation. Support from the British Leprosy Relief Association (LEPRA), and from the IMMLEP component of the UNDP/World Bank/WHO TDR Programme, for the work in Malawi from which data in Figures 3.1b and 3.4b were derived, is gratefully acknowledged. Sue Ashayer helped greatly with the manuscript.

References

Barnes PF, Bloch AB, Davidson PT, Snider DE (1991) Tuberculosis in patients with human immunodeficiency virus infection. *New England Journal of Medicine, 324*, 1644–1650
Beck JS (1988) The tuberculin skin test. *Journal of Pathology, 155*, 1–2
Bloom BR (1986) Learning from leprosy: a perspective on immunology and the third world. *Journal of Immunology, 137*, i–x
Bretscher PA (1992) A strategy to improve the efficacy of vaccination against tuberculosis and leprosy. *Immunology Today, 13*, 342–345
Clemens JD, Guong JJH, Feinstein AR (1983) The BCG controversy: a methodological and statistical reappraisal. *Journal of the American Medical Association, 249*, 2362–2369
Collins FA (1991) Antituberculosis immunity: new solutions to an old problem. *Reviews of Infectious Disease, 13*, 940–950
Comstock GW (1982) Tuberculosis. In: Evans, AS, Feldman HA (eds), *Bacterial Infections*

of Man. Plenum Medical Books, New York. pp. 605–632

Comstock GW (1988) Identification of an effective vaccine against tuberculosis. *American Review of Respiratory Disease, 138*, 479–480

Comstock GW, Livesay VT, Woolpert SF (1974) The prognosis of a positive tuberculin reaction in childhood and adolescence. *American Journal of Epidemiology, 99*, 131–138

Dannenberg AM (1989) Immune mechanisms in the pathogenesis of pulmonary tuberculosis. *Reviews of Infectious Diseases, 11*, S369–S378

Elliott AM, Luo N, Tembo G (1990) Impact of HIV on tuberculosis in Zambia: a cross-sectional study. *British Medical Journal, 301*, 412–415

Etemadi A, Farid R, Stanford JL (1992) Immunotherapy of drug-resistant tuberculosis. *Lancet, 340*, 1360–1361

Fine PEM (1989) The BCG story: lessons from the past and implications for the future. *Reviews of Infectious Diseases, 11*, S353–S359

Fine PEM, Pönnighaus JM (1988) Leprosy in Malawi: 2. Background, design and prospects of the Karonga Prevention Trial, a leprosy vaccine in northern Malawi. *Transactions of the Royal Society of Tropical Medicine and Hygiene, 82*, 810–817

Fine PEM, Sterne JAC, Pönnighaus JM, Rees, RJW, Bliss L. Delayed-type hypersensitivity, mycobacterial vaccines and protective immunity (in preparation).

Fok JS, Ho RS, Arora PK, Harding GE, Smith DW (1976) Host-parasite relationships in experimental airborne tuberculosis. V. Lack of hematogenous dissemination of *Mycobacterium tuberculosis* to the lungs in animals vaccinated with Bacille Calmette-Guérin. *Journal of Infectious Diseases, 133*, 137–144

Frost WH (1939) The age selection of mortality from tuberculosis in successive decades. *American Journal of Hygiene, 30*, 91–96

Hart PD'A, Sutherland I, Thomas J (1967) The immunity conferred by effective BCG and vole bacillus vaccines, in relation to individual variations in induced tuberculin sensitivity and to technical variations in the vaccines. *Tubercle, 48*, 201–210

Horwitz O, Bunch-Christensen K (1972) Correlation between tuberculin sensitivity after 2 months and 5 years among BCG vaccinated subjects. *Bulletin of the World Health Organization, 47*, 49–58

Jackett PS, Bothamely GH, Batra HV, Mistry A, Young DB, Ivanyi J (1988) Specificity of antibodies to immunodominant mycobacterial antigens in pulmonary tuberculosis. *Journal of Clinical Microbiology, 26*, 2313–2318

Jacobs WR, Snapper SB, Tuckman, M, Bloom BR (1989) Mycobacteriophage vector systems. *Reviews of Infectious Diseases, 11*, S404–S410

Kaufmann SHE (1988) CD8⁺ T lymphocytes in intracellular microbial infections. *Immunology Today, 9*, 168–174

Kaufmann SHE and Young DB (1992) Vaccination against tuberculosis and leprosy. *Immunology, 184*, 208–229

Kaufmann SHE (1993) Immunity to intracellular bacteria. *Annual Review of Immunology, 11*, 129–163

Kindler V, Sappino A-P, Grau GE, Piguet P-F and Vassalli P (1989) The inducing role of tumor necrosis factor in the development of bactericidal granulomas during BCG infection. *Cell, 56*, 731–740

Kumararatne DS, Pithie AS, Drysdale P, *et al.* (1990) Specific lysis of mycobacterial antigen-bearing macrophages by class II MHC-restricted polyclonal T cell lines in healthy donors or patients with tuberculosis. *Clinical and Experimental Immunology, 80*, 314–323

Mackaness GB (1971) Delayed hypersensitivity and its significance. In: *International Proceedings No. 14: States of Immunization in Tuberculosis in 1971.* Washington DC, DHEW, pp. 69–89

Medical Research Council. Tuberculosis Vaccines Clinical Trials Committee (1972) BCG and vole bacillus vaccines in the prevention of tuberculosis in adolescence and early adult life [Fourth Report]. *Bulletin of the World Health Organization, 46*, 371–385

National Tuberculosis Institute, Bangalore (1974) Tuberculosis in a rural population of South India: a five-year epidemiological study. *Bulletin of the World Health Organization, 51*, 473–488

Onyebujoh P, Rook G (1991) *Mycobacterium vaccae* immunotherapy. *Lancet, 388*, 1534

Orme IM (1987) The kinetics of emergence and loss of mediator T lymphocytes acquired in response to infection with *Mycobacterium tuberculosis*. *Journal of Immunology, 138*, 293–298

Orme IM (1991) Processing and presentation of mycobacterial antigens: implications for the development of a new improved vaccine for tuberculosis control. *Tubercle, 72*, 250–252

Orme IM, Collins FM (1984) Adoptive protection of the *Mycobacterium tuberculosis* infected lung: Dissociation between cells that passively transfer protective immunity and those that transfer delayed-type hypersensitivity to tuberculin. *Cellular Immunology, 84*, 113–120

Osborn TW (1983) Changes in BCG strains. *Tubercle, 64*, 1–13

Palmer CD (1952) BCG vaccination and tuberculin allergy. *Lancet, i*, 935–940

Palmer CE (1957) Contribution to sympoium on 'value of tuberculin reactions for the selection of cases for BCG vaccination and significance of post-vaccination allergy.' *Bulletin of the International Union Against Tuberculosis, 27*, 106–111

Palmer CD, Long MW (1966) Effects of infection with atypical mycobacteria on BCG vaccination and tuberculosis. *American Review of Respiratory Disease, 94*, 553–568

Rees RJW, Meade TW (1974) Comparison of the modes of spread and the incidence of tuberculosis and leprosy. *Lancet, i*, 47–49

Rodrigues LC, Gill N, Smith PG (1991) BCG vaccination in the first year of life protects children of Indian subcontinent ethnic origin against tuberculosis in England. *Journal of Epidemiology and Community Health, 45*, 78–80

Roelsgaard E, Iversen E, Bløcher C (1964) Tuberculosis in tropical Africa: an epidemiological study. *Bulletin of the World Health Organization, 30*, 459–518

Rook GAW (1990) Mechanisms of immunologically mediated tissue damage during infection. In: Champion RH, Pye RJ (eds.), *Recent Advances in Dermatology*. Churchill Livingstone, London, pp. 193–210

Rook GAW (1991) Mobilising the appropriate T-cell subset: the immune response as taxonomist. *Tubercle, 72*, 253–254

Rook GAW, Al Attiyah R, Filley E (1991) New insights into the immunopathology of tuberculosis. *Pathobiology, 59*, 148–152

Selwyn PA, Hartel D, Lewis VA *et al.* (1989) A prospective study of the risk of tuberculosis among intravenous drug users with human immunodeficiency virus infection. *New England Journal of Medicine, 320*, 545–550

Skamene E (1989) Genetic control of susceptibility to mycobacterial infections. *Review of Infectious Diseases, II*, Suppl 2, S394–S399

Smith DW, Wiegeshaus EH, Edwards ML (1988) The protective effects of BCG vaccination against tuberculosis. In: Bendinelli M, Friedman H (eds.) *Mycobacterium tuberculosis interactions with the immune system*. Plenum Press, New York. pp. 341–370

Smith PG (1982) Retrospective assessment of the effectiveness of BCG vaccination against tuberculosis, using the case control method. *Tubercle, 62*, 23–35

Smith PG (1993) BCG vaccination. In: Davis PDO (ed.) *Tuberculosis*. Chapman and Hall, London (In press)

Stanford JL, Shield MJ, Rook GA (1981) How environmental mycobacteria may predetermine the protective efficacy of BCG. *Tubercle, 62*, 55–62

Stanford JL, Rook GAW, Bahr GM *et al.* (1990) *Mycobacterium vaccae* in immunoprophylaxis and immunotherapy of leprosy and tuberculosis. *Vaccine, 8*, 525–530

Stead WW (1992) Genetics and resistance to tuberculosis. Could resistance be enhanced by genetic engineering? *Annals of Internal Medicine, 116*, 937–941

Stead WW, Bates JH (1971) Evidence of a 'silent' bacillemia in primary tuberculosis. *Annals of Internal Medicine, 74*, 559–561

Styblo K, Meijer J (1976) Impact of BCG vaccination programmes in children and young adults on the tuberculosis problem. *Tubercle, 57*, 14–43

Sutherland I (1976) Recent studies in the epidemiology of tuberculosis, based on the risk of being infected with tubercle bacilli. *Advances in Tuberculosis Research, 19*, 1–63

Sutherland I, Svandová E, Radhakrishna S (1982) The development of clinical tuberculosis following infection with tubercle bacilli. 1. A theoretical model for the development of clinical tuberculosis following infection, linking from data on the risk of tuberculosis infection and the incidence of clinical tuberculosis in the Netherlands. *Tubercle, 63*, 255–268

Sutherland I, Bleiker MA, Meijer J, Styblo K (1983) The risk of tuberculosis infection in the Netherlands from 1967 to 1979. *Tubercle, 64*, 241–253

Ten Dam HGF (1984) Research on BCG vaccination. *Advances in Tuberculosis Research, 21*, 79–106

Ten Dam HG, Pio A (1982) Pathogenesis of tuberculosis and effectiveness of BCG vaccination. *Tubercle, 63*, 225–233

Tuberculosis Prevention Trial, Madras (1980) Trial of BCG vaccines in South India for tuberculosis prevention. *Indian Journal of Medical Research, 72* (Suppl) 1–74

Tuberculosis Program, Public Health Service, USA (1955) Experimental studies of vaccination, allergy, and immunity in tuberculosis: 1. Design for a research programme. *Bulletin of the World Health Organization, 12*, 13–29

Vordermeier H-M, Harris DP, Friscia G *et al.* (1992) T cell repertoire in tuberculosis: selective anergy to an immunodominant epitope of the 38-kDa antigen in patients with active disease. *European Journal of Immunology, 22*, 2631–2637

Wallgren A (1948) The time-table of tuberculosis. *Tubercle, 29*, 245–251

Wiegeshaus EH, Smith DW (1989) Evaluation of the protective potency of new tuberculosis vaccines. *Reviews of Infectious Diseases, 11*, S484–S490

WHO Tuberculosis Research Office (1955) Certain characteristics of BCG-induced tuberculin sensitivity. *Bulletin of the World Health Organization, 12*, 123–141

World Health Organization (1987) Expanded Programme on Immunization: Joint WHO/UNICEF statement on immunization and AIDS. *Weekly Epidemiological Record, 62*, 53–54

Youmans GP (1979) Relationship between hypersensitivity and immunity in tuberculosis. In: Youmans GP (ed) *Tuberculosis*. WB Saunders, Philadelphia. pp. 302–316

Young DB, Kaufmann SHE, Hermand PWM, Thole JER (1992) Mycobacterial protein antigens: a compilation. *Molecular Microbiology, 6*, 133–145

Discussion

Graham A.W. Rook and John L. Stanford

University College London Medical School, UK

In individuals infected with *M. tuberculosis*, growth of the organism is eventually slowed down or halted by one of two mechanisms:

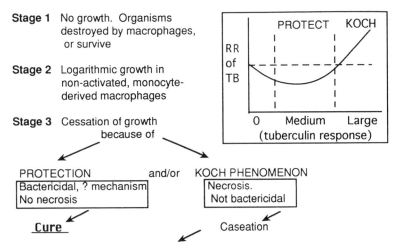

Stage 1 No growth. Organisms destroyed by macrophages, or survive

Stage 2 Logarithmic growth in non-activated, monocyte-derived macrophages

Stage 3 Cessation of growth because of

PROTECTION and/or KOCH PHENOMENON

| Bactericidal, ? mechanism |
| No necrosis |

Necrosis.
Not bactericidal

Cure

Caseation

Stage 4 Liquefaction of caseous centre; cavities; spread.

Figure 3.5 The evolution of mycobacterial lesions (adapted from Dannenberg, 1991, *Immunology Today, 12*, pp 228–233, with permission of Elsevier Science Publishers). The protective and tissue-damaging patterns of response may correlate with the small and large tuberculin skin-test responses respectively. The relationship of these skin-test responses to the relative risk (RR) of tuberculosis is indicated diagrammatically in the insert

1. In a small minority a protective bactericidal mechanism cures the patient.
2. In the majority a tissue-damaging response which is unable to eliminate *M. tuberculosis* creates an environment in which the organism grows poorly, but can lie dormant for many years.

These pathways are illustrated in Figure 3.5, which is adapted from Dannenberg (1991). We still do not know the mechanism of the protective bactericidal mechanism in man, since the only reports of killing of *M. tuberculosis* by human macrophages are unrepeatable in other laboratories (Denis, 1991). Indeed we do not know for certain that protection is mediated by activated macrophages, and other papers in this forum address alternative possibilities such as a role for CD8+ T cells.

Similarly the molecular and cellular basis of the tissue-damaging response is not fully understood, but it is likely that the 'Koch phenomenon' is fundamental to it (Koch, 1891), and that the chronic tissue damage, caseation and fibrosis in clinical tuberculosis are slowly progressive manifestations of a related process (Rook and Al Attiyah, 1991). The problem for the physician is that even when the bacterial load is reduced more than 90% by chemotherapy, this tissue-damaging response fails to destroy the remaining bacteria. Thus prolonged treatment is required and even after such treatment, reactivation by old age, HIV or immunosuppression is likely. An ideal treatment regimen would seek not only to kill bacteria by chemotherapy, but also to correct the immunoregulatory defect, and persuade the immune response to recognize and remove persisters.

There is circumstantial evidence that one component of the Koch phenomenon is cytokine-induced damage in a T cell-mediated lesion which is excessively sensitive to these mediators (Al Attiyah *et al.*, 1992; Rook and Al Attiyah, 1991). This sensitivity to cytokines may be attributable to the activity of inappropriate T helper cell subsets (Barnes *et al.*, 1993), and is exacerbated by the release from *M. tuberculosis* of factors that trigger cytokine release (Moreno *et al.*, 1989) and enhance the local toxicity of TNFα (Filley *et al.*, 1992). Thus although our understanding of the two pathways in Figure 3.5 is vague, attention is focusing on the T cell subsets (TH1, TH2, TH0, α/β, γ/δ), and on the cytokine/endocrine networks that regulate their activation and their effector functions (Rook *et al.*, 1993).

In spite of our lack of precise knowledge of mechanisms, it became apparent some years ago that there are simple epidemiological correlates of the protective and tissue-damaging pathways. As discussed and referenced at length by Paul Fine in his paper, the relative risk of tuberculosis is high not only in individuals with negative tuberculin responses but also in those with very large responses. These large responses (Koch phenomena) may indicate that some of these people are incubating the disease. *Protection*, on the other hand, correlates with *small* (non-necrotizing) positive responses, particularly when not attributable to BCG. These results imply that certain environmental mycobacteria can prime protection. Therefore at least some protection is mediated by responses that are not directed towards species-specific antigens. This is initially surprising, but is well established for leprosy since BCG is protective against this disease (Brown *et al.*, 1966), as Paul Fine has recently confirmed (Fine *et al.*, 1986), and very striking protection has recently been obtained in a mouse mode of tuberculosis using an antigen of *M. leprae* (D.B. Lowrie, personal communication). The variable immunogenicity of environmental mycobacteria also provides one strong candidate explanation for the fact that BCG vaccination is 80% protective in some environments, but ineffective in others (Stanford *et al.*, 1981).

Since environmental mycobacteria can prime protective pathways we must ask ourselves whether this fact has any practical applications. In order to explore this an organism *(Mycobacterium vaccae)* with appropriate properties was isolated (reviewed in Stanford *et al.*, 1990). We initially intended to investigate the possibility that when added as a supplement to BCG it would compensate for the lack of protection-inducing organisms in certain environments. It remains possible that such a supplemented BCG vaccine would be effective everywhere, and trials able to test this hypothesis are needed. However, recently a more important and unexpected property of *M. vaccae* has emerged. An injection of 10^9 autoclaved organisms given to patients with active tuberculosis induces accelerated cure. This implies that the Koch phenomenon is not a stable immunoregulatory state, but can be switched to the protective pathway by suitable regulatory signals. Since the mechanism is immunological it can operate (though less reliably) without the help of chemotherapy, and cure can be induced in a percentage of patients with multiresistant infection. (Full descriptions of these studies have been submitted. Meanwhile, brief statements have appeared as letters to the Lancet (Etemadi *et al.*, 1992; Onyebujoh and Rook, 1991).

An informative trial was performed in Kano, Nigeria, where 50–70% of the drugs are fake, diluted or out-of-date, and must in any case be purchased by the patients since supplies are not available in the hospitals (Ityavyar, 1988). As expected under these conditions, the mortality in the placebo group approached 40% although they took their drugs for an average of 6.8 months. On the other hand mortality in the group receiving *M. vaccae* was 2%, in spite of the fact that the patients stopped taking their drugs after only 2.9 months because they felt well, and wished to save money. Moreover increased survival and accelerated clearance of bacilli from sputum have been observed in fully blinded trials in the Gambia and Vietnam where complete courses of chemotherapy were given (manuscripts in preparation).

Striking immunological changes occur in patients within 2 weeks of receiving *M. vaccae*. One exciting parameter is % agalactosyl IgG, which was first identified as a correlate of immunopathology in Crohn's disease and rheumatoid arthritis (Dube *et al.*, 1990; Rademacher *et al.*, 1988). The proportion of this glycoform of IgG is also raised in tuberculosis (Rook *et al.*, 1991). It tends to rise further for 2 months after patients start chemotherapy, but it falls within 14 days if *M. vaccae* is given (Rook *et al.*, submitted). Not only is this proving to be a reliable marker of the immunotherapeutic effect of *M. vaccae*, highly significant in the Kuwaiti, Gambian, Vietnamese and Nigerian trials, but it also proves that recovery in these trials is due to immunotherapy and not to privileged chemotherapy, since the latter causes a rise rather than a fall in this parameter. The recipients of *M. vaccae* also show changes compatible with a shift from TH2 (or TH0) to TH1 activity, because the rise in antibody to carbohydrate components of *M. tuberculosis* which usually follows chemotherapy is suppressed, and tuberculin positivity at 2–3 weeks is enhanced (Rook *et al.*, submitted).

The results of the trials of *M. vaccae* as an immunotherapeutic supplement to chemotherapy must be regarded as preliminary at present, since at the time of writing this manuscript, they are unpublished, and the trials themselves are imperfect. However, data are striking, and the concept is potentially too important to ignore. Increasing numbers of patients have multiresistant disease, and it is also unlikely that drugs can be designed that will kill persisters. Therefore shorter, more reliable treatment protocols will only be possible if the immune response can be induced to play a more active role in curing the patient. The general scepticism about the potential curative role of the patients' own immune system amongst those involved in tuberculosis control is understandable in an historical sense, but it is a dogma with no factual foundation. If our preliminary observations on the effects of *M. vaccae* are correct, then very much shorter and cheaper treatment protocols will be possible in the future.

References

Al Attiyah R, Morena C, Rook GAW (1992) TNF-alpha-mediated tissue damage in mouse foot-pads primed with mycobacterial preparations. *Research in Immunology, 143,* 601–610

Barnes PF, Abrams JS, Lu S, Sieling PA, Rea TH, Modlin RL (1993) Patterns of cytokine production by mycobacterium-reactive human T cell clones. *Infection and Immunity, 61,* 197–203

Brown JAK, Stone MM, Sutherland I (1966, 1968) BCG vaccination of children against leprosy in Uganda. First results and second follow-up. *British Medical Journal, i,* 7–14 (1966); *i,* 24 (1968)

Dannenberg AM (1991) Delayed-type hypersensitivity and cell-mediated immunity in the pathogenesis of tuberculosis. *Immunology Today, 12,* 228–233

Denis M (1991) Killing of *Mycobacterium tuberculosis* within human monocytes: activation of cytokines and calcitriol. *Clinical and Experimental Immunology, 84,* 200–206

Dube R, Rook GA, Steele J *et al.* (1990) Agalactosyl IgG in inflammatory bowel disease: correlation with C-reactive protein. *Gut, 31,* 431–434

Etemadi A, Farid R, Stanford JL (1992) Immunotherapy for drug-resistant tuberculosis. *Lancet, 340,* 1360–1361

Filley EA, Bull HA, Dowd PM, Rook GAW (1992) The effect of *Mycobacterium tuberculosis* on the susceptibility of human cells to the stimulatory and toxic effects of Tumour Necrosis Factor. *Immunology, 77,* 505–509

Fine PEM, Pönnighaus JM, Maine N, Clarkson JA, Bliss L (1986) The protective efficacy of BCG against leprosy in Northern Malawi. *Lancet, ii,* 499–502

Ityavyar DA (1988) Health service inequalities in Nigeria. *Social Sciences and Medicine, 27,* 1223–1235

Koch R (1891) Fortsetzung über ein Heilmittel gegen Tuberculose. *Deutsch Medizinisch Wochenschrift, 17,* 101–102

Moreno C, Taverne J, Mehlert A *et al.* (1989) Lipoarabinomannan from *Mycobacterium tuberculosis* induces the production of Tumour Necrosis Factor from human and murine macrophages. *Clinical and Experimental Immunology, 76,* 240–245

Onyebujoh P, Rook GAW (1991) (Letter to Lancet). *Lancet, 338,* 1534

Rademacher T, Parekh RB, Dwek RA *et al.* (1988) The role of IgG glycoforms in the pathogenesis of rheumatoid arthritis. *Springer Seminars in Immunopathology, 10,* 231–249

Rook GAW, Al Attiyah R (1991) Cytokines and the Koch phenomenon. *Tubercle, 72,* 13–20

Rook GAW, Al Attiyah RJ, Filley E (1991) New insights into the immunopathology of tuberculosis. *Pathobiology, 59,* 148–152

Rook GAW, Onyebujoh P, Stanford JL (1993) TH1 → TH2 switch and loss of CD4 cells in chronic infections; an immuno-endocrinological hypothesis not exclusive to HIV. *Immunology Today* (in press)

Stanford JL, Rook GAW, Bahr GM *et al.* (1990) *Mycobacterium vaccae* in immunoprophylaxis and immunotherapy of leprosy and tuberculosis. *Vaccine, 8,* 525–530

Stanford JL, Shield MJ, Rook GAW (1981) How environmental mycobacteria may predetermine the protective efficacy of BCG. *Tubercle, 62,* 55–62

4

Of molecules and men: the detection of tuberculosis, past, present and future

Peter Godfrey-Faussett

ZAMBART Project, Lusaka, Zambia and London School of Hygiene & Tropical Medicine, UK

Introduction

'Prevention is better than cure.' Yet for tuberculosis, cure is the best prevention. Transmission of tuberculosis is more likely from those patients with a cough who have many tubercle bacilli in their sputum and live in close association with susceptible contacts (Rouillon *et al.*, 1976). However, transmission often occurs before detection of the index case so that removal of patients with multibacillary disease to hospital for treatment reduces the amount of infection in their immediate families no more than treating them adequately at home (Kamat *et al.*, 1966). The aims of case detection are to render patients non-infectious to protect the community and to return the individual to full health. Although these goals are universal, the appropriate methods will vary with the context. Economic and infrastructural resources, cultural beliefs and behaviour, population density and demography, prevalence of human immunodeficiency viruses (HIVs) and of disease or colonization by atypical mycobacteria will all be essential data for the design of effective programmes.

This chapter will look back at the current strategies for case detection and diagnosis and look forward to the needs and possibilities of measures for the future.

Whom are we trying to detect?

The great majority of tuberculous infection is acquired from patients with many bacilli in their sputum which can be detected by microscopic examination following appropriate staining (smear-positive cases). The most important objective

Tuberculosis: Back to the Future. Edited by J.D.H. Porter and K.P.W.J. McAdam
© 1994 John Wiley & Sons Ltd

is therefore to find as many of these cases and prevent further transmission. However, as mentioned above, much transmission occurs before diagnosis. Smear-positive cases will have passed through a period, of unknown duration, when they had fewer bacilli in the sputum than could be detected microscopically (smear-negative cases) and were less infectious and conversely, many smear-negative cases will in due course become smear-positive (Hong Kong Chest Service, 1984). Although smear positivity correlates well with infectivity, infection is a stochastic process and certainly occurs from paucibacillary smear-negative cases too. A more sensitive technique that detected both smear-positive and smear-negative cases would have an impact on transmission. Furthermore, in regions where the epidemiology of tuberculosis is being transformed by HIV (Slutkin et al., 1988; Harries, 1990) the proportion of new infection attributable to smear-positive cases will fall. Not only will there be an increase in the numbers of smear-negative cases (Elliott et al., 1990) in these areas but susceptibility to infection will also rise (Daley et al., 1992).

The need to diagnose extrapulmonary cases is less urgent since these patients will not generally transmit their disease to others. Nonetheless, many countries with a high prevalence of tuberculosis that have concentrated their resources on finding smear-positive cases are now facing a new wave of disease following the HIV epidemic. There will be many extrapulmonary cases in whom diagnosis is more difficult (Sunderam et al., 1986). Over-treatment is costly and late diagnosis will lead to increased morbidity and mortality and probably an acceleration of the progression of their HIV infection. General clinical features of extrapulmonary disease may also be mistaken for those of HIV disease (Colebunders et al., 1987) and effective treatment may therefore be denied, particularly in regions where the costs of HIV testing preclude its use as a diagnostic tool.

The situation is also difficult in children where tuberculosis is particularly hard to diagnose accurately (Cundall, 1986; Migliori et al., 1992) and where the effects of HIV are less well established (Chintu, manuscript submitted). There is also a problem in distinguishing tuberculosis in infants from infection with HIV.

'First catch your hare'

Much has been written about the new diagnostic possibilities that are emerging for tuberculosis and some of these will be addressed later but before any approach can be tried, the patient needs to be found. Health seeking behaviour varies widely between cultures and will be determined both by traditionally held beliefs and by the perceived effects of local health care provision. Although most patients do have symptoms (Banerji and Anderson, 1963; Allan, 1979), many do not appreciate the serious nature of their illness (Demers et al., 1990). In many cultures adequate treatment will be delayed because people prefer to consult traditional healers or to treat themselves (Allan et al., 1979). Even when patients do come forward, the training and morale of those involved in primary care is vital. In a series of studies of active case finding methods conducted in Kenya more than 80% of those identified by active measures as 'suspects' who required further investigation had already attended a medical facility for symptoms referable to their chest on one or more occasions (Nsanzumuhire *et al.*, 1981; Aluoch *et al.*, 1982). Alarmingly, even with monthly visits from the project team, staff at the primary clinics recorded the names of less than 12.5% of those with cough or chest pain of greater duration than 1 month or with haemoptysis. Improving training and support for such clinics might obviate the need for active case finding. Another approach, in many areas, would be to involve traditional healers, from whom many people seek advice before attending the local clinic.

In other contexts, fewer patients may seek treatment. In low prevalence countries, tuberculosis is a disease of the marginalized (Torres *et al.*, 1990). Drug-users, the homeless, alcoholics and immigrants are less likely to seek help from clinics that are seen to be an integral part of the establishment. The provision of health care facilities aimed specifically at these groups to provide a range of services could also facilitate passive case finding for tuberculosis. An example might be the system established in the USA for migrant labourers (Centers for Disease Control, 1992).

Active case finding is generally costly and yields disappointingly few extra cases. Like all screening programmes, there is a danger that the very population one wishes to reach are those who do not respond to invitations through suspicion of the authorities, lack of comprehension or other needs that are perceived as more pressing. Patients found by active measures may also perceive that they have less wrong and so be less likely to complete treatment (Cassels *et al.*, 1982). Nonetheless, opportunistic screening of groups at high risk such as the immunocompromised, prison inmates or those in residential care (Morris, 1991) may be cost-effective and prevent morbidity and further transmission.

Koch's bacillus

As emphasized above ('Whom are we trying to detect?'), there will be different needs in different situations. The traditional model of history, examination and sputum microscopy has proved itself capable of detecting the majority of infectious cases and in conjunction with adequate case finding and treatment remains the backbone of tuberculosis control. All other techniques need to be compared critically with microscopy and their diagnostic role assessed.

Radiology has always been less useful in the diagnosis of tuberculosis than sputum microscopy. The majority of patients with typical apical cavitatory disease will also have positive sputum microscopy. Sequential radiographs may, however, be useful both in diagnosis and in management of disease.

As discussed earlier (Chapter 2), HIV has had an enormous impact on tuberculosis. Although many patients infected with both pathogens will have a typical history and examination, a substantial number will have unusual symptoms and signs. The number of bacilli found in the sputum will generally be lower and in areas where people with HIV infection commonly develop *Mycobacterium avium* infection either mycobacterium may be found. HIV has also altered the radiological picture and reduced the amount of 'classical' disease whilst increasing the amount of hilar lymphadenopathy and pleural effusions (Pitchenik and Rubinson, 1985). Normal chest radiographs are also recognized in HIV-seropositive patients with confirmed pulmonary tuberculosis (Pedro-Botet *et al.*, 1992).

Microscopic examination of sputum smears stained by the Ziehl–Neelsen method can detect bacilli when there are of the order of 10^4 per ml of sputum (Yeager *et al.*, 1967; Hobby *et al.*, 1973). Although species other than *M. tuberculosis* may have different morphology, these differences are not sufficient to allow speciation by microscopy alone so the specificity of microscopy will depend on the prevalence of colonization or pulmonary disease due to non-tuberculous mycobacteria. In high prevalence countries *M. tuberculosis* predominates to the extent that the specificity of microscopy was 99.8% in another of the Kenyan case finding studies (Aluoch *et al.*, 1984).

Culture of mycobacteria from sputum or other clinical samples is much more sensitive and allows for biochemical identification of species leading to excellent specificity. Unfortunately, the slow doubling time of *M. tuberculosis* on all media so far used makes culture slow, and even with expensive Bactec radiospirometric technology to detect early growth, results take weeks rather than days.

Microscopy and culture can also be applied to specimens other than sputum to provide a definite diagnosis in suspected cases. More invasive techniques for obtaining respiratory secretions such as induction of sputum by hypertonic saline inhalation (Parry, 1992), gastric washing or bronchoscopy with bronchial washing or alveolar lavage (de Gracia *et al.*, 1988) all increase the yield in smear-negative cases but may be impossible in children. Culture of faeces after suitable decontamination may also be useful (Donald, 1992). For extrapulmonary disease biopsy provides both histological and microbiological samples but less invasive methods may be adequate. In hospitals with advanced imaging technology, biopsies of abdominal lymph nodes, bones, kidneys, brains and no doubt others can be made under direct radiological or ultrasonographic guidance without a major operation. In places with fewer expensive facilities, aspiration with a wide bore needle provides material from lymph nodes (Bem, 1992) or from pericardia, synovia pleura, or peritoneum, the last two of which can also be sampled by a percutaneous needle biopsy. Urine can be collected over 24 hours and the bacilli concentrated by centrifugation. Lumbar puncture provides cerebrospinal fluid. A proportion of patients, particularly those with HIV infection, may also have *M. tuberculosis* cultured directly from the blood (Shafter *et al.*, 1989).

All these techniques produce material for routine microbiological examination, but the same limitations apply. Microscopy requires more than 10^4 organisms per ml. and is not specific. Culture requires only a few live organisms but takes too long. There has therefore for some time been considerable interest in developing tests that would either demonstrate specific host responses to *M. tuberculosis* or detect the organisms themselves or some of their constituents.

What do we need?

Most new diagnostic tests are developed in research laboratories, refined until the sensitivity and specificity are as high as possible, assessed on available clinical material, published in the scientific literature and then ignored.

Once again it is vital to consider the context in which a test is going to be used. Specificity is generally more important than sensitivity when considering tests for tuberculosis. The specificity required will depend upon the prevalence of disease amongst those being tested.

If we imagine a new test for the diagnosis of paediatric tuberculosis, we can envisage its use in patients on the paediatric ward in whom tuberculosis is suspected. As many as 50% of patients may actually have tuberculosis. Suppose the test has a specificity of 95% and a sensitivity of 75% (somewhere in the range of many ELISAs). Of each 100 patients investigated, 37.5 will be diagnosed correctly and only 2.5 will be misdiagnosed and put on treatment. If someone then uses this smart new test to screen the contacts of mothers with tuberculosis of whom only 5% have disease, 4 will be diagnosed accurately whilst 5 are started on treatment that at best will be expensive and at worst will be toxic.

In the active case finding studies in Kenya, referred to above (Aluoch *et al.*, 1982, 1984; Nsanzumuhire *et al.*, 1981), the rate of disease amongst groups of suspects variously identified was 1–5%. If we wanted to provide a test for tuberculosis amongst these suspects that would mean that the majority of the treatment available was given to people who actually had tuberculosis, we would have to have developed a test with a specificity of above 98%. Furthermore, when assessing the test in the laboratory we would need at least 200 negative controls to be reasonably confident that the stated specificity was within 1 or 2% of the real value.

Modern approaches

Alternative approaches to the diagnosis of tuberculosis can be divided into those that look at the host's response to infection with *M. tuberculosis* and those that look for constituents of the bacillus itself. Over the past two decades there have been many attempts to use the host's immune response as a specific marker of disease. Most of these have looked at antibodies present in the serum against a range of mycobacterial extracts or purified antigens. Others, notably for bovine tuberculosis, have used cytokines generated by the cellular immune response. Other less specific responses by the host that have been considered as diagnostic markers are adenosine deaminase, an enzyme involved in purine catabolism, whose levels are elevated in tuberculous pleural effusions, and lysozyme, a bacteriolytic enzyme often associated with granuloma activity, for which the ratio of pleural fluid to serum levels is higher in tuberculosis than in other diseases.

Attempts to detect constituents of the bacillus have concentrated either on nucleic acid probes, often using the polymerase chain reaction, or other more recent methods, to amplify small amounts of DNA to detectable levels, or on detecting antigens, either cytoplasmic or secreted, or structural components such as tuberculostearic acid.

The host's response

Serological tests. Although many techniques have been tried for the serodiagnosis of tuberculosis from as early as the 19th century, the development of the enzyme-linked immunosorbent assay (ELISA) and its widespread use in many diagnostic fields over the last two decades has led to a profusion of possible tests (reviewed by Daniel and Debanne, 1987).

There are several inherent difficulties in hunting for antibodies to diagnose tuberculosis. Crude antigen preparations which are likely to share epitopes with most, if not all, wild strains of *M. tuberculosis* are also likely to share some epitopes with non-pathogenic environmental mycobacteria. Purified antigens, on the other hand, may not be expressed by every patient infected with tubercle bacilli. Antibody responses may persist for years, particularly if one accepts the notion of a dormant population of bacilli that are occasionally surfacing to reproduce before hiding away again (Grange, 1992). In high prevalence areas, it may be difficult to distinguish current from old disease. Some assays show rising titres as treatment progresses (Fadda *et al.*, 1992), allowing retrospective confirmation of the diagnosis. Sensitivity tends to be higher in high prevalence countries, presumably because patients tend to seek attention later and with more advanced disease. However, the high prevalence countries tend to be those that are most affected by the HIV epidemic either now or in the next decades and the infection with HIV may cause both failure of specific B cell responses and polyclonal B cell activation which may render antibody based tests useless (van der Werf *et al.*, 1992).

Overall, sensitivities have generally varied between 60 and 80% while specificities have been above 96% with a few exceptions. Depending on the prevalence of disease and the objective sought, these values could be sufficiently high to be useful if they can be reproduced in field conditions.

Why then have serological tests been so slow to enter routine laboratory practice? Part of the explanation may lie in the fact that in the areas where the tests perform best (high prevalence countries) the detection of smear-negative cases is not a priority for limited resources and the relative absence of atypical mycobacteria allows sputum microscopy to remain a highly specific tool. Another explanation is that some promising tests have relied on antigen purified by immunoadsorbent chromatography using antisera that may only be available in limited quantities (Daniel and Anderson, 1978). This allows a useful test to be identified but limits its applicability due to supply or stability of the reagents required. The use of murine monoclonal antibodies, either to purify antigens for a standard ELISA or as competition for epitopes on crude antigen preparation (Wilkins and Ivanyi, 1990), will help make tests more available outside the research laboratory in which they were developed.

Other tests. The cellular response to tuberculosis could also be used to help diagnosis. Lymphocyte proliferative responses to specific mycobacterial antigens can be elicited but require expensive equipment, facilities for radioactive materials and considerable quality control if reproducible results are to be obtained. In the veterinary field, advances have been made with an assay in which the lymphocytes in whole blood are stimulated with purified protein derivative from *M. bovis* and the amount of gamma-interferon produced is measured (Rothel *et al.*, 1990).

Less specific host responses such as adenosine deaminase (Ocana *et al.*, 1983; Voight, 1989) and lysozyme (Verea Hernando, 1987) or both (Fontan Bueso *et al.*, 1988) have also been used and found to be helpful particularly in the diagnosis of pleural and peritoneal effusions. However, these enzymes may be produced in response to other similar pathogenetic mechanisms such as sarcoidosis and also in rheumatoid arthritis, systemic lupus erythematosus and adenocarcinoma (Petterson *et al.*, 1984; Sanchez-Hernandez *et al.*, 1991). The proportion of pleural effusions that are caused by each disease will determine whether or not these are useful tests in a given context.

Detection of bacillary constituents

Serological tests. Detection of antigens from *M. tuberculosis* has been attempted in sputum, cerebrospinal fluid and serum using a variety of immunoassay techniques. Unfortunately, for optimal performance, these tests require a homogeneous distribution of antigen through the sample which has led to technical difficulties with sputum. Several studies have therefore first cultured the sputum in liquid medium for a short time before hunting for antigen with perfect results on small numbers of samples (Strauss *et al.*, 1981; Raja *et al.*, 1988). Studies on uncultured sputum, which would be much more useful in areas with many patients, have been less encouraging with lower sensitivity and some false positive results (Kadival *et al.*, 1982; Yanez *et al.*, 1986; Kansal and Khuller, 1991). Cerebrospinal fluid provides a more convenient sample and, in the diagnosis of tuberculous meningitis, immunoassay of mycobacterial antigens seems rather promising (Krambovits *et al.*, 1984; Kadival *et al.*, 1986; Radhakrishnan and Mathai, 1991a), although one comparative study found antibody detection to be both more sensitive and specific (Radhakrishnan and Mathai, 1991b).

Structural components. It is possible to detect specific components of mycobacterial cell walls using gas chromatography and mass spectrometry. However, the equipment required is expensive and cumbersome and unlikely to become widely available. Tuberculostearic acid is a structural lipid found in mycobacteria and other members of the Actinomycetales (such as *Nocardia* and *Actinomyces*). It has been detected in sputum (Odham *et al.*, 1979; Pang *et al.*, 1989) and cerebrospinal fluid (Mårdh *et al.*, 1983; French *et al.*, 1987) of patients with tuberculosis but was found to be neither sensitive nor specific as a test for pleural disease (Yew *et al.*, 1991).

Molecular approaches

Mycobacteria are not an obvious choice of organism to study in the laboratory. Their tough, waxy cell wall, frustratingly slow growth and the real risk of laboratory acquired infection have pushed investigators towards more user-friendly bacteria. However, despite its short history, the study of mycobacterial molecular genetics is throwing up exciting possibilities to help in the struggle against tuberculosis and has created such enthusiasm that *M. tuberculosis* is now among the organisms whose entire genome will be sequenced in conjunction with the human genome project.

Although whole chromosomal DNA had been used as a probe (Roberts *et al.*, 1987), as particular genes were cloned and sequenced, it became possible to select short segments of DNA that were specific to *M. tuberculosis* and use these to detect complementary sequences in clinical samples (Pao *et al.*, 1988) or early cultures (Peterson *et al.*, 1989). Unfortunately, DNA probes have not lived up to the initial expectations. The mycobacterial cell wall and the rheology of sputum have hindered methods to treat clinical samples in an easy way that releases the mycobacterial DNA. The result has been disappointingly low sensitivity which is little better than microscopy despite needing a lot more work, expertise and expense. DNA probes may still be useful for early identification of routine mycobacterial cultures.

On the other hand, new techniques for amplifying specific DNA fragments could overcome the limitations of sensitivity while maintaining excellent specificity. Using DNA polymerases to copy sequences of interest had already been tried successfully, but the elegant advantage of the polymerase chain reaction (PCR) was to use a thermostable polymerase from the thermophilic bacteria *Thermus aquaticus* (Saiki *et al.*, 1988). This allowed repeated cycles of DNA synthesis to occur by simply cycling the incubation temperature. At lower temperatures (around 50–60 °C) specific oligonucleotide primers, that match a known sequence of *M. tuberculosis* but no other organism, will anneal to any molecules of DNA of the complementary sequence in the reaction mixture. Mismatches will not be stable at the chosen annealing temperature. The temperature is now raised to 72 °C, the optimum for the *Taq* polymerase. Starting from the primers, the polymerase copies the target sequence, creating double-stranded DNA. When the temperature is raised above 94 °C, the complementary strands of DNA separate into two single strands to which the primers are able to bind once more as the temperature falls and the cycle can be repeated without having to add any extra reagents. The amount of DNA rises exponentially until limited by concentrations of reagents. After the first few cycles, the great majority of the synthesized DNA will be exactly the same length, starting from the position of one of the primers and ending at the other. Using PCR it has proved possible within a few hours to amplify a single molecule of target DNA to levels that are detectable by routine techniques (Li *et al.*, 1988).

The PCR has rapidly found uses in many areas of biomedical research and has been used in diagnostic assays for a wide range of pathogens (Stoker, 1990). Other methods for amplifying DNA are also being described that may be just as useful for detecting small quantities of DNA. Some of these require temperature cycling while others can be incubated at a single temperature. Strand displacement amplification for instance can amplify specific sequences from *M. tuberculosis* more than 10^7-fold in 2 hours at 37 °C (Walker *et al.*, 1992).

The PCR has been used by several groups of investigators to hunt for DNA from *M. tuberculosis* and other members of the *M. tuberculosis* complex (Brisson-Noel *et al.*, 1989; Hermans *et al.*, 1990a; Pao *et al.*, 1990; Eisenach *et al.*, 1991; Manjunath *et al.*, 1991). Much of the experience gained will also be relevant to other amplification based systems. It has proved relatively easy to find sequences specific to *M. tuberculosis* and to detect tiny amounts of purified DNA produced by diluting solutions of known concentration. However, when applied directly to clinical material, amplification is less predictable and non-specific amplification may occur, leading to extra bands or smears on ultraviolet transilluminated, ethidium bromide stained agarose gels. In order to be certain that the band visualized represents the correct DNA, it is necessary either to use further specific oligonucleotides in Southern hybridizations (Manjunath *et al.*, 1991) or as 'nested' primers for a second amplification of an internal segment or to digest the fragment with a restriction endonuclease into fragments of predictable size (Pao *et al.*, 1990). 'Nesting' the PCR, by transferring a small aliquot of the product of the first reaction into a second reaction with primers selected to amplify a shorter length of DNA from within the first fragment, not only confirms that the correct fragment has been amplified but also increases sensitivity and reduces the concentration of any substances in the clinical extract that might inhibit the efficiency of amplification (Godfrey-Faussett *et al.*, 1991; Pierre *et al.*, 1991). 'Nesting' can also be achieved in a single tube by using primers of different lengths and raising the annealing temperature for the second set of cycles, to prevent one set of primers binding (Kemp *et al.*, 1990; Wilson *et al.*, 1993a and 1993b). This approach avoids the extra manipulations required with a standard nested technique but does not dilute any inhibitory substances that might be present.

The exquisite sensitivity of the PCR has drawbacks. Because a single target sequence may be amplified to detectable levels, false positive results will occur if such DNA should contaminate reaction mixtures. The most abundant supply of target sequences will be from the PCR itself since the product of the reaction will contain many millions of suitable templates that can be carried back to the next assay on fingertips, pipettes, clothing or in aerosols. However, there are other important sources of contamination too, such as cloning fragments of DNA that include the target sequence into plasmid vectors; sample to sample contamination during extraction of DNA; routine culture of *M. tuberculosis*. Standard laboratory practices for microbiological decontamination may kill mycobacteria but will not generally degrade their DNA, which will remain amplifiable. As expected, false positive results have also been observed with the strand displacement amplification technique (Walker *et al.*, 1992). Several precautions may be taken to minimize problems with carry-over from one reaction to the next (Kwok and Higuchi *et al.*, 1989; Longo *et al.*, 1990) but attention should also be paid to contamination before the sample reaches the laboratory (reusable sample bottles may be sterile but still contain DNA) and during DNA extraction. If low levels of contamination are to be detected, large numbers of negative controls are needed at every stage of the process and not just for the PCR itself. This leads to an exponential amplification in the number of reactions required for each sample, but allows a more confident result to be given.

Contamination is a problem that all PCR laboratories must face, but those involved with mycobacteria have the additional difficulty of extracting the DNA from within the cells. This is probably the limiting factor in determining the sensitivity of PCR assays for *M. tuberculosis* in clinical material.

Although several groups have published encouraging studies involving considerable numbers of samples, routine mycobacteriology laboratories are not yet convinced and the results of a recent study organized by the WHO must make the most dedicated molecular diagnostician pause (G. Noordhoek, personal communication). Batches of 200 samples containing varying numbers of *M. bovis* BCG suspended in water, saliva or sputum were sent, coded, to seven laboratories that had established PCR assays for *M. tuberculosis*. One of these was unable to provide results within 6 months. Three had results with specificities of less than 80% and the three laboratories in which false positives were rare only picked up 60% of samples with 10^3 organisms in 0.2 ml, little improvement on a good microscopy service. All groups were using an insertion sequence that is present in multiple copies in most isolates of *M. tuberculosis* but only once one in *M. bovis* so sensitivity might have been an order of magnitude better had real tubercle bacilli been used.

It is too early to define the role of PCR-based assays but it is clear that future improvements must focus on efficiency of DNA extraction from clinical samples to improve sensitivity and further measures to assess and reduce false positivity. Suggestions that positive results in patients who do not have tuberculosis are due to latent or non-viable organisms (de Wit *et al.*, 1992) are hard to synthesize with the rather unimpressive sensitivity data. In situations where sensitivity is less important and microscopy lacks the necessary specificity, for instance in areas where both *M. tuberculosis* and *M. avium intracellulare* are found in the lungs of HIV-infected patients, a PCR-based test can be used on microscopically positive material to identify the species rapidly.

The applicability of molecular technologies to the diagnosis of tuberculosis in high prevalence areas is also not yet clear. However, some of the principal objections seem reactionary. ELISA technology is now widely distributed and used throughout most of the world, yet at its introduction it seemed complex and unfriendly. Indeed, PCR-based tests are being modified to use multi-well trays and colorimetric end-points (Kemp *et al.*, 1990; Wilson *et al.*, 1993b). Carry-over contamination is not inherently worse in poor countries and many have enough laboratory space physically to separate reagents from amplification products. The cost of a PCR-based test will continue to fall as smaller volumes are used and companies compete for their share of the polymerase market. Already, the film for a chest radiograph is more expensive than the reagents for some assays.

While nobody would suggest that amplifying DNA should replace sputum microscopy, finding suitable uses for the increasingly user-friendly technology may be feasible. Reference laboratories processing large numbers of samples might welcome a method that could run on an automated ELISA reader rather than studying slides for hours on end (Wilson *et al.*, 1993a). The quality of district microscopy services could be checked by sending aliquots of sputum (perhaps on filter paper discs through the post) to a central laboratory (Wilson *et al.*, 1993a). Diagnosis of paediatric and extrapulmonary tuberculosis might be improved which would allow validation of clinical or basic laboratory guidelines that are currently used.

Detection of drug resistance

Infectious cases of tuberculosis can already be rapidly identified by sputum microscopy. Determining which of those cases are spreading drug-resistant strains usually takes a few months with current methods. Molecular mechanisms of resistance to both isoniazid (Zhang *et al.*, 1992) and rifampicin (Telenti *et al.*, 1993) have been established, which should soon lead to rapid methods to demonstrate the genotype of strains and so predict its phenotype.

DNA fingerprinting based on Southern hybridization of chromosomal DNA digested with a restriction endonuclease and probed with the insertion element IS*6110* is proving to be a valuable tool for epidemiological studies in both high (Godfrey-Faussett and Stoker, 1992) and low (Hermans *et al.*, 1990b) prevalence countries. Newer methods that use the polymorphism associated with IS*6110* but are based on DNA amplification allow fingerprints to be generated directly from clinical samples without the need to culture an isolate first (Plikaytis *et al.*, 1993). Although DNA fingerprints do not change during the development of rifampicin resistance (Godfrey-Faussett, *et al.*, 1993), clusters of patients from nosocomial outbreaks can be identified and if the original isolate was drug-resistant it is highly likely that the others will be too (Centers for Disease Control, 1991).

The ability to transfer genetic material into and out of mycobacteria (Snapper *et al.*, 1988) will also find many practical uses in the near future. If one inserts the *lux* gene from the firefly, or some other reporter, into *M. tuberculosis*, living organisms will produce light, or whatever marker has been chosen. If the isolate is now grown in culture with antituberculous drugs the light will be extinguished long before it would be possible to determine that growth had failed.

Post-modernism in the detection of tuberculosis

The detection and diagnosis of tuberculosis is the foundation stone for controlling the disease. The fruits of much of the research work in this area over the last decades will need to be regathered following the arrival of the HIV epidemic. What has been the impact of HIV on the population's perception of the TB control programme? If many people who seek treatment do not survive beyond a year and, worse, some develop dreadful rashes from the drugs, passive case finding may break down. Of those who seek treatment, which will we be able to diagnose with traditional skills?

This chapter has provided an overview of some of the issues involved. The importance of the specific context has been emphasized repeatedly. We have powerful new technologies available but their roles remain obscure. It is easy to be seduced by the femtograms of DNA that PCR can retrieve but until field trials show that the technique offers a real advantage in a given situation it will remain a laboratory wonder.

Each of us should concentrate on specific objectives within our own context. The diagnosis of paediatric and extrapulmonary tuberculosis remain real challenges. Rapid detection of drug-resistant tuberculosis is already a major issue in some countries and will become so in others. Providing a framework of care for the marginalized that is accessible and acceptable is essential if we are to drain the reservoirs of infection.

Exciting new tools will become available but we already have the ability to detect the majority of the infectious cases. We need to concentrate on implementing what we already know as well as seeking to expand the boundaries of our knowledge.

Acknowledgements

I thank my many colleagues involved in the London School of Hygiene & Tropical Medicine/University Teaching Hospital Lusaka's 'Zambian AIDS-related tuberculosis study' (ZAMBART). I gratefully acknowledge the Commission of the European Community, the World Health Organization, the UK Overseas Development Administration, the Enid Linder Foundation and the Commercial Community of Zambia all of whom support ZAMBART.

References

Allan WGL, Girling DJ, Fayers PM, Fox W (1979) The symptoms of newly diagnosed pulmonary tuberculosis and patients' attitudes to the disease and to its treatment in Hong Kong. *Tubercle, 60*, 211–223

Aluoch JA, Edwards EA, Stott H, Fox W, Sutherland I (1982) A fourth study of case-finding methods for pulmonary tuberculosis in Kenya. *Transactions of the Royal Society of Tropical Medicine and Hygiene, 76*, 679–691

Aluoch JA, Babu Swai O, Edwards EA *et al.* (1984) Study of case-finding for pulmonary tuberculosis in outpatients complaining of a chronic cough at a distant hospital in Kenya. *American Review of Respiratory Disease, 129*, 915–920

Banerji D, Anderson S (1963) A sociological study of awareness of symptoms among persons with pulmonary tuberculosis. *Bulletin of the World Health Organization, 29*, 665–683

Bem C, Patil PS, Elliott AM, Namaambo KM, Bharucha H, Porter JDH. (1993) The value of wide needle aspiration in the diagnosis of tuberculous lymphadenitis in Africa. *AIDS* (in press)

Brisson-Noel A, Gicquel B, Lecossier D, Levy-Frebault V, Nassif X, Hance AJ (1989) Rapid diagnosis of tuberculosis by amplification of mycobacterial DNA in clinical samples. *Lancet, ii*, 1069–1071

Cassels A, Heineman E, Le Clerq S, Gurung PK, Rahut CB (1982) Tuberculosis case-finding in Eastern Nepal. *Tubercle, 63*, 175–185

Centers for Disease Control (1991) Nosocomial transmission of multidrug-resistant tuberculosis among HIV-infected persons—Florida and New York, 1988–1991. *Morbidity and Mortality Weekly Report, 40*, 585–591

Centers for Disease Control (1992) Prevention and control of tuberculosis in migrant farm workers: recommendations of the advisory council for the elimination of tuberculosis. *Morbidity and Mortality Weekly Report, 41* (RR-10), 1–15

Chintu C, Luo C, Bhat G, Malek A, DuPont H, Zumla A. Seroprevalence of human immunodeficiency virus type-1 infection in Zambian children with tuberculosis. Manuscript submitted December 1992.

Colebunders R, Mann JM, Francis H *et al.* (1987) Evaluation of a clinical case-definition of acquired immunodeficiency syndrome in Africa. *Lancet, i*, 492–494

Cundall DB (1986) The diagnosis of pulmonary tuberculosis in malnourished Kenyan children. *Annals of Tropical Paediatrics, 6*, 249–255

Daley CL, Small PM, Schecter GF *et al.* (1992) An outbreak of tuberculosis with accelerated progression among persons infected with the human immunodeficiency virus. *New England Journal of Medicine, 326*, 231–235

Daniel TM, Anderson PA (1978) The isolation by immunoadsorbent affinity chromatography and physicochemical characterization of *Mycobacterium tuberculosis* antigen 5. *American Review of Respiratory Disease, 117*, 533–539

Daniel TM, Debanne SM (1987) The serodiagnosis of tuberculosis and other mycobacterial diseases by enzyme-linked immunosorbent assay. *American Review of Respiratory Disease, 135*, 1137–1151

de Gracia J, Curull V, Vidal R *et al.* (1988) Diagnostic value of bronchoalveolar lavage in suspected pulmonary tuberculosis. *Chest, 93*, 329–332

Demers RY, Fischetti LR, Neale AV (1990) Incongruence between self-reported symptoms and objective evidence of respiratory disease among construction workers. *Social Science and Medicine, 30*, 805–810

de Wit D, Maartens G, Steyn L (1992) A comparative study of the polymerase chain reaction and conventional procedures for the diagnosis of tuberculous pleural effusion. *Tubercle and Lung Disease, 73*, 262–267

Donald P (1992) Diagnosis of paediatric tuberculosis by stool culture. Presented at 1992 World Congress on Tuberculosis, Washington

Eisenach KD, Sifford MD, Cave MD, Bates JH, Crawford JT (1991) Detection of *Mycobacterium tuberculosis* in sputum samples using a polymerase chain reaction.

American Review of Respiratory Disease, 144, 1160–1163

Elliott A, Luo N, Tembo G *et al.* (1990) Impact of HIV on tuberculosis in Zambia: a cross-sectional study. *British Medical Journal, 301*, 412–415

Fadda G, Grillo R, Ginesu F, Santoru L, Zanetti S, Dettori G (1992) Serodiagnosis and follow up of patients with pulmonary tuberculosis by enzyme-linked immunosorbent assay. *European Journal of Epidemiology, 8*, 81–87

Fontan Bueso J, Verea Hernando H, Garcia-Buela JP *et al.* (1988) Diagnostic value of simultaneous determination of pleural adenosine deaminase and pleural lysozyme serum/lysozyme ratio in pleural effusions. *Chest, 93*, 303–307

French GL, Teoh R, Chan CY, Humphries MJ, Cheung SW, O'Mahony G (1987) Diagnosis of tuberculous meningitis by detection of tuberculostearic acid in cerebrospinal fluid. *Lancet, ii*, 117–119

Godfrey-Faussett P, Stoker NG (1992) Aspects of tuberculosis in Africa. 3. Genetic fingerprinting for clues to the pathogenesis of tuberculosis. *Transactions of the Royal Society of Tropical Medicine and Hygiene, 86*, 472–475

Godfrey-Faussett P, Wilkins EGL, Khoo S, Stoker N (1991) Tuberculous pericarditis confirmed by DNA amplification. *Lancet, 337*, 176–177

Godfrey-Faussett P, Scott A, Kelly P, Stoker NG, (1993) Development of drug-resistant *Mycobacterium tuberculosis* during treatment. *Tubercle and Lung Disease*, (in press)

Grange (1992) The mystery of the mycobacterial 'persistor.' *Tubercle and Lung Disease, 73*, 249–251

Harries AD (1990) Tuberculosis and human immunodeficiency virus infection in developing countries. *Lancet, 335*, 387–390

Hermans PWM, Schuitema ARJ, van Soolingen D *et al.* (1990a) Specific detection of *Mycobacterium tuberculosis* complex strains by polymerase chain reaction. *Journal of Clinical Microbiology, 28*, 1204–1213

Hermans PWM, van Soolingen D, Dale JW *et al.* (1990b) Insertion element IS*986* from *Mycobacterium tuberculosis*: a useful tool for diagnosis and epidemiology of tuberculosis. *Journal of Clinical Microbiology, 28*, 2051–2058

Hobby GL, Holman AP, Iseman MD, Jones JM (1973) Enumeration of tubercle bacilli in sputum of patients with pulmonary tuberculosis. *Antimicrobial Agents and Chemotherapy, 4*, 94–104

Hong Kong Chest Service/Tuberculosis Research Centre, Madras/British Medical Research Council (1984) A controlled trial of 2-month, 3-month and 12-month regimens of chemotherapy for sputum-smear-negative pulmonary tuberculosis. *American Review of Respiratory Disease, 130*, 23–28

Kadival GV, Sanuel AM, Virdi BS, Kale RN, Ganatra RD (1982) Radioimmunoassay of tuberculous antigen. *Indian Journal of Medical Research, 75*, 765–770

Kadival GV, Mazarelo TBMS, Chaparas SD (1986) Sensitivity and specificity of enzyme-linked immunosorbent assay in the detection of antigen in tuberculous meningitis cerebrospinal fluids. *Journal of Clinical Microbiology, 23*, 901–904

Kamat SR, Dawson JJY, Devadatta S. *et al.* (1966) A controlled study of the influence of segregation of tuberculous patients for one year on the attack rate of tuberculosis in a 5-year period in close family contacts in South India. *Bulletin of the World Health Organization, 34*, 517–532

Kansal R and Khuller GK (1991) Detection of mannophosphoinositide antigens in sputum of tuberculosis patients by dot enzyme immunoassay. *Medical Microbiology and Immunology, 180*, 73–78

Kemp DJ, Churchill MJ, Smith DB *et al.* (1990) Simplified colorimetric analysis of polymerase chain reactions: detection of HIV sequences in AIDS patients. *Gene, 94*, 223–228

Krambovits E, McIllmurray MB, Lock PE, Hendrickse W, Holzel H (1984) Rapid diagnosis of tuberculous meningitis by latex particle agglutination. *Lancet, ii*, 1229–1231

Kwok S, Higuchi R (1989) Avoiding false positives with PCR. *Nature, 339*, 237–238

Li H, Gyllensten UB, Cui X, Saiki RK, Erlich HA, Arnheim N (1988) Amplification and analysis of DNA sequences in single human sperm and diploid cells. *Nature, 335*, 414–417

Longo MC, Berninger MS, Hartley JL (1990) The use of uracil DNA glycosylase to control carry-over contamination in polymerase chain reactions. *Gene, 93*, 125–128

Manjunath N, Shankar P, Rajan L, Bhargava A, Saluja S, Shriniwas (1991) Evaluation of a polymerase chain reaction for the diagnosis of tuberculosis. *Tubercle, 72*, 21–27

Mårdh PA, Larsson L, Høiby N, Engbaek HC, Odham G (1983) Tuberculostearic acid as a diagnostic marker in tuberculous meningitis. *Lancet, i*, 367

Migliori GB, Borghesi A, Rossanigo P *et al.* (1992) Proposal of an improved score method for the diagnosis of pulmonary tuberculosis in childhood in developing countries. *Tubercle and Lung Disease, 73*, 145–149

Morris CD (1991) Sputum examination in the screening and diagnosis of pulmonary tuberculosis in the elderly. *Quarterly Journal of Medicine, 81*, 999–1004

Nsanzumuhire H, Aluoch JA, Karuga WK *et al.* (1981) A third study of case-finding methods for pulmonary tuberculosis in Kenya, including the use of community leaders. *Tubercle, 62*, 79–94

Ocana I, Martinez-Vazquez JM, Segura RM, Fernandez de Sevilla T, Capdevila JA (1983) Adenosine deaminase in pleural fluids: test for diagnosis of tuberculosis pleural effusion. *Chest, 84*, 51–53.

Odham G, Larsson L, Mardh PA (1979) Demonstration of tuberculostearic acid in sputum from patients with pulmonary tuberculosis by selected ion monitoring. *Journal of Clinical Investigation, 63*, 813–819

Pang JA, Chan HS, Chan CY, Cheung SW, French GL (1989) A tuberculostearic acid assay in the diagnosis of sputum smear-negative pulmonary tuberculosis: a prospective study of bronchoscopic aspirate and lavage specimens. *Annals of Internal Medicine, 111*, 650–654

Pao CC, Lin SS, Wu SY, Juang WM, Chang CH, Lin JY (1988) The detection of mycobacterial DNA sequences in uncultured clinical specimens with cloned *Mycobacterium tuberculosis* DNA as probes. *Tubercle, 69*, 27–36

Pao CC, Yen TSB, You J-B, Maa J-S, Fiss EH, Chang C-H (1990) Detection and identification of *Mycobacterium tuberculosis* by DNA amplification. *Journal of Clinical Microbiology, 28*, 1877–1880

Parry C (1992). Nebulised sputum induction for the diagnosis of pulmonary tuberculosis in Malawi. Presented at 1992 World Congress on Tuberculosis, Washington

Pedro-Botet J, Gutierrez J, Miralles R, Coll J, Rubies-Prat J (1992) Pulmonary tuberculosis in HIV-infected patients with normal chest radiographs. *AIDS, 6*, 91–93

Peterson EM, Lu R, Floyd C, Nakasone A, Friedly G, de la Maza LM (1989) Direct identification of *Mycobacterium tuberculosis*, *Mycobacterium avium*, and *Mycobacterium intracellulare* from amplified primary cultures in BACTEC media using DNA probes. *Journal of Clinical Microbiology, 27*, 1543–1547

Pettersson T, Klockars M, Weber T (1984) Pleural fluid adenosine deaminase in rheumatoid arthritis and systemic lupus erythematosus. *Chest, 86*, 273–274

Pierre C, Lecossier D, Boussougant Y *et al.* (1991) Use of a reamplification protocol improves sensitivity of detection of *Mycobacterium tuberculosis* in clinical samples by amplification of DNA. *Journal of Clinical Microbiology, 29*, 712–717

Pitchenik AE, Rubinson HA (1985) The radiographic appearance of tuberculosis in patients with the acquired immunodeficiency syndrome (AIDS) and pre-AIDS. *American Review of Respiratory Disease, 131*, 393–396

Plikaytis BP, Crawford JT, Woodley CL Butler WR, Eisenach KD, Cave MD, Shinnick TM (1993) Rapid, amplification-based fingerprinting of *Mycobacterium tuberculosis. Journal of General Microbiology* 139, 1537–1542

Radhakrishnan VV, Mathai A (1991a) Detection of *Mycobacterium tuberculosis* antigen 5 in cerebrospinal fluid by inhibition ELISA and its diagnostic potential in tuberculous meningitis. *Journal of Infectious Diseases, 163*, 650–652

Radhakrishnan VV, Mathai A (1991b) A dot-immunobinding assay for the laboratory diagnosis of tuberculous meningitis and its comparison with enzyme-linked immunosorbent assay. *Journal of Applied Bacteriology, 71*, 428–433

Raja A, Machicao AR, Morrissey AB, Jacobs MR, Daniel TM (1988) Specific detection of *Mycobacterium tuberculosis* in radiometric cultures by using an immunoassay for antigen 5. *Journal of Infectious Diseases, 158*, 468–470

Roberts MC, McMillan C, Coyle MB (1987) Whole chromosomal DNA probes for rapid identification of *Mycobacterium tuberculosis* and *Mycobacterium avium* complex. *Journal of Clinical Microbiology, 25*, 1239–1243

Rothel JS, Jones SL, Corner LA, Cox JC, Wood PR (1990) A sandwich enzyme immunoassay for bovine interferon-gamma and its use for the detection of tuberculosis in cattle. *Australian Veterinary Journal, 67*, 134–137

Rouillon A, Perdrizet S, Parrot R (1976) Transmission of tubercle bacilli: the effect of chemotherapy. *Tubercle, 57*, 275–299

Saiki RK, Gelfand DH, Stoffel S *et al.* (1988) Primer-directed enzymatic amplification of DNA with a thermostable DNA polymerase. *Science, 239*, 487–491

Sanchez-Hernandez IM, Pantoja C, Ussetti P, Gallardo J, Carrillo F, Cuevas J (1991) Pleural fluid adenosine deaminase and lysozyme levels in the diagnosis of tuberculosis. *Chest, 100*, 1479–1480

Shafer RW, Goldberg R, Sierra M, Glatt AE (1989) Frequency of *Mycobacterium tuberculosis* bacteremia in patients with tuberculosis in an area endemic for AIDS. *American Review of Respiratory Disease, 140*, 1611–1613

Slutkin G, Leowski J, Mann J (1988) The effect of the AIDS epidemic on the tuberculosis problem and tuberculosis programmes. *Bulletin of the International Union against Tuberculosis and Lung Disease, 63*, 21–24

Snapper SB, Lugosi L, Jekkel A *et al.* (1988) Lysogeny and transformation in mycobacteria: stable expression for foreign genes. *Proceedings of the National Academy of Science of the USA, 85*, 6987–6991

Stoker NG (1990) The polymerase chain reaction and infectious diseases: hopes and realities. *Transactions of the Royal Society of Tropical Medicine and Hygiene, 84*, 755–756, 758.

Strauss E, Wu N, Quraishi MAH, Levine S (1981) Clinical applications of the radioimmunoassay of secretory tuberculoprotein. *Proceedings of the National Academy of Science of the USA, 78*, 3214–3217

Sunderam G, McDonald RJ, Maniatis T, Olseke J, Kapila R, Reichman LB (1986) Tuberculosis as a manifestation of the acquired immunodeficiency syndrome (AIDS). *Journal of the American Medical Association, 256*, 362–369

Telenti A, Lowrie D, Matter L, Imboden P, Cole S, Schopfer K, Marchesi F, Colston MJ, Bodmer T (1993) Detection of rifampicin-resistance mutation in *Mycobacterium tuberculosis. Lancet, 341*, 647–650

Torres RA, Mani S, Altholz J, Brickner PW (1990) Human immunodeficiency virus infection among homeless men in a New York City shelter. Association with *Mycobacterium tuberculosis* infection. *Archives of Internal Medicine, 150*, 2030–2036

van der Werf TS, Das PK, van Soolingen D, Yong S, van der Mark TW, van der Akker R (1992) Sero-diagnosis of tuberculosis with A60 antigen enzyme-linked immunosorbent assay: failure in HIV-infected individuals in Ghana. *Medical Microbiology and Immunology, 181*, 71–76

Verea Hernando HR, Masa Jimenez JF, Dominguez Juncal L, Perez Garcia-Buela J, Martin Egaña MT, Fontan Bueso J (1987) Meaning and diagnostic value of determining the lysozome level of pleural fluid. *Chest, 91*, 342–345

Voight MD, Kalvaria I, Trey C, Berman P, Lombard C, Kirsch R (1989) Diagnostic value of ascites adenosine deaminase in tuberculous peritonitis. *Lancet, i*, 751–754

Walker GT, Little MC, Nadeau JG, Shank DD (1992) Isothermal *in vitro* amplification of DNA by a restriction enzyme/DNA polymerase system. *Proceedings of the National Academy of Science of the USA, 89*, 392–396

Wilkins EGL, Ivanyi J (1990) Potential value of serology for diagnosis of extrapulmonary tuberculosis. *Lancet, 336*, 641–644

Wilson SM, Nava E, Morales A, Godfrey-Faussett, P, Gillespie S, Andersson N (1993b) Simplification of the polymerase chain reaction for detection of *Mycobacterium tuberculosis* in the tropics. *Transactions of the Royal Society of Tropical Medicine and Hygiene, 87*, 177-180

Wilson SM, McNerney R, Godfrey-Faussett P, Stoker NG, Voller A (1993a) Progress towards a simplified polymerase chain reaction and its application to the detection of tuberculosis. *Journal of Clinical Microbiology 3*, 776-782

Yanez MA, Coppola MP, Russo DA, Delaha E, Chaparas SD, Yeager H (1986) Determination of mycobacterial antigens in sputum by enzyme immunoassay. *Journal of Clinical Microbiology, 23*, 822–825

Yeager H, Lacy J, Smith LR, LeMaistre CA (1967) Quantitative studies of mycobacterial populations in sputum and saliva. *American Review of Respiratory Disease, 95*, 998–1004

Yew WW, Chan CY, Kwan SY, Cheung SW, French GL (1991) Diagnosis of tuberculous pleural effusion by the detection of tuberculostearic acid in pleural aspirates. *Chest, 100*, 1261–1263

Zhang Y, Heym B, Allen B, Young D, Cole S (1992) The catalase-peroxidase gene and isoniazid resistance of *Mycobacterium tuberculosis*. *Nature, 358*, 591–593

Discussion

Donald A. Enarson

International Union against Tuberculosis and Lung Disease, Paris, France

Dr Godfrey-Faussett has very nicely laid out aspects of TB diagnosis, but has indicated, quite correctly, that many recent developments in the diagnosis of TB are not yet at a point where we can expect them to play a useful role in case finding at a programme level within developing countries, where the bulk of the tuberculosis problem exists at present. Indeed, as noted in his presentation, a recent evaluation of polymerase chain reaction technology as it relates to tuberculosis diagnosis has indicated that the test characteristics, in comparing one laboratory with another, are such that the test is not yet reliable even for use in the clinical setting in Europe and the United States. I am reminded of a National Conference on Tuberculosis held in

Canada in 1988 at which Professor Joe Bates spoke of the use of this technology and indicated that within 6 months we could expect to have a cheap, easily applied test which could be used 'under a palm tree.' We are still waiting.

In considering case finding within national tuberculosis programmes, it is worthwhile to re-examine its basis. The goal of the National Tuberculosis Programme, unlike the goal of clinical medicine, is the cessation of transmission of tuberculosis in the community. Thus, the target of case finding is not the 'case of tuberculosis' (as in clinical medicine), but the 'infectious case of tuberculosis.' This is why case finding in such programmes is based upon sputum smear microscopy, because of its demonstrated ability to identify the infectious case of tuberculosis (Grzybowski et al., 1975) and its stable relationship to other epidemiological indices (Murray et al., 1990). Thus, it is the 'gold standard' in evaluating other tests. If we, then, return to this test, we need to evaluate it as any other test, and determine validity, reliability, sensitivity, specificity and predictive value.

To assess these characteristics, we must evaluate the ability of the test to predict infection with tuberculosis. The test is performed on the source case and the result measured in the contacts. Using the study of Grzybowski et al. (1975), in which 13 472 contacts were evaluated, it is possible to calculate sensitivity, specificity and predictive value of the smear examination of cases in determining who was infected by that case. Thus, of 1668 individuals who were infected by their recent contact 1609 (96.5%) occurred among those in whom the source case was smear-positive (the sensitivity of the test). In those 11 804 without recent infection, 4122 were contacts of the smear-negative cases (specificity of 34.9%). If one assumes, as has been observed in Tanzania, Benin, Mozambique and Nicaragua, that for every smear-positive case detected in the laboratory, there are 10 suspects who are smear-negative (one of whom has active tuberculosis which is smear-negative), it is possible to calculate the predictive value of the test using the 'prevalence' of disease amongst suspects presenting to the health centre for examination (the basis of passive case finding). Thus 1609 of 9291 contacts of smear-positive cases were infected by the contact (for a positive predictive value of 17.3%) and 41 751 of 41 810 contacts of smear-negative cases were not infected by their contact (for a negative predictive value of 99.9%).

Within the context of the IUATLD 'model' programmes, it is also possible to estimate validity and reliability of the smear examination under routine conditions. For example, in Tanzania, sputum cultures have been carried out on a representative sample of patients treated for smear-positive pulmonary tuberculosis. Of 4879 cultures undertaken, 4532 (92.9%) were positive, indicating that a high proportion of those identified in the field as having tuberculosis did indeed have the disease. (The figure is an underestimate of validity as a number of specimens had a very long transit time and some were contaminated.) In determining reliability of the smear examination, it has been possible to read a representative sample of smears on two occasions in the course of an exercise in quality control. Thus, of 495 slides reread by the Central Reference Laboratory, 453 (91.5%) were read as having the same result. Of 250 slides read as negative in the health centre laboratories, 15 (6.0%) were actually positive on evaluation in the Central Reference Laboratory. If three slides are routinely taken and the rate of reading false negative results is maintained, the rate of false negative results would be 0.02% of patients.

Dr Godfrey-Faussett, in his chapter, indicates that, in the presence of HIV infection, the smear-negative cases represent a greater potential source of infection in the community than previously. Undoubtedly this is true to some extent. However, when the contacts of cases are HIV-negative, as most of them are, the 'vector of infectivity' of smear-negative cases or the proportion of all cases which are smear-negative would have to increase considerably in order for this to occur. From the material previously presented (Grzybowski et al., 1975) it is possible to determine the relative 'vector' of each type of case: in the situation of close contact, the smear-positive case is 13.5 times more infectious; with casual contact, 12.5 times. Thus, the effect of HIV infection in the community would have to result in either the smear-negative case becoming more than 10 times more infectious or the proportion of such cases increasing more than 10 times for there to be an equivalent impact from such cases. This possibility is unlikely. Therefore, it is reasonable to suggest that the smear-positive case *must* remain the priority in case finding unless systematic investigations in the future demonstrate otherwise. Of course, where other types of cases can be managed by the health service, they must be found and treated because they are infectious to a certain degree and they may become infectious. However, in many urban settings where HIV is having a marked impact (as is now the case in the 'model' programmes), the capacity of the health service to handle even smear-positive cases is in jeopardy.

How well does passive case finding using smear microscopy function in finding the majority of infectious (smear-positive cases) in the community? If, as proposed (Murray et al., 1990) one uses the average annual risk of infection to evaluate the coverage of case finding in a community, it is possible to estimate the coverage of case finding of sputum smear-positive cases in the 'model' programmes. In utilizing such estimates, however, it must be remembered that the average annual risk of infection is a summary of what has happened over the lifetime of the individuals tested. Thus, for surveys undertaken in children 10 years of age, the estimate is a point estimate of the situation 5 years previously. Thus, in Tanzania, where tuberculin survey results are available over the past 30 years and case finding results for 15 years, an estimate can be made (Enarson et al., 1993). In 1985, prior to the subsequent striking effect of HIV, whereas the expected rate of cases was approximately 48 per 100 000, the rate of notification was around 38 per 100 000 (with an estimated case finding coverage of 79%).

Although these are not precise estimates, they show that the sputum smear examination is a robust test for the purpose of identifying the infectious case of tuberculosis which is the object of the Tuberculosis Control Programme. Moreover, using this test within an organized system of a national tuberculosis programme with the smear examination and passive case finding, it is possible to detect a high proportion of the total number of cases estimated to exist in the community. Sputum smear microscopy is, unquestionably, difficult, cumbersome and time consuming but, nevertheless, performs well under field conditions. Clearly the need of the hour for operations research in programmes is to concentrate on improving this test by making it easier and quicker to perform without losing sensitivity, negative predictive value, validity or reliability.

References

Enarson DA, Chum HJ, Gninafon M, Nyangulu DS, Salamao A (1993) Tuberculosis and human immunodeficiency virus infection in Africa. In: Reichman L, Hershfield E (eds) *Tuberculosis*. Marcel Dekker pp. 395–412

Grzybowski S, Barnett GD, Styblo K (1975) Contacts of cases of active pulmonary tuberculosis. *Royal Netherlands Tuberculosis Association Selected Papers*, 90–106

Murray CJL, Styblo S, Rouillon A (1990) Tuberculosis in developing countries: burden, intervention and cost. *Bulletin of the International Union Against Tuberculosis and Lung Disease, 65*, 6–24

5

'The cure': organization and administration of therapy for tuberculosis

Philip C. Hopewell

University of California, San Francisco, USA

Introduction

During the past 100 years in industrialized countries, 'the cure' for tuberculosis has evolved from the combination of rest, fresh air, sunshine and a healthy diet provided by isolated mountain sanatoria, through progressively more invasive surgical procedures to modern outpatient drug therapy. Although none but the last of these approaches has been shown to be beneficial, in fact, the innovations that marked each of these eras probably improved the likelihood of one's recovery from tuberculosis. Nevertheless, the outlook for the consumptive patient was rather grim until the advent of specific and effective chemotherapeutic agents. Data reviewed by Grzybowski and Enarson (1978) (Figure 5.1) showed that without chemotherapy, 50% of patients with tuberculosis died within 5 years of diagnosis, 32% were spontaneously 'cured;' and 18% established an equilibrium with the disease and were chronically bacteriologically positive. Grzybowski and Enarson also compared the effects of poorly organized and well organized chemotherapy programmes. As is seen in Figure 5.1, there was a dramatic difference based, according to the authors, solely on the organization of drug therapy. This analysis makes the point that while antituberculosis drugs are extremely valuable, their usefulness is substantially decreased by poor systems of drug supply and supervision of therapy. This latter point has to a large extent been lost on many current public health programmes, as will be discussed.

Early reports of the effects of antituberculosis drug therapy were quite dramatic. The first word of the success of isoniazid in treating tuberculosis came from the lay press (Keers, 1978). In pursuit of the story of a rumoured 'miracle drug,' reporters

Tuberculosis: Back to the Future. Edited by J.D.H. Porter and K.P.W.J. McAdam
© 1994 John Wiley & Sons Ltd

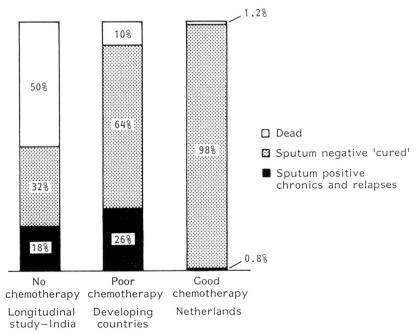

Figure 5.1   Data describing the outcome of tuberculosis 5 years after the diagnosis when there was no therapy, when therapy was poorly organized, and when therapy was given in a well-supervised programme (data from Grzybowski and Enarson, 1978, with permission of the International Union against Tuberculosis and Lung Disease).

gained access to the wards of the Sea View Hospital, the site of a clinical trial of isoniazid. The stories that were then published, complete with photographs, described previously moribund patients dancing in the hallways of the institution after having received the drug. It was certain; tuberculosis was on its way toward being eradicated, at least in the minds of the public. Tuberculosis clinicians and investigators were less sanguine, however. The recent clinical experience with streptomycin—initial improvement of patients followed by worsening caused by streptomycin-resistant organisms—was not forgotten (McDermott, 1947). And, in fact, this experience was repeated in initial clinical trials of isoniazid monotherapy (Medical Research Council, 1952). In the first comparative clinical trial of isoniazid, resistance to the agent developed in 11% of patients by 1 month of therapy and in 52% by 2 months.

The two historical snippets described above present important bases for understanding today's situation vis-à-vis tuberculosis. The first is that public attitudes toward the disease developed because of the success of chemotherapy, translated into progressively less public health attention to tuberculosis (Reichman, 1991). Thus, the infrastructure essential for assuring successful therapy was allowed to deteriorate badly. Second, it was demonstrated that even with powerful antimycobacterial agents, tuberculosis is a difficult disease to treat, and that the emergence of drug resistance is an ever-present threat (David, 1970). Now, in part but not entirely, because of the pandemic of infection with the human immunodeficiency virus (HIV) we are witnessing two frightening phenomena, a worldwide increase in the incidence of tuberculosis and the occurrence of disease caused by organisms that are resistant to multiple antituberculosis drugs (Sudre *et al.*, 1992; Dooley *et al.*, 1992).

This review will focus largely on management decisions related to drug therapy for tuberculosis—who should be treated and how. Simply describing drug regimens and the anticipated success rates extrapolated from clinical trials is insufficient to assist in guiding health care providers. Thus, attention will be paid to the means by which the regimens may be delivered to the patients. The fundamental philosophy that should underlie tuberculosis treatment programmes is that successful completion of therapy is the responsibility of the provider or programme that undertakes to treat patients with tuberculosis. The benefits of effective treatment should be viewed as accruing not only to the patient but to society as well. Thus, providing 'the cure' for tuberculosis is a societal imperative in both industrialized and non-industrialized countries.

Principles of chemotherapy

In the four decades that effective chemotherapy for tuberculosis has existed, clinical trials have established three basic principles upon which successful treatment is based. First, at least two agents to which the organisms are susceptible must be used. Second, treatment requires a relatively long period of time (even with so-called short-course regimens). Third, the drugs must be taken regularly. Adherence to these principles not only maximizes the likelihood of cure but minimizes the chance that drug resistance will develop. The aim of therapy is to provide the most effective treatment in the shortest time, but there are additional considerations that have an impact on the choice of regimens. These considerations include the resources available for drug purchase and for supervision of treatment, and the potential for a regimen causing an adverse reaction.

Successful tuberculosis treatment depends on much more than the science of chemotherapy. Chemotherapy can be successful only within the framework of the overall clinical and social management of patients and their contacts. Moreover, tuberculosis control programmes require an organized network of primary and referral services with cooperation between public and private providers and among the various components of the health care system. Such collaboration and co-operation are especially important in the context of today's tuberculosis—a context in which a substantial number of patients require other services—care for HIV-related illnesses, drug treatment programmes, refugee health care—to name a few. By operating through the relevant services, treatment can be delivered more efficiently with a greater degree of patient compliance.

Who should be treated for tuberculosis?

The answer to this question is simple: persons with tuberculosis should be treated. However, the definitive diagnosis of tuberculosis can be established only by isolation of *Mycobacterium tuberculosis* from the patient in question, but the vast majority of the world's tuberculosis cases are not diagnosed by cultures. Laboratory facilities for cultures are not available in most of the world. Moreover, even if there is access to an equipped laboratory using current standard technology, the results of cultures are not available for 4 to 6 weeks after submission of the specimen, and decisions regarding therapy generally cannot wait that long. Thus, because of the lack of access to cultures and the delay in results, therapeutic decisions commonly are based on the results of microscopic examination of sputum (or other specimens) and in some instances on the clinical and radiographic features of the patient.

The sensitivity of microscopy for identifying acid-fast bacilli (AFB) in the sputum of patients with pulmonary tuberculosis varies depending upon the skill of the microscopist, the number of specimens examined, and the concentration of organisms in sputum. To find 1–2 organisms in 300 oil immersion fields the concentration of organisms must be 5000–10000, the concentration generally taken as the threshold for a positive smear (Smithwick, 1976). Under operational conditions positive smears have been found in 50–70% of patients who subsequently have a positive culture (Toman, 1979). The sensitivity is increased somewhat if a second specimen is obtained. In fact, two smears taken together have approximately the same rate of positivity as culture of a single specimen.

Based on these assessments, using only AFB smears to diagnose tuberculosis for the purpose of treatment will find perhaps as many as 70% of the existing active cases and will identify those who are the most infectious. This approach is the basis for the WHO recommendations for who should have the highest priority for treatment—persons with positive sputum smears. In developing countries this is probably as good as can be hoped for and would be expected to have the greatest epidemiological impact. Nevertheless, waiting until the disease process has become sufficiently advanced to cause a positive sputum smear before a diagnosis can be established, and treatment initiated, results in more new infections than would have occurred if cases were detected at an earlier stage. The potential benefits of using cultures on a selective basis to diagnose tuberculosis in a developing country have not been investigated.

Several studies have examined the role of presumptive treatment of patients who have negative sputum smears and cultures but have radiographic abnormalities suggestive of tuberculosis. In a study of patients with radiographically 'active' tuberculosis in Hong Kong (Hong Kong Chest Service, 1984) it was found that 99 (57%) of 173 untreated patients who had three negative smears and cultures during the initial evaluation developed bacteriologically positive tuberculosis in 5 years. In a similar group of patients who were treated for 3 months with isoniazid, rifampicin, pyrazinamide, and streptomycin, tuberculosis developed in only 4% in

5 years; thus, presumptive treatment based on radiographic findings decreased the number of potentially infectious cases.

In a group of 139 patients in San Francisco who had at least three negative sputum smears but who were given chemotherapy based on a presumptive diagnosis, 66 (48%) were determined to have active tuberculosis; 16 with positive initial cultures, 43 with improvement in chest films and seven because of clinical improvement (Gordin *et al.*, 1989). In a similar study, Dutt and coworkers (1989) reported that 126 (30%) of 414 patients who had negative smears and cultures for *M. tuberculosis* had a radiographic response to antituberculosis treatment.

These studies demonstrate that there are advantages to treatment of 'presumed' tuberculosis in persons with negative sputum smears but who have compatible chest radiographic findings. Thus, ideally, choosing candidates for therapy involves both microbiological and radiographic evaluation. Unfortunately, most programmes that cannot afford to perform cultures for diagnosis also cannot afford radiographic evaluations. Additionally, relying on radiographic findings may result in a large number of misdiagnoses and inefficient use of expensive drugs. Thus, under conditions of limited resources, treatment decisions must be made that balance the use of resources with the gains of using more expensive but sensitive diagnostic studies.

In addition to the standard use of sputum and chest radiographs, under current circumstances clinical evaluation is also an important factor in identifying persons to be treated, especially in areas of high prevalence of HIV infection. Although the data are not consistent, several studies suggest that there is a lower frequency of positive sputum smears among patients with HIV infection (Barnes *et al.*, 1991; Long *et al.*, 1991; Brindle *et al.*, 1993). Thus, in this group examination of sputum may have a greater rate of false negativity. At the same time, data from several sources indicate that tuberculosis is very likely to be the diagnosis in HIV-infected patients who have respiratory symptoms in countries having a high prevalence of both diseases (Daley *et al.*, 1992; Kamanfu *et al.*, 1993). For these reasons patients in developing countries who have respiratory symptoms and who are thought to be HIV-infected would be candidates for antituberculosis chemotherapy. Thus, the physical examination is directed toward trying to identify HIV-infected persons. Symptoms and findings that are predictive of HIV infection are listed in Table 5.1 and include a history of chronic diarrhoea or weight loss, or findings of diffuse lymphadenopathy and/or thrush (Widy-Wirski *et al.*, 1988; Colebunders *et al.*, 1989). As described subsequently, diagnosis of HIV infection also influences the approach to therapy. For this reason either HIV testing or clinical diagnosis is important in all patients with tuberculosis.

In summary, the answer to the question, 'Who should be treated for tuberculosis?' is as follows:

1. Persons with acid-fast organisms seen by microscopy. In developing countries this may be the only diagnostic test available. Although non-tuberculous

Table 5.1   Sensitivity, specificity and positive predictive value for HIV infection of various symptoms and findings

	Sensitivity (%)	Specificity (%)	Positive predictive value (%)
Fever	64	68	59
Weight loss (>10% of body weight)	60	70	59
Diarrhoea	38	92	79
Rash	27	92	71
Thrush	21	97	84
Lymphadenopathy	17	98	85
Herpes zoster	16	100	98

Data from Widy-Wirski *et al.* (1988)

mycobacteria have the same appearance on smears, in most situations a positive sputum smear should be assumed to be *M. tuberculosis*.

2. If cultures for mycobacteria are available, persons with positive cultures should be treated.
3. Persons with radiographic findings consistent with 'active' tuberculosis but who have negative smears and cultures. This indication should be used selectively, depending on resources.
4. Persons with respiratory symptoms and findings suggestive of HIV infection, even with negative sputum smears. This indication is applicable in circumstances where there is a high prevalence of both HIV infection and tuberculosis. This indication may be modified to indicate that cough should be present for more than 2 weeks and that the symptoms are not responsive to a course of antibiotic therapy.
5. Persons with clinical or microbiologic evidence of extrapulmonary tuberculosis.

Initiation of treatment

Once it is decided that treatment for tuberculosis should be started, there are several subsidiary but very important decisions remaining. These decisions include the composition of the regimen, the duration of the administration and the means of treatment supervision. The important variables that must be taken into account in making treatment decisions include the HIV status of the patient, the likelihood that the organisms are drug-resistant, the anticipated difficulty in maintaining patient compliance. In the non-industrialized countries financial constraints largely dictate the composition of the treatment regimen provided by governmental tuberculosis control programmes. Likewise in industrialized countries supervision of therapy and the general organization of care is often suboptimal because of lack of funding and structural deficiencies in public health programmes. A major challenge for the

1990s and beyond is to develop innovative resource-efficient means for supervising tuberculosis treatment (Brudney and Dobkin, 1991).

Initial treatment regimens

During the past 45 years a large number of studies have provided information concerning the use of combinations of antituberculosis drugs and of the roles of the different agents in multidrug regimens. Specific recommendations for therapy have been published by the International Union Against Tuberculosis and Lung Disease (Committee on Treatment, 1988), American Thoracic Society (ATS, in press) and WHO (1991).

It is clear that isoniazid possesses the best combination of effectiveness, patient acceptance and cost of any of the antituberculosis agents. Thus, it should be used for the duration of treatment unless there are adverse effects or the organisms are resistant to the drug. Rifampicin is similar in the degree of efficacy to isoniazid. Both rifampicin and isoniazid are essential in at least the initial phase of any regimen that is less than 12 months in duration. Pyrazinamide in the initial phase of therapy enables regimens of as short as 6 months to be used with a high degree of success.

Currently, for patients with positive cultures the minimum duration of therapy associated with an acceptable cure rate is 6 months. The initial phase of therapy for a 6 month regimen should include isoniazid, rifampicin, and pyrazinamide. In many areas ethambutol or streptomycin is also included in the initial phase because of a concern with isoniazid resistance. The drugs should be ingested daily as a single dose. Alternatively, a thrice weekly dosing schedule may be used in order to provide direct observation of therapy (Hong Kong Chest Service/Tuberculosis Research Centre, 1984). The continuation phase of the 6 month regimen consists of isoniazid and rifampicin given daily, three times a week or twice a week, the last two schedules being used to facilitate direct observation of medication ingestion.

A regimen that has been highly successful in Tanzania and has also been transported to several other African countries consists of an initial phase of isoniazid, rifampicin, pyrazinamide and streptomycin given daily for 2 months followed by 6 months of isoniazid and thiacetazone (Chum, 1989). This regimen has produced high cure rates but has the disadvantage of using streptomycin and thiacetazone. As noted below, both agents are somewhat problematic in the context of HIV infection.

Another option is treating for 9 months with isoniazid and rifampicin. This regimen may be necessary in patients who cannot tolerate pyrazinamide. As noted above either ethambutol or streptomycin should be used in the initial phase if resistance to isoniazid is suspected. Again, isoniazid and rifampicin may be given twice or thrice weekly after an initial 1 to 2 months of daily therapy.

For patients who have radiographic findings suggestive of tuberculosis but have negative sputum smears and cultures, a regimen of 4 months' duration is effective

(Hong Kong Chest Service, 1984). The regimen should consist of isoniazid, rifampicin and pyrazinamide with or without ethambutol or streptomycin given for the initial 2 months followed by isoniazid and rifampicin for 2 months. This assumes that such patients have been evaluated carefully for other possible causes of the radiographic findings, as well as having had appropriate specimens obtained for bacteriological studies.

The use of streptomycin in any of the above regimens is problematic. Because parenteral administration is required, there must be a ready supply of sterile syringes and needles. Facilities for sterilization may not be available and disposable supplies are too expensive (and may be reused although not adequately sterilized). There is also the potential for accidental needle-stick injuries. These factors greatly limit the usefulness of streptomycin.

Thiacetazone in initial treatment regimens

For many years in Africa and South America 'standard' therapy for tuberculosis consisted of an initial 2 month phase of isoniazid, streptomycin and thiacetazone given daily (or 5 days a week), with direct observation being required because of the streptomycin injections, followed by 10 months of either daily self-administered isoniazid/thiacetazone or twice weekly isoniazid/streptomycin. The costs of this regimen are far less than the more potent short-course regimens described subsequently (Table 5.2). In clinical trials of this regimen, rates of successful treatment were well over 90% (Kent et al., 1970). However, in practice rates of cure depended mainly upon the degree of supervision provided to assure medication ingestion; overall rates of programme success in the range of 50% were common (Hopewell et al., 1984; Hopewell et al., 1985). Thus, even prior to the epidemic of HIV infection, the 12 month regimen was clearly suboptimal.

In patients with HIV infection the 12 month regimen has been shown to be

Table 5.2   Costs of antituberculosis drugs (UNICEF prices/100)

Drug	Dose/Form	Price
Isoniazid	300 mg tablets	1.19
Rifampicin	300 mg tablets or capsules	9.87
Isoniazid plus rifampicin	150 mg/300 mg capsules	10.20
Pyrazinamide	500 mg tablets	4.30
Isoniazid plus rifampicin plus pyrazinamide	50 mg/120 mg/300 mg tablets	11.50
Ethambutol	400 mg tablets	2.38
Streptomycin	1 g vial	26.74
(water for injection)	(5 ml vial)	(3.30)
Isoniazid plus thiacetazone	300 mg/150 mg tablets	1.13

Tuberculosis Unit, WHO (1991)

associated with a higher mortality rate and greater rates of treatment failure than is found with regimens containing isoniazid and rifampicin (Perriens *et al.*, 1991; Raviglione *et al.*, 1992). Additionally, HIV-infected patients are subject to severe cutaneous hypersensitivity reactions (Stevens–Johnson syndrome). Nunn and associates (Nunn *et al.* 1991) reported cutaneous hypersensitivity reactions in 20% of HIV-infected persons compared with 1% in HIV seronegative patients.

The ideal solution to the problems associated with thiacetazone-containing regimens is to replace thiacetazone with ethambutol. This, however, is an expensive alternative. Thiacetazone 150 mg per day (combined with isoniazid) costs approximately \$4.14 (US) for one year whereas the cost of ethambutol is approximately \$17.37 (US) for a daily dose of 800 mg for one year (Table 5.2) (WHO, 1991). Additionally there is at least a theoretical concern that incorporating ethambutol into primary treatment regimens will preclude its being used in retreatment of patients who have relapsed tuberculosis.

Another approach to the problem posed by using thiacetazone in HIV-infected patients is to attempt to identify which patients are HIV-infected at the time of diagnosis of tuberculosis. As noted previously, physical findings of thrush, lymphadenopathy or herpes zoster as well as a history of chronic diarrhoea, fever, and weight loss, all criteria in the WHO clinical case definition of AIDS have a high positive predictive value for HIV infection (Widy-Wirski *et al.*, 1988). Thus, by using clinical evaluation in patients with tuberculosis one could select either a thiacetazone or a non-thiacetazone regimen depending on the likelihood of HIV infection. It should be kept in mind, however, that in areas in which both tuberculosis and HIV are highly prevalent, it is common for a majority of patients with tuberculosis to be HIV-infected; thus, there may be few patients who would qualify for a thiacetazone containing regimen (Daley *et al.*, 1992; Kamanfu *et al.*, in press).

Supervision of treatment

Figure 5.2 shows the schedule for clinic visits and laboratory evaluations used in the Tuberculosis Control Programme in San Francisco for initial treatment. Having such a protocol in place systematizes the follow-up and enables operational data to be collected. Because of the crucial importance of the treatment regimen used for patients with newly diagnosed tuberculosis, strong considerations should be given to administering all drug doses under the direct observation of a health worker or other responsible person, including relatives or others with whom the patient has a close relationship (Hopewell, 1986). In an innovative project among homeless persons in San Francisco, supervision of preventive therapy is being provided by 'peer health advisors'—persons largely self-selected from among the residents of homeless shelters. Direct observation is obviously labour-intensive, but by improving rates of cure and decreasing the frequency with which drug resistance develops long-term costs may be reduced. This form of supervision may take place

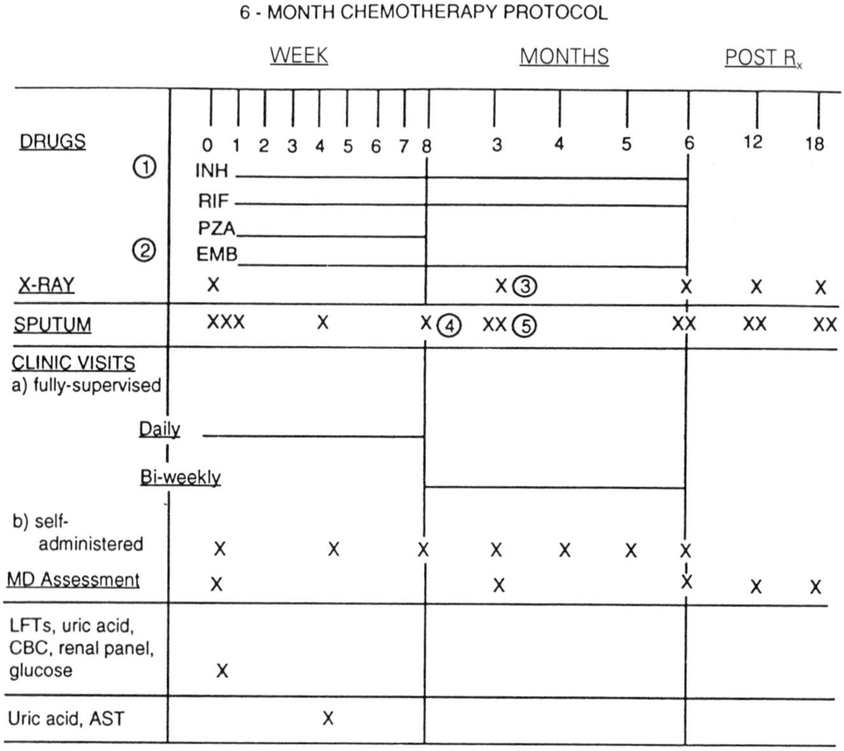

6 - MONTH CHEMOTHERAPY PROTOCOL

		WEEK		MONTHS		POST Rx

DRUGS
① INH ___
RIF ___
PZA ___
② EMB ___

0 1 2 3 4 5 6 7 8   3   4   5   6   12   18

X-RAY   X   X③   X   X   X

SPUTUM   XXX   X   X④ XX⑤   XX   XX   XX

CLINIC VISITS
a) fully-supervised

Daily ___
|
Bi-weekly

b) self-administered   X   X   X   X   X   X   X

MD Assessment   X   X   X   X   X

LFTs, uric acid, CBC, renal panel, glucose   X

Uric acid, AST   X

1. INH, RIF & PZA will be used initially on all patients unless pregnant or with rising LFTs. If the organism is fully susceptible, the course indicated is followed. If INH resistance is documented, at 2 months, the PZA & INH will be dropped and RIF & EMB continued for a total of 1 year treatment.
2. EMB should be used as a fourth drug if there's reasonable suspicion of INH resistance, i.e. previous treatment with INH, or from a country with high incidence of INH resistance. This includes Philippines, South East Asia & Korea, etc.
3. Only if all initial sputums are negative.
4. If 8 week culture positive, continue INH/RIF for 6 mos. after first negative culture & supervise treatment.
5. If one negative sputum not yet documented.

INH = isoniazid, RIF = rifampin, PZA = pyrazinamide, EMB = ethambutol
LFT = liver function tests, CBC = complete blood count, AST = aspartate aminotransferase

Figure 5.2 Flow sheet that schematically describes the management of patients receiving a 6 month regimen of antituberculosis therapy

in a variety of settings—clinic, home, place of employment, school, shelter, drug treatment programme, etc. The rendezvous point may vary from day to day depending on the patient's wishes and schedule.

At the time therapy is initiated patients should be carefully evaluated to determine the likelihood of difficulties in completion of the treatment programme. Although assessments of potential compliance problems are known to be inaccurate, there are several patient characteristics that are predictive of difficulty in

Table 5.3 Ranking of factors thought to be predictive of need for increased time and effort to complete therapy by personnel in urban tuberculosis clinics, United States

Variable	Score[a]
Homelessness	7.52
Chronic substance abuser	7.08
History of missed appointments	6.96
Emotional disturbance	6.22
Lack of transportation	6.05
Recurrent tuberculosis (relapse)	5.11
No family or social support	5.01

From Judd K, Hopewell P, unpublished data
[a]Ranked on a scale of 0 to 9

patient management: these include use of alcohol, young age, and being unmarried (Darbyshire *et al.*, 1984). Additional variables that have been identified by surveying health care providers in urban tuberculosis clinics in the United States are shown in Table 5.3.

In a retrospective review of the costs and outcomes of treatment for tuberculosis in the United States, Judd and coworkers (1989) found that the cost of directly observed therapy for 6 months was no more than the less intensive and less successful modes of treatment supervision. The cost per case treated under direct observation from the outset was $2084 (US) whereas waiting until the patient demonstrated non-compliance before initiating direct supervision cost $2857 (US). Treatment supervision in which the patient was seen only monthly was less expensive, $1958 (US) per patient, but was also less successful. Given these data, at least in the United States, the use of the costlier means of supervision actually produced costs savings. Moreover, if it is assumed that non-compliant patients are infectious for a longer period of time, the cost of an increased number of tuberculous infections should be taken into account. Likewise, as has been dramatically demonstrated in recent years, non-compliance fosters drug resistance. The cost of treatment of drug-resistant tuberculosis is at least an order of magnitude greater than providing directly observed therapy to patients with newly discovered tuberculosis.

Compliance among tuberculosis patients in developing countries poses a major barrier to implementation of successful chemotherapy programmes (Hopewell *et al.*, 1984; Hopewell *et al.*, 1985; Chaulet, 1987). Non-compliant behaviour is reinforced by erratic supply of drugs and supplies for diagnosis and by variable job performance and commitment by health care workers. Use of short duration regimens is likely to enhance patient adherence to a regimen but close supervision and an effective administrative/management system are still essential. In some ways the use of directly observed therapy is more easily accomplished in a developing country where 'hospitalization' during the initial intensive phase is feasible. However, the remoteness and inaccessibility of some areas virtually preclude any centralized form of supervision. In such situations local village health workers may be used for supervision. If health workers are not available school teachers and village leaders can be called on in some cases. Under these circumstances a community-based approach in which there is endorsement of and participation in the tuberculosis control programme by the community would seem to have the best chance of succeeding (Solórzano and Álvarez, 1991).

Also of great concern for tuberculosis control programmes is erratic or selective compliance, that is taking antituberculosis drugs irregularly or taking only one agent to which the organisms are susceptible. Such behaviour would be likely to foster drug resistance and treatment failure. This is presumably the basis for the high prevalence of resistance to isoniazid in many developing countries (Kleeberg and Oliver, 1984). One approach to the problem of selective drug taking is using combination preparations—isoniazid and rifampicin or isoniazid, rifampicin and pyrazinamide. According to the UNICEF price list for 1991 (WHO, 1991), the costs of combination preparations are no greater and may be less than the total costs of the individual drugs in a regimen (Table 5.2).

Management of patients who have failed therapy or who have relapsed

With modern regimens of chemotherapy used in an organized tuberculosis control programme treatment, failures and relapses are very uncommon both in industrialized and non-industrialized countries (Slutkin *et al.*, 1988; Judd *et al.*, 1989; Chum, 1989). However, with less well organized programmes, failures and relapses are frequent (Hopewell, 1984). As noted previously retreatment regimens that require the use of second-line antituberculosis drugs are very expensive. Additionally, when the organisms are resistant to both isoniazid and rifampicin the likelihood of a successful outcome is only in the range of 50% (Goble *et al.*, 1993).

Treatment failure is defined as continued or recurrent active disease, indicated by positive sputum smears, cultures or radiographic worsening, in a patient who is currently receiving therapy. With regimens that contain isoniazid and rifampicin 85–95% of patients whose sputum was positive when treatment was initiated should have negative sputum after 2 months of therapy and nearly 100% will be negative after 4 months. Patients who continue to have positive sputum by 2 to 4 months of treatment should be reassessed carefully. Repeat susceptibility studies should be performed and if the patient has not been receiving directly observed therapy, this should be started. If resistance is found the treatment regimen should be reformulated to include at least two and preferably three agents to which the organisms are susceptible. Treatment should be continued under direct observation. If microbial resistance is not found, the initial treatment regimen should be continued under direct observation. If sputum conversion has not occurred by 4 to 6 months of treatment drug susceptibilities should again be determined but, even prior to the results being obtained, the regimen should be changed to include at least two new agents.

In geographic areas or in patient populations having a high prevalence of multidrug-resistant tuberculosis, failure of a patient to respond quickly to a usually effective regimen should be viewed with alarm. Depending on the epidemiologic circumstances—the likelihood that the disease is caused by multidrug-resistant organisms—failure to respond or worsening should be assumed to be caused by multidrug-resistant organisms (Edlin *et al.*, 1992; Fischl *et al.*, 1992;). In this situation choices of antimycobacterial agents should be based on prevailing community patterns of resistance. Again, at least two and preferably three agents to which the organisms are presumed to be susceptible should be used. Often such regimens must include agents such as the fluoroquinolones that currently are experimental with regard to tuberculosis.

Relapse is defined as recurrence of active disease after apparently successful completion of a full course of therapy. Information from several sources shows that if relapse occurs in a patient who was treated with and complied with a regimen that contained isoniazid and rifampicin, the organisms are likely to retain susceptibility to the agents that were used (Mitchison and Nunn, 1986). Thus, successful retreatment can usually be accomplished using the original regimen. However, drug susceptibilities should be determined and if resistance is encountered, the regimen should be modified. In persons who relapse and are severely ill with tuberculosis, the better part of valour would be to begin with at least two new agents while continuing the previously used drugs.

In most of the non-industrialized countries, options for retreatment are limited because of the cost and availability of second-line antituberculosis agents (WHO, 1991). The current WHO recommendation for retreatment of smear-positive patients consists of an initial daily phase of isoniazid, rifampicin, pyrazinamide, ethambutol and streptomycin given for 2 months followed by the same drugs minus streptomycin for 1 month. The continuation phase consists of 5 months of isoniazid, rifampicin and ethambutol given either three times a week or daily. For optimal efficacy all doses should be given under direct supervision.

Monitoring for adverse effects and for response

The frequency and type of monitoring for adverse drug reactions depends on the capabilities of the programme (Figure 5.2). Where resources permit, it is recommended that baseline measurements of liver enzymes, bilirubin, serum creatinine, complete blood count and platelet count be obtained. If pyrazinamide is to be used serum uric acid should be measured, and when ethambutol is used visual acuity and red–green discrimination should be evaluated. All patients should be evaluated clinically during the course of chemotherapy. It is desirable to have a standard checklist of symptoms that can be reviewed with the patient at least on a monthly basis (Table 5.4). In addition, patients should be educated as to the signs and symptoms to which they should be alert and report if noted. Some studies have

Table 5.4   Checklist for monitoring for adverse effects of antituberculosis drugs

Date:		Date:		Date:	
Meds:	Weight	Meds:	Weight	Meds:	Weight
INH ○	Alcohol use	INH ○	Alcohol use	INH ○	Alcohol use
RIF ○	↓ Appetite	RIF ○	↓ Appetite	RIF ○	↓ Appetite
PZA ○	Nausea/vomiting	PZA ○	Nausea/vomiting	PZA ○	Nausea/vomiting
EMB ○	Weakness/ fatigue	EMB ○	Weakness/ fatigue	EMB ○	Weakness/ fatigue
SM ○	Fever/chills	SM ○	Fever/chills	SM ○	Fever/chills
Other ○ Specify	Yellow eyes	Other ○ Specify	Yellow eyes	Other ○ Specify	Yellow eyes
	Dark urine		Dark urine		Dark urine
	Numbness		Numbness		Numbness
	Rash		Rash		Rash
	Joint pain		Joint pain		Joint pain
	Blurred vision		Blurred vision		Blurred vision
	Other—specify		Other—specify		Other—specify
	Bilirubin		Bilirubin		Bilirubin
	Creatinine		Creatinine		Creatinine
	SGOT		SGOT		SGOT
	Uric acid		Uric acid		Uric acid
	Visual acuity		Visual acuity		Visual acuity
	Pills left		Pills left		Pills left
	Initials of interviewer		Initials of interviewer		Initials of interviewer

suggested that adverse drug reactions (in addition to reactions to thiacetazone) occur more commonly among HIV-infected patients (Chaisson *et al.*, 1987). For this reason and because of the additional medical problems HIV-infected patients may have, they should be followed more closely.

The response to therapy is measured largely on bacteriological and clinical grounds. For patients who had positive smears pretreatment, sputum examinations should be performed at least at the end of the second, fourth and sixth months of treatment. When cultures can be performed, specimens collected at the above intervals should be cultured as well as examined microscopically. If the resources are available response to therapy may be assessed by radiographs as well as by microbiological examination. For patients who had negative smears and cultures (if available), the chest film should be repeated 2 to 3 months after the initiation of therapy. If the film has improved, consistent with a response to therapy, treatment should be continued for a total of 4 months as described previously. A finding of no change on the chest film would be consistent with either the process being inactive tuberculosis or another disease while a worsened film would indicate that, probably, another disease was causing the abnormality.

Special problems in treatment

Children

The basic principles that apply in the management of adults with pulmonary tuberculosis are equally applicable in children. Although children have been excluded from nearly all clinical trials of short durations of chemotherapy, there are several reports documenting the usefulness of 6 and 9 month regimens in children (Ibanez-Quevado and Ross-Bravo, 1980; Abernathy *et al.*, 1983). At least in younger children, sputum specimens for bacteriological evaluations cannot usually be obtained. Consequently, the response to treatment is assessed by clinical and radiographic criteria. For this same reason drug susceptibility or resistance must often be inferred from the pattern of the presumed source case or community data rather than being determined in the laboratory.

Pregnancy and lactation

Active untreated tuberculosis represents a far greater hazard to a pregnant women and her fetus than does treatment for the disease. In a pregnant woman or mother of a young infant, it is important that the most effective therapy for tuberculosis be given. Streptomycin is the only antituberculosis drug documented to have harmful effects on the fetus (Snider *et al.*, 1980). Streptomycin interferes with development of the ear and may cause congenital deafness (Robinson and Cambon, 1964). This potential is presumably shared by kanamycin and capreomycin; however, there is little or no specific information on the fetal effects of these two drugs, nor of cycloserine, ethionamide or pyrazinamide.

Although several antituberculosis drugs are present in breast milk, their concentrations and the total amounts that could possibly be ingested by a nursing infant are such that adverse effects would be unlikely (Snider and Powell, 1984). Thus, no modifications of treatment regimens are necessary in nursing mothers.

Associated diseases

Tuberculosis commonly occurs in association with other diseases. The association may exist either because an underlying disorder alters immune responsiveness, thereby predisposing to tuberculosis, or because the accompanying condition may occur frequently in the same social and cultural milieu as tuberculosis. Examples of the former class of disorders include haematological or reticuloendothelial malignancies, immunosuppressive therapy, HIV infection, chronic renal failure and malnutrition. The latter group includes, among others, chronic alcoholism and its secondary effects and neuropsychiatric disturbances. All of these conditions may influence therapy. The response to treatment of the impaired host may not be as satisfactory as that of a person with normal host responsiveness. For this reason, therapeutic decisions must be made on a much more individualized basis and, when possible, steps taken to correct the immunosuppression. In patients with impaired renal function, streptomycin, kanamycin and capreomycin should be avoided if at all possible. If there is severe impairment of renal function, reduction of doses of drugs such as ethambutol and isoniazid may be necessary and measurement of blood concentrations may be helpful (Andrew *et al.*, 1980). Liver disease, particularly alcoholic hepatitis and cirrhosis, is commonly associated with tuberculosis. In general the complications of potentially hepatotoxic antituberculosis drugs have not been greater in patients with liver disease (Girling, 1982). However, detecting such adverse effects if they occur may be difficult because of the pre-existing disorder of hepatic function. In this group, routine testing of liver function should be performed. Finally, in patients with neuropsychiatric disorders, close supervision of treatment, often with direct observation of medication ingestion, is necessary.

Treatment of known or presumed multidrug-resistant tuberculosis

Microbial resistance to antituberculosis drugs is usually a consequence of poorly constructed treatment regimens or poor supervision of therapy. As a result of both of these errors resistance to isoniazid is very high, reaching 25–30% of new cases, in many parts of the world (Kleeberg and Oliver, 1984). Of far less importance numerically but much more dramatic have been the explosive outbreaks of multidrug-resistant tuberculosis that have occurred among HIV-infected patients in the United States. In some instances these organisms have been resistant to as many as seven antituberculosis drugs. In part because of the drug resistance, case fatality rates have reached 85% in from 1 to 4 months after diagnosis (Dooley *et al.*, 1992).

In communities or in population groups in which multidrug resistance is prevalent, initial drug treatment regimens should be based on the prevailing patterns of drug susceptibility within the community. In many instances drug regimens will of necessity involve experimental agents, such as the fluoroquinolones, as well as second-line antituberculosis drugs. There are no specific guidelines beyond those stated previously concerning the basic principles of management. No regimen or agent has been proven to be superior to any other agent.

Potentially useful but unproven agents for treating tuberculosis

Because of the long hiatus in drug development for tuberculosis there are few new agents that are known to have antimycobacterial activity and to be potentially useful in multidrug regimens. Agents that are currently licensed in the United States or are currently being investigated include the following:

Amikacin Amikacin is highly bactericidal against *M. tuberculosis*. The minimal inhibitory concentration (MIC) is 4 to 8 mg/kg for a wide range of strains. The usual daily dose is 15 mg/kg given either intravenously or intramuscularly. The dose should be reduced in older persons. Like other aminoglycoside antibiotics amikacin has both nephro- and ototoxicity. Dosing can be guided by serum levels with a peak target of 35–45 mg/ml. The optimum dose and duration of amikacin in treating tuberculosis are not known.

Fluoroquinolones Both ofloxacin and ciprofloxacin are marketed in the United States for a variety of indications but not for tuberculosis. These agents as well as other agents of this class are bactericidal for *M. tuberculosis*. Usual doses are 750 mg twice daily for ciprofloxacin and 400 mg/day for ofloxacin. Side effects are minimal but long-term toxicity studies have not been performed.

Rifabutin Rifabutin is a rifamycin derivative that has a longer tissue half time and perhaps better ability to penetrate the organism. There is cross resistance between rifampicin and rifabutin, although this is variable. The MIC for rifabutin for most strains of *M. tuberculosis* is 0.6 mg/ml. The toxicity of rifabutin is essentially the same as that of rifampicin.

Betalactam–clavulanic acid combinations Semisynthetic betalactam antibodies such as amoxycillin plus clavulanic acid have *in vitro* activity against *M. tuberculosis*. The MIC of the combination is approximately 4 mg/l, a level that can be achieved with an oral dose of 500 mg of amoxycillin.

As stated previously there are not reports that describe using any of these agents in multiple drug regimens; thus, their role is not known. The fluoroquinolones seem the most promising by virtue of their being orally administered and not being subject to cross resistance. Amikacin is useful when a parenteral agent is needed. The rifamycin derivatives are limited in usefulness because of the high level of cross resistance with rifampicin. There is so little experience with the betalactam agents that their potential usefulness is not known.

Changes in tuberculosis control policy and procedures made necessary by HIV infection

Infection with HIV has caused a telescoping of the natural history of tuberculosis. No longer can it be assumed that only approximately one-third of close contacts of new cases will be infected. As noted previously there is inferential evidence that HIV-infected persons are more likely to acquire infection with *M. tuberculosis* than is the general population (Daley *et al.*, 1992). Perhaps of more importance, it is quite clear that an HIV-infected person who acquires a new infection with *M. tuberculosis* is much more likely to progress rapidly to have clinical tuberculosis as was described by DiPerri and coworkers (1989) and Daley and associates (1992). As a consequence of the rapid progression, case fatality rates for tuberculosis are much higher than in non-immunocompromised patients with the vast majority of fatalities occurring before treatment is started or in the first month of therapy (Small *et al.*, 1991). Contributing to the higher case fatality rates is the occurrence of tuberculosis caused by multiple drug-resistant organisms. Superimposed on these changes in the nature of the disease is the fact that the HIV-infected patients in whom tuberculosis is of greater likelihood are also more difficult to maintain on a regular treatment regimen. Thus, while because of the immunosuppression there is less of a 'margin of safety' in treating such patients, doing so requires labour intensive schemes such as directly observed therapy described earlier.

The implications of the foregoing are that basic tuberculosis control measures must be applied more quickly and with greater intensity as follows:

1. At least in hospitals and clinics providing care for HIV-infected persons rapid radiometric means of detecting growth of mycobacteria should be used with speciation of organisms by DNA probes or other rapid techniques. If such technology is not available in a given institution, strong consideration should be given to using another laboratory in which they are available.
2. Sensitivity testing should likewise be performed as quickly as possible using techniques described above.
3. Contact investigation should be initiated immediately upon identification of a presumed (positive smear) or confirmed case. The contact interview should be performed by a person who has some familiarity with the life-style of the new patient in order to identify unsuspected settings in which transmission of *M. tuberculosis* may have occurred.
4. All contacts identified should be evaluated promptly. If it is thought that either the case or his/her contacts are at risk of HIV infection, the contact should be

asked his/her HIV status or be advised to have the test performed. If the contact is known or thought to be at risk of being HIV infected, decisions about preventive therapy should not be based on skin test results; rather, preventive therapy should be given to contacts regardless of the skin test results. Preventive therapy for persons suspected of having been infected with drug-resistant organisms should be based on prevailing sensitivity patterns.

If it is suspected or known that the contact is HIV-infected, careful questioning regarding possible symptoms of tuberculosis should be undertaken and the patient should have a thorough physical examination and chest film to exclude current tuberculosis.

5. HIV-infected patients with tuberculosis should be treated initially with isoniazid, rifampicin, ethambutol and pyrazinamide. The last two drugs can be discontinued after 2 months. The duration of therapy (6 or 9 months) is probably less important than the compliance with therapy (Small et al., 1991). For this reason directly observed therapy is the preferable treatment scheme. As with the contact investigation, supervision of therapy is best done by a health care worker familiar with the patient's lifestyle.

If there are problems with compliance or if the response to therapy, judged clinically, radiographically or bacteriologically, is suboptimal, therapy should be prolonged. It should be kept in mind, however, that apparent treatment failure or relapse may be caused by another HIV-related disease, not tuberculosis. As noted previously, if drug resistance is known or proven, appropriate regimens based on prevailing susceptibility patterns of determined sensitivities should be used. In these situations more prolonged therapy should be used.

References

Abernathy RS, Dutt AK, Stead WW, Moers DJ (1983) Short-course chemotherapy for tuberculosis in children. *Pediatrics, 72*, 801–806

American Thoracic Society (in press) Treatment of tuberculosis and tuberculosis infection in adults and children. *American Review of Respiratory Disease*

Andrew OT, Schoenfeld PY, Hopewell PC, Humphrey MH (1980) Tuberculosis in patients with end-stage renal disease. *American Journal of Medicine, 68*, 59–65

Barnes PF, Bloch AB, Davidson PT, Snider DE, Jr (1991) Tuberculosis in patients with human immunodeficiency virus infection. *New England Journal of Medicine, 324*, 1644–1650

Brindle RN, Nunn PP, Githul W, Allen BW, Githua S, Walyaki P (1993) Quantitative bacillary response to treatment in HIV-associated pulmonary tuberculosis. *American Review of Respiratory Disease 147*, 658–663

Brudney K, Dobkin J (1991) Resurgen tuberculosis in New York City: Human immunodeficiency virus, homelessness, and the decline of tuberculosis control programs. *American Review of Respiratory Disease, 144*, 745–749

Centers for Disease Control, Advisory Committee for the Elimination of Tuberculosis (1989) Recommendation for the elimination of tuberculosis. *Morbidity and Mortality Weekly Report, 38*, 236–250

Chaisson RE, Schecter GF, Theuer CC, Rutherford GW, Echenberg DS, Hopewell PC (1987) Tuberculosis in patients with the acquired immune deficiency syndrome (AIDS): a population based study. *American Review of Respiratory Disease, 136*, 570–574

Chaulet P (1987) Compliance with antituberculosis chemotherapy in developing countries. *Tubercle, 68* (Suppl), 19–24

Chum HJ (1989) Ten years of the National Tuberculosis/Leprosy Programme in Tanzania. *Bulletin of the International Union Against Tuberculosis and Lung Disease, 64*, 34–36

Colebunders RL, Braun MM, Nzila N, Dikilu K, Muepu K, Ryder R (1989) Evaluation of the World Health Organization clinical case definition of AIDS among tuberculosis patients in Kinshasa, Zaire (letter). *Journal of Infectious Diseases, 160*, 902–903

Committee on Treatment, International Union Against Tuberculosis and Lung Disease (1988) Antituberculosis regimens of chemotherapy. *Bulletin of the International Union Against Tuberculosis and Lung Disease, 63*, 60–64

Daley CL, Chin LL, Small PM *et al.* (1992) Pulmonary complications of HIV infection in Tanzania. *American Review of Respiratory Disease, 145*, A821

Darbyshire JH, Aber VR, Nunn AJ (1984) Predicting a successful outcome in short-course chemotherapy. *Bulletin of the International Union Against Tuberculosis, 59*, 22–23

David HL (1970) Probability distribution of drug-resistant mutants in unselected populations of *Mycobacterium tuberculosis*. *Applied Microbiology, 20*, 810–814

DiPerri G, Danzi MC, DeChecci G *et al.* (1989) Nosocomial epidemic of active tuberculosis among HIV-infected patients. *Lancet, ii*, 1502–1504

Dooley SW, Jarvis WR, Martone WJ, Snider DE, Jr (1992) Multidrug-resistant tuberculosis. *Annals of Internal Medicine, 117*, 257–259

Dutt AK, Moens D, Stead WW (1989) Smear and culture-negative pulmonary tuberculosis: Four-month short-course chemotherapy. *American Review of Respiratory Disease, 139*, 867–870

Edlin BR, Tokars JI, Grieco MH (1992) Nosocomial transmission of multidrug-resistant tuberculosis among patients with the Acquired Immune Deficiency Syndrome patients: Epidemiological studies and restriction fragment length polymorphism analysis. *New England Journal of Medicine, 326*, 1514–1521

Fischl MA, Uttamchandani RB, Daikos GL (1992) An outbreak of tuberculosis caused by multiple-drug-resistant tubercle bacilli among patients with HIV infection. *Annals of Internal Medicine, 117*, 177–183

Girling DJ (1982) Adverse effects of antituberculosis drugs. *Drugs, 23* (1–2), 56–74

Goble M, Iseman MDR, Masden L, Waite D, Ackerson L, Horsburgh CRJr (1993) Treatment of 171 patients with pulmonary tuberculosis resistant to isoniazid and rifampin. *New England Journal of Medicine, 238*, 527–532

Gordin FM, Slutkin G, Schecter G, Goodman PC, Hopewell PC (1989) Presumptive diagnosis and treatment of pulmonary tuberculosis based on radiographic findings. *American Review of Respiratory Disease, 139*, 1090–1093

Grzybowski S, Enarson DA (1978) Results in pulmonary tuberculosis patients under various treatment program conditions. *Bulletin of the International Union Against Tuberculosis, 53*, 70–75

Hong Kong Chest Service/Tuberculosis Research Centre, Madras/British Medical Research Council (1984) A controlled trial of 2-month, 3-month, and 12-month regimens of chemotherapy for sputum smear negative pulmonary tuberculosis: Results at 60-months. *American Review of Respiratory Disease, 130*, 23–28

Hong Kong Chest Service/Tuberculosis Research Centre, Madras/British Medical Research Council (1984) A controlled trial of 3-month, 4-month and 6-month regimens of chemotherapy for sputum-smear negative tuberculosis: Results at 5 years. *American Review of Respiratory Disease, 130*, 871–876

Hopewell PC (1986) Factors influencing the transmission and infectivity of *Mycobacterium tuberculosis*: Implications for clinical and public health management of tuberculosis. In: Sande MA, Hudson LD, Root RK (eds) *Respiratory Infections*. Churchill Livingstone, New York, pp. 191–216

Hopewell PC, Sanchez-Hernandez M, Baron RB, Ganter B (1984) Operational evaluation of treatment for tuberculosis: Results of a "standard" 12-month regimen in Peru. *American Review of Respiratory Disease, 129*, 439–443

Hopewell PC, Ganter B, Baron RB, Sanchez-Hernandez M (1985) Operational evaluation of treatment for tuberculosis: results of an 8-month regimen in Peru. *American Review of Respiratory Disease, 132*, 737–741

Ibanez-Quevado S, Ross-Bravo G (1980) Quimioterapia abreviada de 6 meses en tuberculosis pulmonar infantil. *Revista Chilena de Pediatría, 51*, 249–252

Judd K, Miller R, Luft H, Hopewell PC (1989) Outcomes and costs of tuberculosis treatment strategies in the United States. *American Review of Respiratory Disease, 139*, A 314 (Abstract)

Kamanfu G, Mlika-Cabanne N, Girard P-M, *et al.* (1993) Pulmonary complications of HIV infection in Bujumbura, Burundi. *American Review of Respiratory Disease, 147*, 658–663

Keers RY (1978) The rainbow's end: Streptomycin, PAS and isoniazid. In: Keers RY (ed.) *Pulmonary Tuberculosis: A Journey Down the Centuries*. MacMillan Publishing, New York, pp. 209–226

Kent PW, Fox W, Miller AB, Nunn AF, Fall R, Mitchison DA (1970) The therapy of pulmonary tuberculosis in Kenya: A comparison of the results achieved in controlled clinical trials with those achieved by the routine treatment services. *Tubercle, 51*, 24–43

Kleeberg HH, Oliver MS (1984) *A World Atlas of Initial Drug Resistance*. US Department of Health and Human Services, Atlanta

Long R, Scalcini M, Manfreda J *et al.* (1991) Impact of human immunodeficiency virus type 1 on tuberculosis in rural Haiti. *American Review of Respiratory Disease, 143*, 69–73

McDermott W, Muschenheim C, Hadley SJ, Bunn PA, Gorman RV (1947) Streptomycin in the treatment of tuberculosis in humans. I. Meningitis and generalized hematogenous tuberculosis. *Annals of Internal Medicine, 27*, 769–822

Medical Research Council (1952) The treatment of pulmonary tuberculosis with isoniazid. *British Medical Journal, ii*, 735–746

Mitchison DA, Nunn AJ (1986) Influence of initial drug resistance on the response to short-course chemotherapy of pulmonary tuberculosis. *American Review of Respiratory Disease, 133*, 423–430

Nunn P, Kibuga G, Gathua S *et al.* (1991) Cutaneous hypersensitivity reactions due to thiacetazone in HIV-1 seropositive patients treated for tuberculosis. *Lancet, 337*, 627–630

Perriens JH, Colebunders RL, Karahunga C *et al.* (1991) Increased mortality and tuberculosis treatment failure rate among human immunodeficiency virus (HIV) seropositive compared with seronegative patients with pulmonary tuberculosis treated with 'standard' chemotherapy in Kinshasa, Zaire. *American Review of Respiratory Disease, 144*, 750–755

Raviglione MC, Narain JP, Kochi A (1992) HIV-associated tuberculosis in developing countries: Clinical features, diagnosis and treatment. *Bulletin of the World Health Organization, 70*, 515–526

Reichman LB (1991) The u-shaped curve of concern. *American Review of Respiratory Disease, 144*, 741–742

Robinson GC, Cambon KG (1964) Hearing loss in infants of tuberculous mothers treated with streptomycin. *New England Journal of Medicine, 271*, 949–951

Slutkin G, Schecter GF, Hopewell PC (1988) The results of nine month isoniazid-rifampin therapy for pulmonary tuberculosis under program conditions in San Francisco. *American Review of Respiratory Disease, 138*, 1622–1624

Small PM, Schecter GF, Goodman PC, Sande MA, Chaisson RE, Hopewell PC (1991) Treatment of tuberculosis in patients with advanced human immunodeficiency virus infection. *New England Journal of Medicine, 324*, 289–294

Smithwick RW (1976) *Laboratory Manual for Acid-fast Microscopy.* Centers for Disease Control, Atlanta

Snider DE, Jr, Powell KE (1984) Should women taking antituberculosis drugs breast-feed? *Archives of Internal Medicine, 144*, 589–590

Snider DE, Jr, Layde PM, Johnson MW, Lyle MA (1980) Treatment of tuberculosis during pregnancy. *American Review of Respiratory Disease, 122*, 65–79

Solórzano Moguel JJ, Álvarez Cuevas ME (1991) Atención del enfermo tuberculoso a nivel comunitario en el estado de Chiapas, México. *Boletin de la Oficina Sanitaria Panamericana, 111*, 432–438

Sudre P, ten Dam HG, Kochi A (1992) Tuberculosis: A global overview of the situation today. *Bulletin of the World Health Organization, 70*, 149–159

Toman K (1979) Tuberculosis case finding. In *Tuberculosis Case-Finding and Chemotherapy.* World Health Organization, Geneva, pp. 6–8

Widy-Wirski R, Berkley S, Downing R *et al.* (1988) Evaluation of the WHO clinical case definition for AIDS in Uganda. *Journal of the American Medical Association, 260*, 3286–3289

World Health Organization, Tuberculosis Unit (1991) Guidelines for tuberculosis treatment in adults and children in national tuberculosis programmes. *WHO/TUB, 91*, 161

Discussion

Jacques H. Grosset

Groupe Hospitalier Pitie-Salpetrière, Paris, France

It is clear that drug therapy is capable of curing nearly 100% of tuberculosis patients but, in practice, the real availability of drugs to the patients is the key issue for success. Two of the points made by Philip Hopewell, namely 'successful completion of therapy is the responsibility of the provider or programme that undertakes to treat patients with tuberculosis' and 'chemotherapy can be successful only within the framework of the overall clinical and social management of patients and their contacts' are crucial. In that respect, I should like to amplify the implications of these two points. Both mean that, not only should the tools for diagnosis and drugs be available including adequate salaries for both medical and paramedical officers, but also they should be free of charge, and the patients should be in a position to benefit from them. (That is the reason why, in many if not all the so-called industrialized countries, patients may accede free of charge to all means of diagnosis and treatment for tuberculosis). To overcome the potential conflict that the patient may experience between the requirements of his (or her) treatment and the financial support of his (or her) family, society usually ensures the patient's full salary during the whole course of treatment. Such organization has not been developed in industrialized countries by generosity but because it was needed for the success of patient treatment. This does not mean that there is no other way to succeed in the control of tuberculosis. It means, however, that an effective chemotherapy programme requires significant social, financial and operational support as well as a reliable supply of drugs.

In the same line of thoughts, the paper has rightly emphasized the absolute need for a regular intake of drugs and the importance, in many settings, of the close supervision of drug delivery and intake. It should be emphasized that the important matter is not that the treatment is ambulatory or institutional but that regular intake of drugs is ensured wherever the patient is treated. For example, in regions where the population is scattered, some kind of institutional treatment, like Styblo's hostellization, might well be a solution whereas in large cities, intermittent, fully supervised ambulatory treatment might be the solution of choice.

Another important issue in Philip Hopewell's presentation is that dealing with the methods for the diagnosis of tuberculosis. In an industrialized country, the standard procedure for diagnosing pulmonary tuberculosis is the X-ray screening of symptomatic patients followed by sputum smear and culture from those patients with X-ray abnormalities. In many other places of the world, microscopic examination of sputum is the only available tool. As infectious cases of pulmonary tuberculosis are usually smear-positive, microscopic examination of sputum may permit their diagnosis. However, to detect one case of tuberculosis the microscopist has to scan numerous smear-negative specimens from symptomatic though not tuberculous patients. The diagnosis of tuberculosis by smear only is therefore a time-consuming, not very motivating procedure, highly dependent upon the quality of sputum collection and smearing, and the skill and patience of the microscopist. For these reasons, a simple and inexpensive screening procedure for those patients who should be submitted to smear examination is highly desirable. Ideally, a robust, autopower, miniature X-ray-apparatus would be the solution, if feasible. Again it is clear that the problem is not medical but political and financial.

Finally, if I had to discuss one point in the paper, I would choose to make clear that to set up and run a laboratory for culture of mycobacteria is much more complicated, and expensive than to set up a radiological service.

As for the new promising microbiological techniques—rapid detection of growth, use of molecular biology techniques—their cost-effectiveness has to be determined before recommending their use in developing as well as in industrialized countries.

6
Drug supply:
meeting a global need

Diana E.C. Weil

World Health Organization, Geneva, Switzerland

Introduction

Tuberculosis control depends on the ability of health personnel to identify quickly and cure newly infectious tuberculosis patients. Six to eight months of chemotherapy, with four to six drugs, is needed to ensure that a patient is rendered non-infectious and cured. If drug supply is unreliable or chronic shortages exist, patients could be given inadequate treatment thereby increasing their risk of developing and spreading drug resistant tuberculosis; they could lose confidence in health services and default from treatment; or they could be denied treatment altogether. Therefore, without reliable drug supply, a control programme may not only fail to reduce the tuberculosis burden, it may exacerbate it.

Four objectives in supplying drugs for a tuberculosis control programme stand out:

1. Accurate forecasting of drug needs.
2. Adequate financing for drug supply.
3. Efficient procurement of drugs of good quality.
4. Timely distribution of drugs to TB patients.

The following is a discussion of some of the most important obstacles confronting national tuberculosis programmes in seeking to achieve these objectives and of steps that need to be taken to resolve these problems. Focus is given here to drug supply issues in developing countries, where an estimated 95% of tuberculosis cases occur and where drug supply problems are most serious.

In 1991 the Tuberculosis Programme of the World Health Organization selected anti-TB drug supply as one of the major issues to be addressed in promoting revitalized global efforts to control tuberculosis. The programme began to

Tuberculosis: Back to the Future. Edited by J.D.H. Porter and K.P.W.J. McAdam
© 1994 John Wiley & Sons Ltd

investigate which problems were most serious and to consider what steps it could take to address them in collaboration with governments, other agencies and disease control programmes, and the pharmaceutical industry (Weil, 1992).

The following discussion draws on the preliminary results of a survey on drug supply issues distributed to national tuberculosis programmes by the WHO programme in 1992. The survey questionnaire included 23 questions. At the time of the drafting of this paper, responses had been received from 74 developing countries.[1]

Responses were received from 31 of 45 WHO member states in the WHO Africa region (AFRO), 14 of 36 member states in the region of the Americas (AMRO), 9 of 22 member states in the Eastern Mediterranean region (EMRO), 5 of 11 member states in the South-east Asia region (SEARO), and 15 of 23 member states or associate members in the Western Pacific region (WPRO).

Drug stock-outs (exhaustion of supply) provide a strong indicator of the impaired effectiveness of a drug supply system; 49% of the survey respondents noted that national stock-outs of some or all antituberculosis drugs had occurred in their country in 1991. These survey results suggest that urgent attention is needed to identify what elements of these systems may not be functioning.

Antituberculosis drugs

There are three antituberculosis drugs available today that have proven bactericidal or sterilizing power: rifampicin, isoniazid and pyrazinamide. Three others are important because they are either bacteriostatic or prevent resistance: streptomycin sulphate, ethambutol and thiacetazone.[2] All of these drugs are out of patent and all are included on essential drug lists where they exist.

Tuberculosis chemotherapy generally involves four to six of these drugs. Rifampicin, the last of the drugs to be developed (nearly two decades ago), is now included in all recommended short-course regimens. Seventy of 74 respondents (95%) to the WHO survey reported that they now supply short-course regimens to at least some portion of their newly diagnosed patients.

In the last decade, an increasing number of fixed combinations have been marketed (rifampicin–isoniazid, thiacetazone–isoniazid, ethambutanol–isoniazid, and triple combinations of rifampicin, isoniazid and pyrazinamide). Use of these combined preparations is advocated to improve the ease of administration, to

---

[1] It is not possible to include an analysis of drug survey results for industrialized countries due to the small number of countries responding, and the difficulty of those that did respond in offering information on national practices because of the decentralization or privatization of health service delivery.

[2] A number of 'second-line' drugs are used mainly in industrialized countries. They are important in the treatment of patients who have primary or acquired resistance to rifampicin, isoniazid or pyrazinamide. The WHO Tuberculosis Programme has recommended that treatment of chronic cases with these drugs remains a low priority for national tuberculosis programmes in developing countries due to their high cost and the limited prospect for cure of these cases.

reduce the risk of the development of drug resistance, and to discourage diversion of drugs for other uses. However, responses to the WHO survey suggest that only 30 of the 74 respondents (41%) use the combined form of isoniazid and rifampicin, although it is generally no more expensive than purchasing the individual formulations. Far fewer (12 (16%)) of the programmes reported using the triple formulation, which is still substantially more expensive than its equivalent in individual preparations.

New classes of antimicrobials have been developed that may eventually play a role in the treatment of tuberculosis, including quinolones, macrolides, rifamycins and betalactams. However, their action against *M. tuberculosis* has not yet been adequately studied in animal models or in clinical trials in humans (Snider, 1991).

WHO and federal agencies in the United States have cooperated in bringing together pharmaceutical industry representatives and researchers to discuss strategies for the development of new antituberculosis drugs. While progress in this initiative has been slow, it is apparent that the public attention accorded the resurgence of tuberculosis in industrialized countries and the rising threat of multidrug-resistant strains has increased industry interest. New government funds for research, tax incentives for product development, and the possible inclusion of antituberculosis agents in the Food and Drug Administration (FDA) orphan drug programme in the United States, may also facilitate action in this field (Snider, 1991). It is too early to predict when any new drugs will be ready for marketing or what the costs of such drugs might be. Therefore, in order to achieve progress in tuberculosis control in the short term, improving access to existing antituberculosis agents must remain a top priority.

Drug production

Based on industry databases providing manufacturer selling prices, it has been estimated that the world market for tuberculostatics in 1990/91 was 250 million deutsche marks (approximately US$177 million).[3] However, these figures may substantially underestimate total market volume because the database does not include non-commercial production and distribution of anti-TB drugs. Information is not available to determine what proportion of these sales were made to disease control programmes.

The private sector plays a far larger role in anti-TB drug procurement than national TB programmes in many countries. One major anti-TB drug supplier estimated that approximately 80% of its sales in developing countries were to the private sector. Few developing countries regulate the sale of antituberculosis drugs, and those few that do lack resources for enforcement. The public health and financial implications of private sector sales warrant attention.

Three companies, two located in the United States and one in Switzerland,

[3]Information received from Bayer AG.

control approximately 50% of the commercial market in tuberculostatics. Other top producers are located in Japan, Germany, Korea as well as the United States. Although a small number of firms control a large share of the global market, control programmes in developing countries appear to be relying on a large number of suppliers, including many generic firms. As part of the WHO survey, national tuberculosis programmes were asked to provide a list of suppliers from whom antituberculosis drugs had recently been purchased. Thirty-three respondents were able to supply names. In all, the lists included 33 different suppliers of isoniazid, 32 suppliers of rifampicin, 27 suppliers of streptomycin, 21 suppliers of pyrazinamide, and 27 suppliers of ethambutol.

Firms in only a few developing countries have significant capacity to produce anti-TB drugs including bulk raw product.[4] Among these are Korea, China and India, where government incentives have improved the environment for product development and joint ventures. However, it is unclear whether expanded production in these countries will immediately offset reduced production in industrialized countries.

Manufacturers of anti-TB drugs rely on a decreasing number of firms in industrialized countries that produce bulk product. The loss of bulk product suppliers could threaten the overall supply of tuberculostatics. The problem is that few firms possess the technical capability to produce bulk product for some drugs, such as rifampicin. Suppliers suggest that firms are leaving the market because antituberculosis drug production is no longer an attractive investment due to its low profit margin and limited sales. Generic firms producing final formulations appear to enter and exit the market to respond to individual orders, but few have a sustained presence in the market.

For example, local tuberculosis control programmes in the United States experienced acute shortages of rifampicin, streptomycin and several second-line drugs in 1991–92. Factors contributing to the shortages included the departure of sole approved suppliers of bulk drugs and final formulations due to limited financial incentives, problems in the generic pharmaceutical industry, and rapid increases in demand (Miller, 1992). Although, the US Centers for Disease Control and the FDA quickly worked to identify new suppliers and stimulate renewed production, this supply crisis signals the need to develop an early warning system to prevent future shortages. The public health threat posed by tuberculosis means that such systems are necessary even in countries, such as the United States, where no national agency handles drug supply financing or distribution.

In recent years, East European countries with high tuberculosis incidence rates, such as Romania, Bulgaria and Poland, have suffered from chronic drug supply shortages. Some of these countries had been important exporters of antituberculosis drugs but production suffered as the result of economic crises in the 1980s. If

---

[4] 26 of 67 (39%) respondents to the WHO survey reported that there was some local anti-TB drug formulation in their country.

planned external assistance for the revival of the pharmaceutical sector in these countries includes renewed production of tuberculostatics, both export markets and local tuberculosis control efforts should benefit.

As the supply crises in the USA and Europe indicate, control programmes will need to work with the pharmaceutical industry to ensure that the supply of drugs keeps up with rising demand accompanying the spread of HIV–TB coinfection and the revitalization of TB control activities in many countries. However, the question remains whether the need for drugs in developing countries, as demonstrated by rising TB notification levels, can be translated into market demand given severely limited financing for drug procurement, as discussed below.

A 1992 tender offered by the government of China, perhaps the largest ever offered for anti-TB drugs, demonstrates that if financing is provided, the market for these drugs can grow enormously. The drug tender was made possible with a loan from the World Bank and aims to meet the anti-TB drug supply needs for the first year of a 5 year control project serving half of China's one billion population.

Drug need forecasting

The estimation of yearly drug needs for treatment of tuberculosis patients is an essential step in planning for accurate drug purchasing and distribution. However, drug need forecasting in tuberculosis control can be complicated, due to the number of drugs involved and the number of different regimens required for different categories of patients: smear-positive, smear-negative, extrapulmonary, and retreatment cases.

The WHO anti-TB drug survey requested information on the methods used by national tuberculosis programmes in quantifying drug needs. Fifty-two of 74 respondents (70%) reported that they used the previous year's case notification figures as the basis for drug need quantification; 21 of these respondents included a buffer (5–10%) to account for possible increased demand. The general information provided by the survey does not offer sufficient insight into the strengths and weaknesses in forecasting, or whether programmes themselves evaluate whether their forecasting methods are accurate.

Some national tuberculosis programmes, such as those assisted by the International Union against Tuberculosis and Lung Disease (IUATLD), have carefully designed worksheets for drug need quantification. In these programmes, drug need estimations are made at district, provincial and national levels, and forecasting is closely linked to monitoring of drug stocks and usage at each level.

Other programmes have no means of monitoring usage in order to evaluate whether notification figures accurately predict future consumption and to correct maldistribution problems. Until recently in Zimbabwe, for example, the tuberculosis programme was required to develop a yearly estimate of all drug needs based on the predicted case load, but this planning tool was not used as a basis for distributing drug supplies. Instead, distribution was dictated by stock-levels and supply requests made by health services, without regard to reported cases.

The degree of conflict between morbidity-based methods of drug forecasting and consumption-based methods of drug distribution may be closely linked to the level of integration of tuberculosis treatment in primary health care systems. Countries that have tuberculosis control officers at the national level but which lack communication with services directly providing treatment may have greater problems in accurately forecasting drug needs. The correlation between drug use forecasts and actual usage might be improved if more essential drug lists and/or national formularies included standardized treatment guidelines provided by national tuberculosis programmes and if these lists were distributed to all health services.

Many national tuberculosis programmes are having difficulty in predicting year-to-year changes in drug needs due to rising TB incidence accompanying the spread of HIV–TB coinfection. In some countries, such as Zimbabwe, estimates of drug needs since the late 1980s have failed to keep pace with increases in the TB case load. To alleviate this problem, programme planners and drug procurement officers will need to work closely with epidemiologists following tuberculosis trends in order to improve forecasting, both at the national level and at the international level. The processes and precision of drug forecasting in national tuberculosis programmes require much closer scrutiny and evaluation.

Financing

Accurate quantification of drug supply requirements is useless unless it is accompanied by timely financing for drug procurement. Drugs represent a substantial element (probably between 20–40%) of the costs of operating national tuberculosis programmes (Murray *et al.*, 1990). This share is expected to decline eventually because treatment, especially early treatment, interrupts transmission and should ultimately lead to a decrease in incidence. However, in the short term, financing for drug supplies will need to increase as many control programmes improve their case finding and treatment activities and HIV infection contributes to larger case loads.

Inadequate or delayed drug financing appears to be one of the most serious problems inhibiting operation of many national tuberculosis programmes. Fifty-eight of 74 WHO survey respondents provided an indication of what they believed to be the greatest weakness in their drug supply system. Of these, 59% noted that lack of adequate financing or their dependence on donors was their major weakness; 68% of AFRO countries responded in this way. Some respondents expressed dismay that national tuberculosis programmes were often not directly involved in any of the drug procurement steps and therefore could not provide detailed information on prices or the process.

Drug financing may be the responsibility of a national tuberculosis programme,

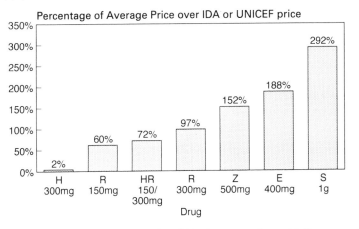

Figure 6.1 Anti-TB drug differentials in 1991. Average price paid (by respondents to WHO survey) vs. IDA or UNICEF price. H: Isoniazid; R: Rifampicin; Z: Pyrazinamide; E: Ethambutol; S: Streptomycin

the Ministry of Health, a non-governmental organization or donor agency, or local governments.[5] Seventy-three of the respondents to the WHO survey indicated who was reponsible for financing anti-TB drug procurement in their country; 19% said that an external donor or non-governmental organization provided all support, with 32% of respondents from AFRO reporting this to be the case, 23% from AMRO, and 7% from WPRO. No respondents from SEARO or EMRO countries suggested that external agencies were the sole source of support for supplies (see Figure 6.1).

An additional 48% of AFRO respondents noted that they were partially dependent on donor support for antituberculosis drug supplies; 23% of respondents from AMRO were in this position, 22% in EMRO, and 40% in SEARO and WPRO countries. Therefore, 57% of all respondents reported that they were wholly or partially dependent on external assistance to meet their current drug supply needs. Thirty-nine per cent of respondents reported that they did not have sufficient and/or secure financing for their 1992 drug supply needs.

There is a wide range of factors that are likely to contribute to limited government financing for anti-TB drug supplies:

1. Low priority accorded tuberculosis control due to lack of information demonstrating the severity of the problem or to a belief that it is a vertical programme that should be externally supported.
2. Lack of convertible currency for drug importation.
3. Individual states or provinces may be responsible for partial or total financing

---

[5]Cost recovery from tuberculosis patients for drug costs is almost always prohibited in the public sector due to the public health threat associated with failure to treat the disease.

for supplies, may have different health priorities or simply lack revenue-generating capacity to cover costs.

4. National tuberculosis programmes may lack the administrative capability to prepare adequate programme budgets or supply requests.[6]

Responses to the WHO survey did not provide sufficient information to suggest which of these factors may contribute most to financing problems. Further investigation of drug financing processes and problems is needed. Some of the likely problems suggested above do not exclusively affect tuberculosis control efforts but afflict essential drug programmes and public health initiatives in general in developing countries. Therefore, collaboration among control programmes, public health policy-makers, financing authorities and donors is urgently needed.

Although donor agencies often decline to cover the recurrent costs of health programmes, there is significant precedent for donor support of provision for anti-TB drugs, possibly because drug treatment for tuberculosis can also be seen as a means of preventing transmission of the disease. A substantial number of donor agencies are currently providing some assistance for anti-TB drug supply. Thirty-six respondents to the WHO survey provided the names of the donor agencies supporting drug supply for their programmes. In total, six international agencies, 12 bilateral aid agencies, and 24 non-governmental organizations were listed. Among these are several leprosy control associations which are playing an increasing role in supporting TB control activities as the incidence of leprosy is rapidly diminishing.

In some countries, national tuberculosis programmes are now seeking to collaborate with AIDS programmes as a means of expanding resources for drug supplies. With the rapid rise in tuberculosis cases associated with HIV–TB coinfection and no treatment for AIDS sufferers available in most developing countries, AIDS experts are now advocating assistance for tuberculosis treatment. WHO is working to foster collaboration between national AIDS and tuberculosis control programmes, although it has not yet helped to arrange subsidies for anti-TB drug supplies.[7]

At the global level, WHO and other agencies will need to work with national tuberculosis programmes to foster increased government and donor commitment to financing drug supplies and to identifying innovative approaches to improve the financial sustainability of programmes as well as the efficiency of drug procurement.

---

[6]51% of the WHO survey respondents noted that the national tuberculosis programme staff were responsible for preparing a preliminary budget for drug supply needs. 63% of the African respondents said the national programme was responsible. At the other extreme, only one in five respondents in the South-east Asia region affirmed this.

[7]Support from the WHO Global Programme on AIDS has been provided for drugs needed to test the efficacy and feasibility of providing TB preventive therapy to HIV-infected persons.

Procurement costs

Short-course chemotherapy for tuberculosis has been shown to be a highly cost-effective health intervention (Murray *et al.*, 1990). However, many countries have been delayed in adopting use of short-course regimens due to the cost of their components drugs. Other countries have been prevented from extending these regimens to more patients due to high costs and limited financing. Many national tuberculosis programme managers have suggested that even if financing for drug supplies improves, high drug prices prohibit obtaining adequate funding for all drug needs. Foreign exchange fluctuations and currency devaluations create further obstacles.

Drug costs have concerned national tuberculosis programmes for many years. The IUATLD organized a working group in 1978 to investigate drug costs. The principal finding of this working group was the wide variation in prices charged for the same drugs in different countries surveyed (Chaulet *et al.*, 1978). Although anti-TB drug prices have fallen substantially in the last decade, particularly for rifampicin and pyrazinamide (Weil, 1992), responses to the WHO drug survey suggest that this country-to-country variation persists. The entry into the market of many generic manufacturers has helped decrease drug prices in the past, but may now also be contributing to these dramatic price variations.

Figure 6.2 shows that the average price paid in 1991 by respondents to the WHO survey for each of the first-line anti-TB drugs was higher than the price available from the UNICEF Supply Division or from the International Dispensary Associates

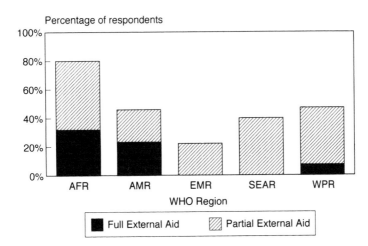

Figure 6.2 TB programmes dependent on external aid for drugs. Information provided by 74 respondents to WHO survey. AFR: African region; AMR: American region; EMR: Eastern Mediterranean region; SEAR: South-East Asian region; WPR: Western Pacific region

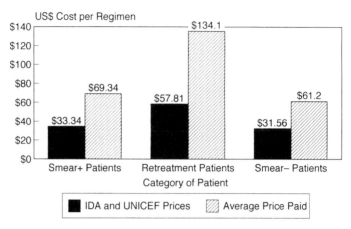

Figure 6.3 Cost differences for WHO-recommended regimens using IDA and UNICEF prices vs. average prices paid for component drugs by respondents to WHO survey. Smear+ regimen: $2HRZE/4H_3R_3$; Smear− regimen: $2HRZ/2H_3R_3$; Retreatment regimen: $2HRZES/1HRZE/5H_3R_3E_3$

(IDA), in some cases dramatically higher. Figure 6.3 shows that these price differences can significantly affect the cost of treating a TB patient.

More investigation is needed to determine why many tuberculosis programmes or central medical stores are paying such high prices.[8] Among the possible contributing factors:

1. Procurement officials lack access to information on suppliers and on prices available in the international market.
2. Procurement agencies such as the UNICEF Supply Division, IDA or reimbursable procurement programmes offered by WHO and the Pan American Health Organization (PAHO), which obtain lower prices through higher volume purchases and other economies of scale are underutilized.
3. Delay in obtaining funding for drug needs may mean that emergency delivery of supplies is required and therefore costs are increased.
4. Government regulations prohibit drug importation in order to stimulate local industry despite the often high price of local procurement.[9]

Drug costs may be prohibiting national tuberculosis programmes from offering the safest therapeutic regimens to their patients. National tuberculosis programmes

---

[8]Only six of the respondents reported that their national tuberculosis programme was directly responsible for procurement. More often, the central medical store or donor handled all procurement matters.

[9]Generally, prices for locally produced drugs in developing countries have been found to be as much as two to three times higher than for imported drugs (Foster, 1991).

in countries where HIV infection is spreading quickly are unsure whether they can afford to make the transition from regimens employing thiacetazone, which can cause severe toxic reactions in HIV-infected TB patients, to short-course regimens that replace thiacetazone with the more expensive drug, ethambutol.[10] Analyses of the cost-effectiveness of these regimens may be needed to justify requests for additional local or external funding to cover the incremental costs. Research is also needed to assess whether lower-cost treatment regimens for smear-negative tuberculosis patients are efficacious, in the light of rising smear-negative case loads with TB–HIV coinfection.

Figures provided by national tuberculosis programmes on drug expenditures in 1990 or 1991 suggest that average per case drug treatment expenditures vary widely. It is difficult to interpret these costs without information on the proportion of patients treated with different regimens. In the absence of this information, we can only roughly calculate the average per case drug expenditure using cost data provided by respondents to the WHO survey and data on yearly tuberculosis case notifications for each country.[11]

Of the 74 countries responding to the survey, 52 provided data on recent drug expenditures (19 from AFRO; 12 from AMRO; 7 from EMRO; 4 from SEARO; and 10 from WPRO). For the countries responding from the African region, drug costs varied from US$9 per case to US$289 per case. In the region of the Americas, expenditures varied from US$12 per case to US$667 per case. In the Eastern Mediterranean, expenditures per case varied from US$15 to US$1142. The range for South-east Asian respondents was US$27 per case to US$67 per case. In the Western Pacific, the range was from US$7 per case to US$420.

This information does not accurately represent the real drug cost for treating a tuberculosis case. However, the figures do indicate the variability in the resources available to different programmes and suggest that some programmes may be highly inefficient in the use of resources, whereas others have insufficient resources to treat the patients they notify.[12]

Drug supply expenditures comprise more than only the costs of the required drugs. Additional resources are required to cover the cost of service fees sometimes levied by procurement agencies, the cost of insurance and freight expenses, customs duties and other port charges (sometimes applied even to importation of essential drugs). Overall procurement expenses may be 20% to almost 100% more than the prices of the drugs alone, not including the cost of in-country distribution

---

[10]Researchers in Kenya estimated that if treatment with a 12 month regimen (2STH/10TH) were replaced by a short-course regimen excluding both streptomycin and thiacetazone (2 EHRZ/6EH), the price would increase by 148%. If a short-course regimen appropriate for non- HIV-infected individuals (2SHRZ/6TH) were replaced by the new regimen for HIV-infected patients, the price would increase by 25% (Nunn *et al.*, in press).

[11]Where necessary, conversion into US dollars was done using exchange rates for mid-November 1991.

[12]As a reference, if UNICEF drug prices are used to develop estimates of what it should cost to treat TB patients using WHO-recommended treatment regimens, per case drug treatment costs generally range from approximately US$30 to US$ 60.

of drugs (Foster, 1991; Chaulet, 1992). Reduction in these burdens must also be addressed if drug supply is to become more affordable.

The responses to the WHO survey suggest that procurement could be made more efficient in many countries if the authorities responsible for purchasing were provided with more information on drug prices available in the international market and if they were better trained in preparing tender documents, in negotiating with suppliers, and in administration.

Longer term objectives to improve anti-TB drug procurement could include assessing the feasibility of joint procurement by neighbouring countries (to increase the volume of orders) and the creation of a revolving fund, or similar mechanism, to improve access to convertible currency for regular drug purchases.

Quality assurance

The objective of keeping drug expenditures low should not override concern for assuring the quality of the drugs procured. For anti-TB drugs, the most important drug quality concern is to ensure that fixed combinations that include rifampicin provide adequate bioavailability of this drug. Recent research suggests that not all of the fixed combination products available in the market fulfil this criteria (Acocella, 1989).

Responses to the WHO anti-TB drug survey suggest that few developing countries have the capacity to assess the quality of the drugs they receive. Only 39% of respondents noted that they have direct means of assessing the quality of drugs procured, usually through a national drug control laboratory. However, access to these facilities varies substantially by region. Only 17% of the respondents from the Africa region reported access to quality control facilities, whereas 40% of those from South East Asia and the Western Pacific reported the same. Sixty-nine per cent of the respondents from the region of the Americas confirmed access to facilities, as did 75% of the Eastern Mediterranean respondents.

Several respondents noted that they relied on receipt, through the WHO Certification Scheme, of licensing certificates from exporting countries and confirmation of use of Good Manufacturing Practices.

More widespread use of the WHO certification scheme and more carefully prepared tender specifications should improve decision-making on drug purchases, but a long-term objective must be to establish local drug control laboratories.

Distribution

The drug supply process is not complete when drug shipments arrive in port or to the central drug warehouse. Distribution of drugs to health services and then to diagnosed patients is the last critical step. Thirty-five of 71 (49%) respondents to the WHO survey reported that their national tuberculosis programme was directly responsible for the distribution of antituberculosis drugs to health services. However, a majority of programmes did not provide a clear indication of what methods they used to determine how much should go where. As noted in the discussion of forecasting above, the lack of a systematic approach to drug supply planning and distribution is likely to contribute to supply stock-outs and threatens the welfare of patients.

In IUATLD mutually-assisted tuberculosis programmes, such as in Tanzania, antituberculosis drug distribution is tightly controlled and drug stocks are closely monitored. These programmes have historically prohibited the distribution of rifampicin beyond the district level to prevent pilfering and misuse. However, with fewer hospital beds now available for inpatient care, more patients will need to be treated in the initial phase in the rural areas where they live.

Measures that have been recommended for improving anti-TB drug distribution and administration include blister packing of daily dosages, and preparation of patient drug kits so that supply of all drugs for a notified case are assured at the initiation of therapy. The cost-effectiveness of using blister packs in TB treatment has not yet been assessed, although valuable information should be obtained from their use in the World Bank-sponsored TB project under way in China.

Because few countries prohibit the private sale of anti-TB drugs, research is needed on the scope and nature of the private sector market for these drugs (particularly in countries where control programmes are weak), and on improving their rational use.

In some countries, new drug distribution systems may need to be developed as tuberculosis control is further integrated into the primary health care infrastructure. These systems will need to rely on collaboration between national tuberculosis programmes and central drug authorities and essential drug programmes.

Conclusion

In order to reduce the public health threat posed by tuberculosis, national tuberculosis programmes must secure the necessary drugs not just for next year but they must sustain regular supply over the long term. To do this, governments, donors, technical experts and pharmaceutical producers must acknowledge that although effective treatment regimens exist and are free in most countries, many patients are not cured because the drugs are simply not there when they need them.

We can go a long way in ensuring uninterrupted supply of anti-TB drugs by pursuing these six strategies:

1. Informing governments, donors and pharmaceutical producers of the burden of tuberculosis and the cost-effectiveness of its control so that financing is increased and production to meet rising demand is assured.
2. Training the staff of national TB programmes in estimating drug needs, preparing drug budgets and tender documents, and managing distribution.
3. Increasing the collaboration of TB programmes, essential drug programmes,

central medical stores, and local non-governmental organizations, in developing and managing anti-TB drug supply systems within the context of primary health care.

4. Fostering collaboration between countries, supply agencies, donors and financing experts to develop new procurement mechanisms that increase the availability of hard currency for purchases, increase the volume of orders and reduce delays in supply.

5. Widely disseminating treatment guidelines so that the rational use of available drugs is improved.

6. Conducting research to develop new drugs, depot preparations, and regimens that increase the ease of drug administration, reduce the length of treatment, and/or reduce the risk of spreading drug-resistant strains.

Acknowledgements

The views expressed in this paper are solely the responsibility of the author and not of the World Health Organization. The author would like to acknowledge the assistance of the WHO Tuberculosis Programme Secretariat, the Tuberculosis and Communicable Disease Advisers in each of the WHO regional offices and WHO country representatives, for their assistance in obtaining responses to the survey on antituberculosis drug supply issues.

References

Acocella G (1989) Human bioavailability studies. *Bulletin of the International Union Against Tuberculosis and Lung Disease, 64*, 38–40

Chaulet P (1992) The supply of antituberculosis drugs and national drugs policies. *Tubercle and Lung Disease, 73*, 295–304

Chaulet P, Benachenhou A, Virot JP *et al.* (1978) Resultats de l'enquete cooperative international sur le cout des medicaments antituberculeux. *Bulletin de l'Union International contre la Tuberculose, 53*, 264–269

Foster S (1991) Supply and use of essential drugs in Sub-Saharan Africa: some issues and possible solutions. *Social Science and Medicine, 32*, 1201–1218

Management Sciences for Health. *International Drug Price Indicator Guide, 1989, 1990, 1991*. Management Sciences for Health, Boston, 1990, 1991, 1992

Miller B (1992) Assessment of anti-tuberculosis drug shortages, U.S., 1991. *Abstracts of the World Congress on Tuberculosis*. Fogarty Center for International Health, Washington, DC

Murray CJL, Styblo K, Rouillon A (1990) Tuberculosis in developing countries: burden, intervention and cost, *Bulletin of the International Union Against Tuberculosis and Lung Disease, 65*, 16–20

Nunn P, Gathua S, Kibuga D *et al.* (1992) The impact of HIV on resource utilization by patients with tuberculosis in a tertiary referral hospital, Nairobi, Kenya. *Tubercle and Lung Disease* (In press)

Snider D (1991) Shortages of antituberculosis drugs, outbreaks of multidrug-resistant disease and new drug development in the US Presentation at the Second Meeting of the Coordination, Advisory and Review Group of the Tuberculosis Programme, World Health Organization, Geneva, Switzerland, 22 November, 1991

Weil (1992) *Issues in Anti-tuberculosis Drug Supply*. WHO Document WHO/TB/92.164. World Health Organization, Geneva

Discussion

Richard O. Laing, *Management Sciences for Health, Boston, MA, USA*

The changing face of tuberculosis in the world requires changes in approach to drug supply for tuberculosis treatment. Tuberculosis drugs have not significantly increased in price over the last 5 years, and dramatic savings can be achieved through efficient procurement methods. Other aspects of drug management, such as selection, quality assurance, distribution and promotion of rational use, need to be incorporated into tuberculosis programmes.

This paper on issues in antituberculosis drug supply reflects a change in the WHO Tuberculosis Unit to give emphasis to drugs as an integral and critical component of tuberculosis management. A review of the supply of antituberculosis drugs and rational drug policies has been published recently (Weil 1992).

Drug supply for tuberculosis can be assured at a cost countries can afford, through efficient drug management within countries and after requiring a degree of integration with existing programmes. In fact, the potential public health costs of not treating tuberculosis effectively are far greater than the direct drug costs. However, efficient drug management can only occur when clinicians become involved in drug selection, procurement, distribution, financing and rational use issues. Thus, it is important that clinicians become aware of the drug management issues to which they can contribute.

Drug management issues

Drug management is usually thought of in terms of four specific areas (Figure 6.4). These are:

1. Selection.
2. Procurement.
3. Distribution.
4. Use.

For the drug management cycle to function, *all* elements must be in place. Too often, a donor or a programme regards drug management in terms of one or two elements, and neglects other critical areas. For example, a drug shortage may arise if different drugs are *selected* in new treatment regimens, or if the *procurement* of drugs is inefficiently organized, or if drugs are *distributed* to where they are not needed, or if when the drugs are delivered they are *used* inappropriately (e.g. rifampicin to treat chlamydial infections). Finally, necessary financial arrangements may not be possible, due to inflation, foreign exchange constraints, or terms of structural adjustment packages.

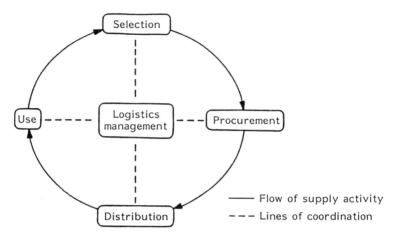

Figure 6.4   The logistics cycle

Selection

Drug selection is a complex issue because it involves balancing clinical efficacy, side effects, drug costs, and inpatient care costs. The issue of thiacetazone is an instructive one. This drug was introduced in the early 1960s as a combination with isoniazid to prevent the emergence of isoniazid resistance. The drug is now associated with severe, sometimes fatal, drug reaction in HIV-positive patients. Clearly, thiacetazone should only be used after HIV screening. In high HIV prevalence areas, thiacetazone should be withdrawn. Streptomycin, previously a mainstay of treatment, is more expensive than alternative therapies and requires syringes, needles and regular medical attention. This is usually provided through inpatient care, with consequent costs. Streptomycin should be changed to be a second-line therapy for relapsing cases.

In general, essential drugs programmes avoid the use of combination drugs. However, a strong case can be made for the combination of rifampicin with isoniazid. Firstly, the combination drug is cheaper than the components. Secondly, combining rifampicin with isoniazid would improve the security of the rifampicin. Thirdly, it will reduce the emergence of rifampicin or isoniazid resistance.

Procurement

The quantification of requirements has been simply documented in a WHO manual (World Health Organization, 1988). In summary, there are two methods:

1. Morbidity-based.
2. Consumption-based.

To be useful, the morbidity method requires notification of all cases, standard treatment guidelines which are generally adhered to, and a means of estimating future increases in demand. The consumption method is based on stock records of drugs and assumes that records reflect actual use; projected consumption must still be adjusted for anticipated changes in case mix or treatment practices. Both methods are useful, but each requires the involvement of clinicians, epidemiologists and procurement specialists.

The most important information needed by a procurement specialist is a listing of available suppliers and comparative prices. Management Sciences for Health (MSH) produces such a list of non-profit suppliers for about 500 drugs, although the MSH list does not necessarily reflect current prices for any of the suppliers listed. The tuberculosis drug price comparisons for the MSH list are given in Annex 1. Price comparisons for pyrazinamide are given in Table 6.1.

Reviewing these comparative drug price lists it is clear that none of these suppliers is consistently the cheapest; this is also true in the marketplace at large. Also, the ratio between maximum and minimum prices is usually between 2 and 5 times. While WHO usually quotes UNICEF prices when calculating costs of tuberculosis treatment regimens, it is instructive to compare minimum, maximum

Table 6.1 Price comparison: pyrazinamide 1992

Pyrazinamide 500 mg tablet (PO)			Cost/tablet 1.5 g
ZEDAP[a]	1000 tab	18.63	0.0186
PAHO	1000 tab	23.75	0.0275
ORBI	1000 tab	27.03	0.0270
IDA	1000 tab	27.35	0.0274
UNICEF	100 tab	3.21	0.0321
UNICEF	100 tab	3.24	0.0324
INMED	1000 tab	35.47	0.0355
ECHO	1000 tab	35.68	0.0357
ACTION	1000 tab	37.57	0.0380

Source: Management Sciences for Health. International Drug Price Indicator Guide, 1992 (forthcoming).[a] ZEDAP is a tender price.

Table 6.2 Treatment cost comparison

Drug	Daily dose	Duration (days)	Cost Min MSH	Cost Max MSH	US 1986 CDC	US 1990 CDC	US 1992 CDC
Isoniazid	300 mg	180	$0.31	$1.93	$5.04	$6.50	$8.50
Rifampicin	600 mg	180	$21.24	$58.14	$106.20	$159.30	$165.30
Pyrazinamide	2 g	60	$4.46	$12.84	$98.00	$160.00	$179.20
			$26.01	$72.91	$209.24	$325.80	$353.00

and US prices. In 1992 the Centers for Disease Control (CDC) compared US drug prices for a fairly standard intensive therapy regimen for 1986, 1990, and 1992 (CDC 1992). This same regimen has been compared for the MSH International Price Guide—minimum and maximum prices (Table 6.2).

From this example and the comparative prices tables, it is clear that savings of two to over ten times can be made through improved procurement. Such savings could affect the decision as to whether to change to short-course therapy.

Prices over time

Considerable concern has been expressed in the USA over the increase in the cost of tuberculosis drugs. In the USA the cost of isoniazid 300 mg has increased by 69%, rifampicin by 56%, and pyrazinamide by 83% between 1986 and 1992 (Centers for Disease Control figures). Internationally, the changes in prices have been far less. Without correcting for inflation, a basket of six drugs (ethambutol, isoniazid, isoniazid (INH) + thiacetazone, pyrazinamide, rifampicin, and streptomycin) are now only 1% higher than they were in 1988. See the Table 6.3 and Figure 6.5.

Quality assurance

Quality assurance is always a concern. However, if efficient procurement practices, particularly pre-qualification of suppliers, are followed, drug quality can generally

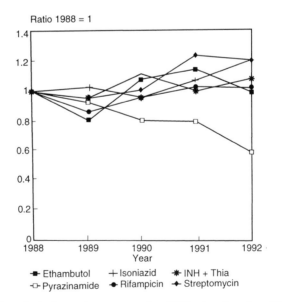

Figure 6.5 Tuberculosis drug prices compared to 1988 prices based on MSH average drug prices. Note: prices not corrected for inflation

Table 6.3   Average tuberculosis drug prices comparative over time (MSH price list)

Drug	Price in US$ per tablet				
	1988	1989	1990	1991	1992
Ethambutol 400 mg	0.0249	0.0196	0.0268	0.0283	0.0247
Isoniazid 100 mg	0.0036	0.0037	0.0034	0.0038	0.0043
INH + Thia 300 + 150 mg	0.0118	0.0111	0.0130	0.0117	0.0126
Pyrazinamide 500 mg	0.0568	0.0524	0.0458	0.0445	0.0333
Rifampicin 300 mg	0.1059	0.0901	0.1008	0.1086	0.1075
Streptomycin 1 g	0.1600	0.1500	0.1615	0.1960	0.1917

be assumed. The Food and Drug Administration (FDA) are at present working on a very simple thin layer chromatography kit which will detect drugs between 85% and 115% of potency at a price of about $0.50 a test. The testing apparatus and disposable equipment for 40 tests will cost about $100.00 (Flinn *et al.*, 1992).

Distribution

The distribution of tuberculosis drugs is often neglected and relegated to junior clerical staff. This can be a mistake, as major problems may exist.

When the tuberculosis drugs arrive in the country, controversy may arise as to where they should be stored, whether in a tuberculosis drugs only warehouse or in a general medical store. Where the general medical store is in a chaotic situation, tuberculosis drugs may need to be kept separately, but in the long term, integration into a single drug distribution system is desirable.

Kit systems have been used in some countries to distribute drugs to the most peripheral units. If tuberculosis drugs are to be included in kits, full course of therapy packs should be included. These packs should be labelled for a specific individual and therapy given only to him/her. This would avoid patients being started on therapy and then running out of drugs.

Rational use of drugs

The rational use of drugs has been a neglected aspect of drug management, and the International Network for the Rational Use of Drugs has been established to address this issue.

Rational drug use depends on being able to make the correct diagnosis, prescribe the correct drugs, dispense these drugs, and foster compliant patients. Prescribing performance is determined by a range of influences, of which knowledge developed through training is but one.

Dispensing is an area of drug management that has been seriously neglected. In a number of indicator studies in Asian and African countries, average dispensing times as low as 12 to 25 seconds have been regularly observed. Correct dispensing depends on having the correct drugs and dispensing materials available and appropriately trained staff actually dispensing. Too often, the process of dispensing is left to a cleaner or nurse aid. Frequently, expensive drugs are dispensed into a scruffy piece of newspaper because no containers are available.

Patient compliance is a complex issue and depends on the patient *and* relatives understanding what effect the drugs can have. Patients should be warned of both good and bad side effects and what they should do. Rigorous adherence to treatment regimens is necessary, but implementation, particularly in relation to admission or domiciliary care, can be flexible.

Financing issues

In many countries, 'cost recovery' in curative programmes has become common. Many health facilities depend on cost recovery for survival. Tuberculosis programmes have traditionally been exempt from charges on the basis that curing tuberculosis has public health benefits. But when countries or programmes are desperate for funds, exemptions may be forgotten.

The private sector in many countries plays a major role in drug supply. Frequently, national tuberculosis programmes do not relate to the private sector providers. In the future, the trend toward privatization is likely to increase. How will tuberculosis programmes respond to the new challenge?

Collaboration with other programmes

As mentioned above, tuberculosis programmes have traditionally been autonomous, independent vertical programmes. As is pointed out in the paper, however, there has recently been more effective collaboration with AIDS programmes and with essential drugs programmes (EDPs). Such collaboration is desirable and necessary.

Future actions

Clearly, tuberculosis drugs can be provided more efficiently and cheaply than at present. However, to achieve this policy-makers need to be informed as to what their options are, and programme implementation staff need to acquire the appropriate skills and expertise.

Conclusion

Tuberculosis as a world health problem is clearly going to increase. Drug supply to address this problem will become more important. The issues related to drug supply are not technically difficult, but implementation of sustained drug delivery systems requires well trained, committed managers who plan well in advance, implement sensibly, and monitor and evaluate their drug supply situation.

Too often, tuberculosis control programmes have neglected drug supply issues with adverse consequences. The means to improve drug supply exist. The lead taken by WHO to address this issue is to be praised.

References

American Public Health Association: Special Initiative on AIDS (November 1992). *Tuberculosis and HIV Disease*. American Public Health Association, Washington DC

Centers for Disease Control (1992) Tuberculosis therapy in USA. Poster presentation. American Public Health Association, Washington DC

Flinn PE, Kenyon AS, Layloff TP (1992) A simplified TLC system for qualitative and semiquantitative analysis of pharmaceuticals. *Journal of Liquid Chromatography, 15*(10), 1639–1653

Laing RO (1990) Rational drug use: an unsolved problem. *Tropical Doctor, 20*, 101–103

Weil DEC (1992) *Issues in Antituberculosis Drug Supply*. World Health Organization, Geneva (WHO/TUB/92.164)

World Health Organization (1988) *Estimating Drug Requirements: a Practical Manual*. World Health Organization, Geneva (WHO/DAP/88.2)

Annex 1

Tuberculosis drugs (includes all suppliers)

Item description / Vendor	Package	Package cost (US$)	Unit cost (US$)	Defined daily dose	WHO EDL	Shelf life	Stability	Storage temp (°C)
Ethambutol HCl 200 mg tablet (PO)								
3993 PAHO	1000 tab	13.22	Cost/tablet 0.0132	1.2 g	E	4 yrs	S	+15–30°C
Ethambutol HCl 400 mg tablet (PO)			Cost/tablet	1.2 g	E	4 yrs	S	+15–30°C
1993 ZEDAP	500 tab	7.59	0.0152					
1993 PAHO	1000 tab	19.80	0.0198					
1992 WHO	1000 tab	20.45	0.0205					
1993 IDA	1000 tab	20.86	0.0209					
1993 UNICEF	500 tab	11.66	0.0233					
1992 IDA	1000 tab	23.83	0.0238					
1993 UNICEF	500 tab	11.94	0.0239					
1993 ORBI	1000 tab	23.87	0.0239					
1993 ECHO	1000 tab	24.29	0.0243					
1993 INMED/WE	1000 tab	25.07	0.0251					
1993 ACTION	1250 tab	34.81	0.0278					
Average cost/tablet =			0.0226	Ratio max/min = 1.83				
Isoniazid (INH) 100 mg tablet (PO)			Cost/tablet	0.3 g	E	2–4 yrs	S	
1993 ZEDAP	1000 tab	1.66	0.0017					
1993 PAHO	1000 tab	2.82	0.0028					
1992 WHO	1000 tab	3.15	0.0032					
1993 ORBI	1000 tab	3.18	0.0032					
1993 UNICEF	1000 tab	3.26	0.0033					
1992 IDA	1000 tab	3.64	0.0036					
1993 UNICEF	1000 tab	3.64	0.0036					
1993 IDA	1000 tab	3.62	0.0036					

Year	Supplier	Pack	Price	Cost/tablet	Dose		Age	
1993	ECHO	1000 tab	3.89	0.0039				
1993	INMED/WE	1000 tab	4.32	0.0043				
1993	ACTION	3200 tab	15.82	0.0049				
1993	HCI	1000 tab	7.47	0.0075				
1993	INMED/US	1000 tab	10.74	0.0107	0.3 g	E	2–4 yrs	S
	Average cost/tablet =			0.0043				
			Ratio max/min = 6.47					

Isoniazid (INH) 300 mg tablet (PO)

Year	Supplier	Pack	Price	Cost/tablet
1992	WHO	1000 tab	5.73	0.0057
1993	PAHO	1000 tab	6.34	0.0063
1993	ORBI	1000 tab	8.11	0.0081
1993	UNICEF	1000 tab	9.65	0.0097
1993	UNICEF	1000 tab	10.00	0.0100
1993	INMED/WE	1000 tab	13.66	0.0137
1993	INMED/US	500 tab	7.97	0.0159
1993	ECDS	1000 tab	24.60	0.0246
	Average cost/tablet =			0.0118
			Ratio max/min = 4.29	

Pyrazinamide 500 mg tablet (PO)

Year	Supplier	Pack	Price	Cost/tablet	Dose		
1993	ZEDAP	1000 tab	18.63	0.0186			
1993	PAHO	1000 tab	23.75	0.0238			
1993	ORBI	1000 tab	27.39	0.0274			
1993	IDA	1000 tab	27.75	0.0278			
1992	IDA	1000 tab	30.00	0.0300			
1993	ECHO	1000 tab	31.14	0.0311			
1993	UNICEF	100 tab	3.21	0.0321			
1993	UNICEF	100 tab	3.24	0.0324	1.5 g	E	S
1992	WHO	1000 tab	32.80	0.0328			
1993	INMED/WE	1000 tab	35.47	0.0355			
1993	ACTION	1000 tab	38.61	0.0386			
	Average cost/tablet =			0.0300			
			Ratio max/min = 2.07				

Item description Vendor	Package	Package cost (US$)	Unit cost (US$)	Defined daily dose	WHO EDL	Shelf life	Stability	Storage temp (°C)
Rifampicin 150 mg tablet (PO)		Cost/tablet		0.6 g	E		S	
1993 ZEDAP	1000 tab	42.57	0.0426					
1993 IDA	100 tab	4.32	0.0432					
1993 ECHO	100 tab	4.67	0.0467					
1992 WHO	100 tab	4.76	0.0476					
1992 IDA	100 tab	4.77	0.0477					
1993 UNICEF	100 tab	5.20	0.0520					
1993 UNICEF	100 tab	5.31	0.0531					
1993 ORBI	100 tab	5.39	0.0539					
1993 PAHO	100 tab	5.43	0.0543					
1993 INMED/WE	100 tab	5.71	0.0571					
1993 KCR	100 tab	7.40	0.0740					
1993 ECDS	1000 tab	78.40	0.0784					
1993 ACTION	100 tab	11.39	0.1139					
Average cost/tablet =			0.0588					
Ratio max/min = 2.68								
Rifampicin 300 mg tablet (PO)		Cost/tablet		0.6 g	E		S	
1993 PAHO	100 tab	6.90	0.0690					
1993 IDA	100 tab	7.63	0.0763					
1992 IDA	100 tab	8.13	0.0813					
1993 UNICEF	100 tab	8.55	0.0855					
1992 WHO	100 tab	9.00	0.0900					
1993 UNICEF	100 tab	9.16	0.0916					
1993 ECHO	100 tab	9.34	0.0934					
1993 ORBI	100 tab	9.79	0.0979					
1993 INMED/WE	100 tab	10.48	0.1048					
1993 ECDS	1000 tab	124.00	0.1240					
1993 KCR	100 tab	13.65	0.1365					

1993	ACTION	100 tab	15.82	0.1582		E	S
			Average cost/tablet =	0.1007		Ratio max/min = 2.29	

Rifampicin + Isoniazid 150/100 mg tablet (PO)

				Cost/tablet			
1993	IDA	1000 tab	47.66	0.0477			
1992	IDA	1000 tab	55.79	0.0558			
			Average cost/tablet =	0.0517		Ratio max/min = 1.17	E	S

Rifampicin + Isoniazid 350/150 mg tablet (PO)

				Cost/tablet			
1993	ACTION	1000 tab	79.11	0.0791			
1993	IDA	1000 tab	79.06	0.0791			
1993	PAHO	1000 tab	84.25	0.0843			
1992	IDA	1000 tab	89.43	0.0894			
1993	ORBI	1000 tab	105.57	0.1056			
			Average cost/tablet =	0.0875		Ratio max/min = 1.34	E	S

Streptomycin Sulfate 1 g vial (INJ)

				Cost/vial			
1993	IDA	50 vial	3.48	0.0695			
1992	IDA	50 vial	3.73	0.0746			
1992	WHO	50 vial	3.97	0.0794			
1993	PAHO	1 vial	0.08	0.0800			
1993	ECHO	100 vial	8.87	0.0887			
1993	ORBI	100 vial	8.87	0.0887			
1993	INMED/WE	100 vial	10.25	0.1025			
1993	KCR	1 vial	0.25	0.2500			
1993	UNICEF	50 vial	13.74	0.2748			
1993	UNICEF	50 vial	14.31	0.2862			
1993	ACTION	98 vial	28.48	0.2906			
1993	ECDS	50 vial	19.15	0.3830			
			Average cost/vial =	0.1723	1 g	Ratio max/min = 5.50	E	S	refrig

Water for injection not included

Item description / Vendor	Package	Package cost (US$)	Unit cost (US$)	Defined daily dose	WHO EDL	Shelf life	Stability	Storage temp (°C)
Streptomycin Sulfate 5 g vial (INJ)			Cost/vial					
1993 PAHO	1 vial	0.07	0.0700	1 g	EP		S	refrig
1993 IDA	50 vial	13.88	0.2775	Water for injection not included				
1992 IDA	50 vial	14.72	0.2944					
1993 ORBI	100 vial	32.13	0.3213					
1993 ZEDAP	1 vial	0.50	0.4980					
	Average cost/vial =		0.2927					
				Ratio max/min = 7.14				
Thiacetazone + Isoniazid 50/100 mg tablet (PO)			Cost/tablet					
1993 ZEDAP	1000 tab	2.53	0.0025		C		S	
1992 WHO	1000 tab	4.51	0.0045					
1993 UNICEF	1000 tab	4.63	0.0046					
1993 UNICEF	1000 tab	4.72	0.0047					
1993 IDA	1000 tab	4.68	0.0047					
1993 ECHO	1000 tab	5.14	0.0051					
1993 INMED/WE	1000 tab	5.47	0.0055					
1992 IDA	1000 tab	5.58	0.0056					
	Average cost/tablet =		0.0047					
				Ratio max/min = 2.21				
Thiacetazone + Isoniazid 75/150 mg tablet (PO)			Cost/tablet					
1993 IDA	1000 tab	7.40	0.0074		CP		S	
1992 IDA	1000 tab	8.13	0.0081					
	Average cost/tablet =		0.0078					
				Ratio max/min = 1.10				
Thiacetazone + Isoniazid 150/300 mg tablet (PO)			Cost/tablet					
1993 ZEDAP	1000 tab	5.78	0.0058		C		S	
1992 WHO	1000 tab	10.28	0.0103					
1993 PAHO	1000 tab	10.47	0.0105					

1993	IDA	1000 tab	10.49	0.0105
1992	IDA	1000 tab	11.05	0.0110
1993	ORBI	1000 tab	11.02	0.0110
1993	ECHO	1000 tab	11.21	0.0112
1993	UNICEF	1000 tab	11.15	0.0112
1993	UNICEF	1000 tab	11.37	0.0114
1993	INMED/WE	1000 tab	11.75	0.0118
1993	ACTION	1600 tab	26.58	0.0166
		Average cost/tablet =		0.0110

Ratio max/min = 2.87

WHO Essential Drug List = (E)ssential, ⟨C⟩omplementary, ⟨P⟩resentation, ⟨N⟩ot on the list
Stability = ⟨S⟩table, ⟨D⟩egradable
Source: International Drug Price Indicator Guide, Management Sciences for Health, 1993

7
Preventive therapy for tuberculosis

Richard J. O'Brien

World Health Organization, Geneva, Switzerland

Introduction

Preventive therapy for tuberculosis is generally understood as the treatment of asymptomatic persons infected by *Mycobacterium tuberculosis* in order to prevent the development of active disease. In this regard, the intervention is not truly prophylaxis but rather the treatment of latent tuberculosis. Thus, in this chapter the term preventive therapy will be used rather than 'chemoprophylaxis'.

Soon after the development of isoniazid, it became apparent that preventive therapy with the drug might be an important control measure. As tuberculosis incidence began to fall in developed countries and the risk of new infection substantially decreased, the majority of new tuberculosis cases developed among those persons infected in the past rather than arising from recent infection. Thus, neither of the two available control measures, i.e. treatment of active cases and BCG vaccination, could have an immediate impact on tuberculosis morbidity.

Isoniazid was of interest because the drug was inexpensive and apparently free of serious toxicity. Following the demonstration that the drug was effective in preventing tuberculosis in infected persons at risk of tuberculosis, there was great enthusiasm for this intervention, especially in the United States, and hope that its widespread application might lead to the rapid elimination of tuberculosis. This dream was never realized, and for a variety of reasons, preventive therapy with few exceptions has never been widely applied outside of North America.

This chapter will review the scientific basis for preventive therapy, outline its current application and limitations, and discuss a number of issues concerning the use of preventive therapy in persons with HIV infection. The latter topic is especially important and timely. It is precisely because of the HIV epidemic and the critical problem of HIV-associated tuberculosis that preventive therapy is receiving increased attention today. The chapter will conclude with a brief discussion of experimental approaches in this area.

Tuberculosis: Back to the Future. Edited by J.D.H. Porter and K.P.W.J. McAdam
© 1994 John Wiley & Sons Ltd

Scientific basis for preventive therapy

Before clinical trials of isoniazid preventive therapy were undertaken, the efficacy of the drug was first demonstrated in animals. In a series of studies in guinea pigs conducted in the United States, it was shown that isoniazid at the dose of 5 mg/kg prevented death in animals challenged with a virulent dose of tubercle bacilli (Ferebee and Palmer, 1956). This dose was then selected for human studies.

A large number of randomized, placebo-controlled clinical trials have been conducted in both developed and developing countries (Ferebee, 1970). These studies involved over 100 000 participants at risk of tuberculosis, including children with primary tuberculosis, contacts of active cases, tuberculin skin test convertors, institutionalized patients with mental disease, and persons with inactive tuberculosis. The effectiveness of preventive therapy, defined as the reduction in the incidence of tuberculosis among persons receiving isoniazid compared with that among those receiving placebo, varied between 25 and 92% (Table 7.1). However, among persons with good compliance efficacy was 90% or greater, indicating that preventive therapy conferred substantial protection. Those who took medication irregularly were also protected against tuberculosis; this finding suggested the possibility that intermittent isoniazid preventive therapy might also be effective. However, the only randomized study of intermittent preventive therapy failed to show protection, probably because the dose of isoniazid chosen was too small. Analysis of data from trials in Alaska has suggested that 6 to 12 months of therapy is required for good efficacy but that taking medication beyond 12 months is not associated with increased protection, at least in the absence of continued exposure to tuberculosis (Comstock and Ferebee, 1970). Long-term follow-up of populations in the same studies have shown that this protection lasts at least 19 years and is probably life-long (Comstock et al., 1979). A more recent study of isoniazid preventive therapy among persons with fibrotic lesions on chest radiograph indicated that 6 months of therapy gave substantial protection, especially for persons with small lesions (International Union Against Tuberculosis, 1982).

Because of the significant limitations of preventive therapy with isoniazid (see below), there has been recent interest in the use of alternative drugs. Early animal studies of rifampicin indicated that this drug was probably a more effective sterilizing agent than isoniazid (Grumbach and Rist, 1967). More recent animal studies of rifampicin alone and in combination with other drugs have confirmed this finding and also suggested that the combination of rifampicin and pyrazinamide might be especially effective (Lecoeur et al., 1989). An interesting finding from this study was the apparent inhibiting effect of isoniazid on the combination of rifampicin and pyrazinamide.

There are also limited clinical data suggesting that rifampicin, alone or in combination with other drugs, might be effective as preventive therapy. Two months of multidrug therapy was shown to be quite effective in reducing the emergence of bacteriologically positive tuberculosis among persons with

Table 7.1 Summary of results of controlled clinical trials of tuberculosis preventive therapy with isoniazid

Type of subjects	Number	Outcome	Years of observation	% reduction
US children with primary tuberculosis	2 750	Tuberculosis complications	10	88
French children with primary tuberculosis	2 970	Tuberculosis complications	3–10	64
Household contacts to old cases, USA	2 814	Tuberculosis disease	4	54
Household contacts to new cases, USA	27 847	Tuberculosis disease	10	60
Household contacts to new cases, Japan	2 238	Tuberculosis disease	1	30
Household contacts, Kenya	764	Positive bacteriology	3	80
Household contacts, Philippines	327	Abnormal chest X-rays	2	41
Shipboard contacts, Netherlands	261	Tuberculosis disease	7	92
Railway workers, Japan	548	Tuberculosis disease	6–12	62
Greenland villagers	8 801	Tuberculosis disease	6	31
Alaskan villagers	6 064	Positive bacteriology	6	59
Tunisian villagers, urban residents	15 910	Positive bacteriology	1	25
Mental institutions, USA	25 210	Tuberculosis disease	10	62
Alaskan schools	1 670	Tuberculosis disease	6–10	67
New York mental institutions	513	Active tuberculosis	6	43
US health departments	1 992	Active tuberculosis	5	60
Chest clinic patients, India	317	Positive bacteriology	6	83
Chest clinic patients, Canada	2 405	Active tuberculosis	7–13	53
US veterans' hospitals	2 389	Positive bacteriology	5	59

radiographically active but smear- and culture-negative tuberculosis (Hong Kong Chest Service, 1984). The only published clinical trial of rifampicin preventive therapy, involving tuberculin-positive persons with silicosis, indicated that 3 months of rifampicin conferred equivalent protection to 6 months of isoniazid; furthermore, the combination of rifampicin/isoniazid was not more effective than rifampicin alone (Hong Kong Chest Service, 1992). The largest published experience with rifampicin preventive therapy was from a programme in Blackburn, England, where the administration of rifampicin/isoniazid to high risk children was associated with a decrease in childhood tuberculosis in the community (Ormerod, 1987).

Application and limitations of preventive therapy

Preventive therapy is most extensively applied in North America, and the most detailed recommendations on the use of preventive therapy have been issued by the American Thoracic Society and the US Centers for Disease Control (American Thoracic Society, 1986; Centers for Disease Control, 1990). These recommendations target those persons most likely to develop tuberculosis and are based both on the probability of tuberculosis infection in a person with a positive tuberculin skin test and on the likelihood that an individual with infection will develop tuberculosis. These recommendations include different definitions of a positive tuberculin skin test for different groups (Table 7.2).

Table 7.2 Persons for whom preventive therapy is recommended

Category	Skin test reaction	Therapy recommended
Persons with HIV infection	5 mm or greater[a]	12 months isoniazid
Close contacts of TB cases	5 mm or greater[b]	6+ months isoniazid[c]
Persons with abnormal chest X-rays[d]	5 mm or greater	12 months isoniazid
Recently infected persons	10 mm or greater[e]	6+ months isoniazid
Other high risk conditions[f]	10 mm or greater	6+ months isoniazid
High risk group, <35 year age[g]	10 mm or greater	6+ months isoniazid

[a] Anergic persons whose estimated risk of tuberculosis infection is 10% or greater should also be considered for preventive therapy.
[b] Children, especially those under age 5, with negative tuberculin skin tests should be placed on preventive therapy and retested 2 months after contact with infection is broken.
[c] Paediatric authorities recommend 9 months of therapy for children.
[d] Persons with stable fibrotic lesions consistent with previously untreated tuberculosis and those with silicosis.
[e] Recent infection is documented by conversion of a negative tuberculin skin test to positive (with at least a 10 mm increase in induration) within a 2 year interval.
[f] Other high risk medical conditions include: chronic renal failure, insulin dependent diabetes mellitus, prolonged immunosuppressive therapy, leukaemias and lymphomas, and conditions associated with rapid weight loss or chronic undernutrition (e.g. chronic alcoholism, malabsorption syndromes following gastrectomy and jejunal–ileal bypass).
[g] Including foreign-born persons from countries where tuberculosis is prevalent, medically underserved low-income populations, and residents of facilities for long-term care.

For those at greatest risk of tuberculosis, such as close contacts of infectious, smear-positive tuberculosis cases, persons with HIV infection, and those with stable fibrotic lesions on chest radiography and no previous treatment for tuberculosis, a reaction of 5 or more millimetres of induration to 5 TU of PPD tuberculin (or 2 TU of RT-23) is considered positive. For persons with other medical conditions known to increase the risk of tuberculosis and other recently infected persons (i.e. those whose tuberculin skin test has converted from negative to positive within the past 2 years), a 10 mm reaction is considered positive. For low risk persons, a positive test is defined by a reaction of at least 15 mm. BCG vaccination complicates the interpretation of a tuberculin skin test, and for persons with a history of BCG higher cut-off points might be chosen (Snider, 1985). However, for HIV-infected persons and child contacts of infectious cases, the 5 mm cut-off point is recommended regardless of BCG status.

Isoniazid preventive therapy is recommended in the USA for all tuberculin-positive, high risk persons. In addition, tuberculin-positive, low risk persons under age 35 in the following high incidence groups are also considered for preventive therapy: foreign-born persons from high prevalence countries; medically underserved low-income persons from high prevalence populations and residents of facilities for long-term care (e.g. correctional institutions, nursing homes, and mental institutions). In some circumstances persons with negative skin tests are also considered for preventive therapy. These include children who are close contacts of infectious cases and anergic HIV-infected persons at increased risk of tuberculosis.

Isoniazid is given at the daily dose of 5 mg/kg, up to 300 mg, for both adults and children. For persons requiring supervised therapy, isoniazid may be given at the dose of 15 mg/kg (up to 900 mg) twice weekly. Twelve months of preventive therapy is recommended for persons with HIV infection and those with stable, abnormal chest radiographs. Based on cost-benefit analysis, at least 6 months of preventive therapy is recommended for all other persons (Snider et al., 1986). Paediatric authorities in the United States have recommended that children receive 9 months of isoniazid preventive therapy (American Academy of Pediatrics, 1992). Tuberculin-negative children who are close contacts of infectious cases and who were started on preventive therapy should have a repeat skin test 2 months after the contact has been broken; those remaining tuberculin negative should stop preventive therapy. Some authorities have suggested that tuberculin-positive persons with abnormal chest films that show fibrotic lesions probably representing old healed tuberculosis and those with silicosis should receive 4 month multidrug chemotherapy rather than isoniazid preventive therapy (D.E. Snider, personal communication). For persons probably infected by isoniazid-resistant bacilli, rifampicin preventive therapy has been recommended (Koplan and Farer, 1980). Rifampicin may also be considered for persons intolerant of isoniazid who have an especially great chance of developing tuberculosis if not given preventive therapy.

These recommendations would also apply to other countries with well-functioning tuberculosis programmes and adequate resources to undertake preventive therapy. As noted above, preventive therapy has not been considered for resource poor countries. However, both the International Union against Tuberculosis and Lung Disease and the World Health Organization's Tuberculosis Programme recommend isoniazid preventive therapy for children under 5 years of age living in households with infectious cases (International Union against Tuberculosis and Lung Diseases, 1991; World Health Organization, 1992). This recommendation is based on the increased risk of life-threatening tuberculosis in these children, the safety of isoniazid in children, its low cost, and the ease of treating children whose family members are also receiving treatment for active tuberculosis.

In 1965 when preventive therapy was first recommended for use in the United States, it was believed to be free of serious toxicity. This belief was based on findings of the clinical trials of preventive therapy which showed that the frequency of adverse events was similar among those receiving isoniazid and those receiving placebo treatment. In 1967 US recommendations on preventive therapy were broadened to include all persons with positive tuberculin tests in the hope that this measure would be widely implemented and would lead to the rapid elimination of tuberculosis. However, in the early 1970s the first hepatitis deaths associated with isoniazid were reported among several employees at the US Capitol in Washington. This finding which received widespread publicity led to a large comprehensive study of more than 14000 persons receiving isoniazid preventive therapy in the United States (Kopanoff et al., 1978). In this study the overall risk of isoniazid-related hepatitis was approximately 1%; however, the risk was clearly age related with its occurrence being rare in younger persons and increasing with age to over 2% in those over age 50. Alcohol use was also a risk factor for hepatitis. Data from the IUAT study found much lower rates of hepatitis but the same relationship to age (International Union against Tuberculosis, 1982). In the US study, eight persons died from hepatitis, seven of them in Baltimore, Maryland. A later study of mortality data from Maryland found that during the study period there had been a marked increase in hepatitis deaths in Baltimore which did not occur in other parts of the state. This suggested that a cofactor had contributed to the isoniazid-related mortality in Baltimore (Comstock, 1986).

Following these findings the recommendations on the use of isoniazid preventive therapy in the USA were changed to exclude low risk reactors over age 35 and to recommend that all persons receiving preventive therapy be educated about the risk of hepatitis and be interviewed at least monthly for symptoms of hepatitis. Despite these changes hepatitis deaths continue to be reported among persons receiving preventive therapy with isoniazid, and more recent information suggests that women, especially those in the postpartum period, may be especially at risk (Snider and Caras, 1992). Because of the more recent findings and the continuing controversy surrounding the use of isoniazid preventive therapy in low risk tuberculin reactors, recent recommendations have excluded these low risk reactors from preventive therapy.

The other major limitation to isoniazid preventive therapy is non-adherence with treatment. It is especially difficult for persons who are healthy and asymptomatic to take medication for a long period of time to prevent an illness that not only is unlikely to occur in the absence of preventive therapy but is also readily treatable should it occur. The available information indicates that non-adherence with therapy is common. In the US study of isoniazid hepatitis, only 22% of persons collected all 12 months of drug supplies (D. Kopanoff, personal communication), and fewer than two-thirds of persons now starting preventing therapy in US tuberculosis programmes complete the recommended course of treatment (D. Brown, personal communication). In other settings the results have been even poorer (Alcabes et al., 1989; Wobeser et al., 1989), and supervised preventive therapy has failed to achieve acceptable results in at least one programme targeting homeless men in the USA (Nazar-Stewart and Nolan, 1992).

Preventive therapy in HIV infection

It is now clearly established that HIV infection is the strongest risk factor yet identified promoting the development of active tuberculosis in persons with HIV and tuberculosis coinfection. Studies have shown that the risk of active tuberculosis in persons with coinfection is in the order of 3–8% per year, with a lifetime risk of perhaps 50% or more (Selwyn, 1989). In areas where coinfection is common, such as certain large urban centres in the United States and a number of countries in sub-Saharan Africa, HIV infection has had critical impact on the tuberculosis problem with a more than doubling of cases in some of these countries in the last few years (Murray, 1991). Tuberculosis control programmes which had been reasonably effective are now at the point of collapse because of the burden of HIV-associated tuberculosis. As HIV infection spreads to countries in Asia where over half of the world's tuberculosis-infected persons reside, the potential impact of HIV infection on tuberculosis is staggering.

Of available control measures, tuberculosis preventive therapy with isoniazid is the only practical one which might reduce the occurrence of HIV-associated tuberculosis. There are some data indicating that isoniazid preventive therapy might be effective. An observational study of intravenous drug users in the New York City suggested substantial protection from isoniazid against the development of tuberculosis (Selwyn et al., 1989). A placebo-controlled study in Zambia also found a substantial degree of protection from the administration of 6 months of daily isoniazid (Wadhawan et al., 1992). However, the degree of protection appears to have lessened with time, suggesting either decreasing efficacy or reinfection. Moreover, there was no difference in mortality between the active treatment and placebo groups. A similar study conducted in Haiti has not only demonstrated the protective effect of isoniazid against tuberculosis but has also found decreased mortality and fewer HIV-related illnesses among those receiving the drug (J. Pape, 1993).

Assuming that isoniazid preventive therapy is efficacious in reducing HIV-associated tuberculosis, there are major impediments to its widespread implementation and important questions about its use which must first be addressed. The following are the most pressing questions which should be addressed by research: (1) Does preventive (mono)therapy lead to the development of drug resistance in coinfected persons? (2) What is the optimal duration of preventive therapy and what drug(s) should be given? (3) What is the optimal preventive treatment for persons infected by drug-resistant bacilli? (4) What is the role of tuberculin testing in preventive therapy programmes? And a related question, how should anergic persons be managed? (5) Are there alternative regimens which will improve the efficacy of preventive therapy? (6) What is the potential impact of preventive therapy programmes on the tuberculosis problem? (7) Can preventive therapy programmes be implemented in the countries experiencing the most serious impact of HIV-associated tuberculosis and is the intervention cost-effective?

Does preventive (mono)therapy lead to the development of drug resistance in coinfected persons

Regarding the first issue, there is no evidence from numerous clinical trials that tuberculosis preventive therapy leads to the development of drug-resistant disease, even among those with fibrotic lesions on chest radiograph or those with silicosis. However, because of the increased difficulty of diagnosing active tuberculosis in persons with HIV infection, there is the theoretical possibility that drug resistance might develop when persons with HIV infection and undiagnosed, active tuberculosis are given a single drug as tuberculosis preventive therapy. This possibility is one argument in favour of multidrug preventive therapy which is much less likely to lead to acquired drug resistance if mistakenly given to persons with active disease. However, this question can only be answered in properly designed clinical trials which are underway. Certainly, when it comes to implementation of preventive therapy programmes, it is essential that adequate diagnostic facilities be available to screen HIV-infected persons for tuberculosis prior to administration of preventive therapy.

What is the optional duration of preventive therapy and what drugs should be given?

The optimal duration of therapy is not known. Because of the suspicion that the efficacy of isoniazid preventive therapy would be reduced in the presence of severe immunosuppression, authorities in the United States have recommended that coinfected persons be treated with 12 months of therapy (Centers for Disease Control, 1989). Hypothetically, the most appropriate therapy depends upon the epidemiological situation. For the treatment of infected persons with little likelihood of reinfection, a regimen which rapidly kills dormant tubercle bacilli is most desirable; for this, isoniazid is probably not the optimal treatment. For persons who have a high probability of continued exposure to persons with active tuberculosis, a regimen which can be given for life and which suppresses the development of disease may be preferred. In this case, it may be reasonable to consider isoniazid. However, these hypotheses must be addressed by research studies.

What is the optimal preventive treatment for persons infected by drug-resistant bacilli?

The question of the optimal treatment of persons infected by drug-resistant organisms is an important one. Primary resistance to isoniazid is common in countries where tuberculosis treatment programmes have been poorly controlled, with rates of 20 or more being reported (Kleeberg and Olivier, 1984). The efficacy of isoniazid preventive therapy would be expected to be reduced in such a setting. Recently, this question has been the concern of authorities in the United States where an epidemic of multidrug-resistant tuberculosis among HIV-infected persons has been noted (Centers for Disease Control, 1991a). In this case, the organisms are resistant to at least isoniazid and rifampicin and often to other first-line drugs such as ethambutol and streptomycin. Although no consensus has emerged about the correct approach to immunosuppressed persons infected by these multidrug-resistant strains, some authorities have suggested that the combination of pyrazinamide and ethambutol or pyrazinamide and ofloxacin might be used (Villarino *et al.*, 1992).

What is the role of tuberculin testing in preventive therapy programmes?

Anergy to PPD-tuberculin and to other delayed-type hypersensitivity skin test (DTH) antigens may occur before signs and symptoms of HIV infection develop. DTH anergy becomes increasingly common as HIV infection progresses, making the diagnosis of tuberculosis infection difficult. Anergy testing with two DTH skin test antigens (*Candida albicans*, mumps, or tetanus toxoid) in conjunction with tuberculin testing has been recommended in the United States to identify anergic persons at risk of tuberculosis (Centers for Disease Control, 1991b). Preventive therapy is recommended for anergic persons whose likelihood of tuberculosis is estimated to be at least 10%. Recent studies have shown that the risk of tuberculosis in anergic, HIV-infected injecting drug users in New York City approximates the risk of those who are tuberculin positive (Selwyn *et al.*, 1992), and a cost-benefit analysis applied to injecting drug users in New York City suggests that the routine use of isoniazid preventive therapy in selected persons at risk of both HIV and tuberculosis infections without either PPD or HIV testing would be cost-effective (Jordon *et al.*, 1992). Studies are needed to determine the cost-effectiveness of the routine use of isoniazid preventive therapy without tuberculin testing for persons with HIV infection in developing countries where HIV-associated tuberculosis is common. Because of the cost and complexity of tuberculin testing, the added difficulty of testing for anergy, and the likely high rate of false negative tuberculin skin tests in HIV-infected persons in these countries, this policy has intuitive appeal.

Are there alternative regimens which will improve the efficacy of preventive therapy?

As has been suggested, there are a number of rifampicin-containing regimens which might improve the efficacy of preventive therapy, and several of these are being assessed in clinical trials. The combination of rifampicin and pyrazinamide is being evaluated in several studies, given either daily or intermittently for 2 or 3 months. Although a preliminary report from one study indicates good tolerance with therapy (Clermont *et al.*, 1991), because of its cost it is unlikely that this regimen would have applicability in resource-poor countries most affected by the problem of HIV-associated tuberculosis.

The combination of rifampicin and isoniazid may have more applicability. There is clinical experience with this combination in a 4-month regimen of chemotherapy, and it has been used as preventive therapy in England. The use of multidrug therapy decreases the risk of acquired drug resistance, and may also be effective in persons infected by isoniazid-resistant organisms. The three-drug combination of rifampicin, isoniazid and pyrazinamide may also be effective, but its application also limited by possible increased toxicity and higher cost. Finally, monotherapy with rifampicin is also of interest and might be well-tolerated and quite effective. However, there is justifiable concern about the use of rifampicin monotherapy in countries, such as those in sub-Saharan Africa, where well managed and tightly controlled preventive therapy programmes would be difficult to implement.

A number of the studies are also examining if intermittent preventive therapy would be effective. Based on the use of intermittent therapy in the treatment of tuberculosis, this method of treatment would probably be efficacious, while reducing cost and toxicity. However, the usual requirement for supervision of intermittently administered regimens may restrict the settings in which this type of treatment is feasible.

What is the potential impact of preventive therapy programmes on the tuberculosis problem?

More practical questions are being asked about the potential impact of preventive therapy programmes in reducing the occurrence of HIV-associated tuberculosis, whether or not these programmes may be cost-effective, and even if they are feasible to implement in countries where they are most urgently needed. Finally, the question of the role of the National Tuberculosis Programme (NTP) in preventive therapy must be defined.

Can preventive therapy programmes be implemented in the countries experiencing the most serious impact of HIV-associated tuberculosis and is the intervention cost-effective?

Theoretically, preventive therapy programmes targeting HIV-infected persons might have a substantial impact on reducing cases of tuberculosis. In some areas of sub-Saharan Africa, over 60% of newly diagnosed tuberculosis cases are HIV-positive. Moreover, there is good reason to believe that programmes would be much more cost-effective (i.e. far less costly) than waiting to treat both the new cases of HIV-associated tuberculosis and the secondary cases arising from increased transmission. Unfortunately, it is unlikely that such programmes will have any substantial impact on the tuberculosis situation in the near future. The entry point for a programme is HIV testing, and few voluntary HIV counselling and testing (VCT) centres have been established in developing countries where HIV-associated tuberculosis is epidemic. Obviously, the cost of the programme is a most important factor, and the cost of HIV-testing alone might exceed the cost of treatment with preventive therapy. Thus, finding the resources and developing the infrastructure in which the majority of persons at risk of both HIV and tuberculosis could receive HIV testing and, if HIV positive, be screened for tuberculosis and given preventive therapy if tuberculosis-free would be a prodigious undertaking. However, in the short term, preventive therapy may be quite attractive, especially if shown to have a positive benefit in prolonging disease-free survival, for individuals and certain groups. These include those undergoing voluntary HIV testing in VCTs and STD clinics, armed forces, and industrial settings. While public health impact might be difficult to demonstrate, the programmes might well have a demonstrable positive economic impact.

It is crucial to determine under what circumstances and in what settings, preventive therapy programmes are feasible. To date only one feasibility study has been conducted, this is at a VCT site in Kampala, Uganda. The preliminary results of this study indicated that compliance with preventive therapy among those offered treatment was over 60% (Aisu *et al.*, 1992). However, significant barriers to the programme, such as tuberculin skin testing and the lack of information about tuberculosis prevention, were found. The results of this study will be helpful in designing other pilot projects in other settings. An important associated finding was that nearly 6% of those being screened to determine eligibility for preventive therapy were found to have smear-positive tuberculosis, again illustrating the significance of the problem and the need for careful screening to exclude those with active disease from preventive therapy. Information on cost-effectiveness of this programme is currently being analysed.

Finally, there is a need to determine the role of the NTP in provision of preventive therapy to persons with HIV infection. A strong argument can be made that NTPs, especially those in countries where HIV-associated tuberculosis is on the rise, will have all they can do to identify and treat active tuberculosis cases and that any diversion of resources from treatment programmes would probably have an adverse effect on the tuberculosis situation (Styblo, 1991). However, NTPs should certainly be actively involved, at least through provision of technical assistance and review, for both feasibility studies of preventive therapy and implementation programmes. On the other hand, any facilities providing counselling and testing for HIV infection should at a minimum educate persons being tested about the signs and symptoms of tuberculosis and refer HIV-positive persons with suspect tuberculosis (i.e. consistent signs and symptoms) for further evaluation. These programmes might also consider including an assessment of the feasibility of preventive therapy into their programmes. In this endeavour, National AIDS Control Programmes (NACP) might be instrumental in ensuring the HIV testing conforms to standard guidelines. NTPs and NACPs should collaborate to the fullest extent possible in these programmes.

Experimental approaches to preventive therapy

Experimental approaches to preventive therapy include innovations in the provision of drugs and the development and assessment of new therapeutic interventions. Innovative approaches in administration of treatment aim to reduce non-adherence. Among the new measures which might be useful are blister pack therapy and use of depot preparations of drugs. Blister pack therapy may be especially useful for drugs given intermittently but not supervised. This would be of great interest should intermittent therapy prove effective and be less toxic and less costly than daily therapy. It is unlikely that supervised, intermittent therapy would ever have widespread applicability in either developed or developing countries. Preliminary studies of a depot preparation of isoniazid in mice are promising (Gangadharam *et al.*, 1991). In these studies, therapeutic levels of the drug for up to 6 weeks were provided by a single implant of isoniazid incorporated into a biodegradable polymer. Should this application prove useful and acceptable, it might have significant potential for use in preventive therapy.

Several new compounds related to rifampicin may be highly effective as tuberculosis preventive therapy, and two of these, rifapentine and rifabutin, are of particular interest. Rifapentine is a cyclopentyl rifamycin derivative with a long half-life and good activity against *M. tuberculosis*. In studies in mice, rifapentine administered once weekly appeared as active as daily rifampicin (Truffot-Pernot *et al.*, 1983). Rifabutin, a spiro-piperidyl-rifamycin, has recently been approved in the United States for the prophylaxis for *M. avium* complex in severely immunocompromised persons with HIV infection (O'Brien *et al.*, 1987). Its activity against *M. tuberculosis* is comparable to rifampicin, and its long half-life and high tissue levels suggest that it may be an effective chemoprophylactic drug. Recent studies in an animal model of chronic tuberculosis infection have indicated that these two agents given intermittently may be as effective as daily rifampicin (Ji *et al.*, 1993). Among the new quinolone antibiotics with antimycobacterial activity, sparfloxacin has been found to have excellent sterilizing activity in mice, comparable to rifampicin and isoniazid (Lalande, 1993). This drug may also be useful for preventive therapy.

Clinical studies of these new drugs which might shed light on their usefulness in preventive therapy are limited. However, placebo-controlled clinical studies of rifabutin in the United States have demonstrated this drug's usefulness in preventing disseminated *M. avium* complex disease in severely immuno-compromised patients with HIV infection (Gordin *et al.*, 1992). In these studies, which involved over 500 participants, three cases of tuberculosis occurred among those receiving placebo treatment, but none among those receiving the active drug (P. Olliaro, personal communication). Because of this drug's long half-life and high tissue and macrophage levels, it may be an excellent agent for preventive therapy, especially in regimens given intermittently.

Finally, an argument has been made that the situation of HIV-associated tuberculosis is so grave that radical solutions should be sought (Stanford *et al.*, 1991). Among these are the application of immunotherapy, perhaps equivalent to the administration of a vaccine to infected persons to prevent the development of active tuberculosis. Studies of adjuvant immunotherapy with killed *M. vaccae* are underway. Should the careful clinical trials suggest any efficacy of this intervention, its use in preventive therapy, either alone or in combination with chemotherapy, might then be assessed.

References

Aisu, Raviglione MC, Van Praag E *et al.* (1992) Feasibility of isoniazid preventive chemotherapy for HIV-associated tuberculosis in Uganda: preliminary results. Presented at the World Congress on Tuberculosis, Bethesda, Maryland, 16–19 November

Alcabes P, Vossenas P, Choen R *et al.* (1989) Compliance with isoniazid prophylaxis in jail. *American Review of Respiratory Disease, 140*, 1194–1197

American Academy of Paediatrics (1992) Chemotherapy for tuberculosis in infants and children. *Paediatrics, 89*, 161–165

American Thoracic Society/Centers for Disease Control (1986) Treatment of tuberculosis and tuberculosis infection in adults and children. *American Review of Respiratory Disease, 134*, 355–363

Centers for Disease Control (1989) Tuberculosis and human immunodeficiency virus infection: recommendations of the Advisory Committee for the Elimination of Tuberculosis. *Morbidity and Mortality Weekly Report, 38*, 236–238, 243–250

Centers for Disease Control (1990) The use of preventive therapy for tuberculosis infection in the United States. Recommendations of the Advisory Committee for the Elimination of Tuberculosis. *Morbidity and Mortality Weekly Report, 39* (RR-6), 9–12

Centers for Disease Control (1991a) Nosocomial transmission of multidrug-resistant tuberculosis among HIV-infected persons—Florida and New York, 1988–1991. *Morbidity and Mortality Weekly Report, 40*, 585–591

Centers for Disease Control (1991b) Purified protein derivative-tuberculin anergy in persons with HIV infection. Guidelines for anergy testing and management of anergic persons at risk of tuberculous infection. *Morbidity and Mortality Weekly Report, 40,* 27–33

Clermont H, Johnson M, Coberly J *et al.* (1991) Tolerance of short course TB chemoprophylaxis in HIV infected individuals. International Conference on AIDS (7th: 1991 Florence). Abstracts. Vol 2. Rome: Istituto Superiore de Sanita p. 272 (Abstract)

Comstock GW (1986) Prevention of tuberculosis among tuberculin reactors: maximizing benefits, minimizing risks. *Journal of the American Medical Association, 256,* 2729–2730

Comstock GW, Ferebee SH (1970) How much isoniazid is needed for prophylaxis? *American Review of Respiratory Disease, 101,* 780–782

Comstock GW, Baum C, Snider DE (1979) Isoniazid prophylaxis among Alaskan Eskimos: a final report of the Bethel isoniazid studies. *American Review of Respiratory Disease, 119,* 827–830

Ferebee SH (1970) Controlled chemoprophylaxis trials in tuberculosis. *Advances in Tuberculosis Research, 17,* 28–106

Ferebee SH, Palmer CE (1956) Prevention of experimental tuberculosis with isoniazid. *American Review of Tuberculosis, 73,* 1–18

Gangadheram PRJ, Ashlekar DR, Falin DC, Wise DL (1991) Sustained release of isoniazid in vivo from a single implant of a biodegradable polymer. *Tubercle, 72,* 115–122

Gordin F, Nightingale S, Wynne B *et al.* (1992) Rifabutin monotherapy prevents or delays *Mycobacterium avium complex* (MAC) bacteremia in patients with AIDS. VIII International Conference on AIDS/III STD World Congress, Amsterdam, 19–24 July, Vol 2, B100 [Amsterdam 3: CONGREX]

Grumbach F, Rist N (1967) Activate antituberculeuse experimentale de la rifampicine, derive de la rifamycine SV. *Review de la Tuberculose et de Pneumocologie, 31,* 749–762

Hong Kong Chest Service/Tuberculosis Research Center, Madras/British Medical Research Council (1984) A controlled trial of 2-month, 3-month and 12-month regimens of chemotherapy for sputum-smear-negative pulmonary tuberculosis: Results at 60 months. *American Review of Respiratory Disease, 130,* 23–28

Hong Kong Chest Service/Tuberculosis Research Center, Madras/British Medical Research Council (1992) A double-blind placebo-controlled clinical trial of three antituberculosis chemoprophylaxis regimens in patients with silicosis in Hong Kong. *American Review of Respiratory Disease, 145,* 36–41

International Union Against Tuberculosis Committee on Prophylaxis (1982) Efficacy of various durations of isoniazid preventive therapy for tuberculosis: five years of follow-up in the IUAT trial. *Bulletin of the World Health Organization, 60,* 555–564

International Union Against Tuberculosis and Lung Disease (1991) Tuberculosis in children—guidelines for diagnosis, prevention and treatment. *Bulletin of the International Union Against Tuberculosis and Lung Disease, 66,* 61–67

Ji B, Truffot-Pernot C, Lacroix C *et al.* (1993) Effectiveness of rifampin, rifabutin and rifapentine for preventive therapy of tuberculosis in mice. *American Review of Respiratory Disease* (in press)

Jordon TJ, Lewit EM, Montgomery RL, Reichman LB (1991) Isoniazid as preventive therapy in HIV-infected intravenous drug abusers. A decision analysis. *Journal of the American Medical Association, 265,* 2987–2991

Kleeberg HH, Olivier MS (1984) *A World Atlas of Initial Drug Resistance.* US Department of Health and Human Services, Atlanta, Georgia

Kopanoff DE, Snider DE, Caras GJ (1978) Isoniazid-related hepatitis. A US Public Health Service cooperative surveillance study. *American Review of Respiratory Disease, 117,* 991–1001

Koplan JP, Farer LS (1980) Choice of preventive treatment for isoniazid-resistant tuberculosis infection. Use of decision analysis and the Delphi Technique. *Journal of the*

American Medical Association, 244, 2736–2740

Lecouer HF, Truffot-Pernot C, Grosset JH (1989) Experimental short-course preventive therapy of tuberculosis with rifampin and pyrazinamide. *American Review of Respiratory Disease, 140,* 1189–1193

Lalande V, Truffort-Pernot C, Pacealy-Moulin A, Grosset J, Ji B (1993) Powerful bacterial activity of sparfloxacin (AT-4140) against *Mycobacterium tuberculosis* in mice. *Antimicrobial Agents and Chemotherapy, 37,* 407–413

Murray JF (1991) Tuberculosis and human immunodeficiency virus infection during the 1990's. *Bulletin of the International Union Against Tuberculosis and Lung Disease, 66,* 21–25

Nazar-Stewart V, Nolan CM (1992) Results of a directly observed intermittent isoniazid preventive therapy program in a shelter for homeless men. *American Review of Respiratory Disease, 146,* 57–60

O'Brien RJ, Lyle MA, Snider DE (1987) Rifabutin (ansamycin LM427): a new rifamycin-S derivative for the treatment of mycobacterial disease. *Reviews of Infectious Diseases, 9,* 519–530

Ormerod LP (1987) Reduced incidence of tuberculosis by prophylactic chemotherapy in subjects showing strong reactions to tuberculin testing. *Archives of Disease in Childhood, 62,* 1005–1008

Pape JW, Jean SS, Mo JL, Hafner A, Johnson WD (1993) Effect of isoniazid prophylaxis on incidence of active tuberculosis and progression of HIV infection. *Lancet, 342,* 268–272

Selwyn PA, Hartel D, Lewis VA *et al.* (1989) A prospective study of the risk of tuberculosis among intravenous drug users with human immunodeficiency virus infection. *New England Journal of Medicine, 320,* 545–550

Selwyn PA, Sckell BM, Alcabes P, Friedland MD *et al.* (1992) High risk of active tuberculosis in HIV-infected drug users with cutaneous anergy. *Journal of the American Medical Association, 268,* 504–509

Snider DE (1985) Bacille Calmette-Guérin vaccination and tuberculin skin tests. *Journal of the American Medical Association, 253,* 3438–3439

Snider DE, Caras GJ (1992) Isoniazid-associated hepatitis deaths: a review of available information. *American Review of Respiratory Disease, 145,* 494–497

Snider DE, Caras GJ, Koplan JP (1986) Preventive therapy with isoniazid. Cost-effectiveness of different durations of therapy. *Journal of the American Medical Association, 255,* 1579–1583.

Stanford JL, Grange JM, Pozniak A (1991) Is Africa lost? *Lancet, 338,* 557–558

Styblo K (1991) Preventive chemotherapy for tuberculosis control in developing countries. The case against preventive chemotherapy. *Bulletin of the International Union Against Tuberculosis and Lung Disease, 66* (suppl 1990/91), 27–28

Truffot-Perot C, Grosset J, Bismuth R, Lecouer H (1983) Activité de la rifampicine administrée de manière intermittente et de la cylopentyl rifamycine (ou DL 473) sur la tuberculose experimentale de la souris. *Revue Française des Maladies Respiratories, 11,* 875–882

Villarion ME, Dooley SW, Geiter LJ, Castro KG, Snider DE (1992) Management of persons exposed to multidrug-resistant tuberculosis. *Morbidity and Mortality Weekly Report, 41* (RR–11), 59–71

Wadhawan D, Mira S, Mwansa N, Perine P (1992) Preventive tuberculosis chemotherapy with isoniazid among persons infected with HIV. Presented at the Eighth International Conference on AIDS. Amsterdam, 19–24 July 1992

Wobeser W, To T, Hoeppner VH (1989) The outcome of chemoprophylaxis on tuberculosis prevention in the Canadian Plains Indians. *Clinical and Investigative Medicine, 12,* 149–153

World Health Organization (1992) *Managing Tuberculosis at the District Level.* WHO Tuberculosis Programme, Geneva.

Discussion

Alwyn G. Mwinga, *University of Zambia, Lusaka*

It is quite clear that the effectiveness of preventive therapy is based on the premise that persons exposed to *Mycobacteria tuberculosis* may develop a latent infection with the possibility of developing clinical disease at a later stage.

I would like to focus on the use of tuberculous preventive therapy in the light of HIV infection in developing countries where the most dramatic effects have been observed.

Tuberculous preventive therapy has never been considered as a viable option for developing countries for various reasons, not least because of the high prevalence of infection and because of the limited resources available to these countries. Indeed, despite the availability of effective chemotherapy and BCG vaccination, up to the beginning of the HIV epidemic, very few developing countries had managed to make any significant impact in the control of tuberculosis even with the setting up of national tuberculosis control programmes. Why then does any developing country need to think of preventive therapy when other methods of tuberculosis control have failed? Will the research being done in these countries merely serve to shed more light on the effectiveness of isoniazid prophylaxis in the HIV-infected individual for the benefit of the developed countries?

As Dr O'Brien has mentioned, preventive therapy for tuberculosis has mainly been used with success in North America. It has only been in the last few years with the emergence of the HIV epidemic and its interaction with tuberculosis that there has been interest in the use of preventive therapy in developing countries. Quite clearly, however, it is not possible to approach the use of preventive therapy in these countries in exactly the same manner as in North America. In countries with a high incidence of tuberculosis, HIV infection has simply made a bad situation worse. Indeed, these countries may well thank HIV for the renewed interest in tuberculosis that has been generated as a result of its 'unholy alliance' with tuberculosis.

I would now like to highlight some of the practical constraints and problems that are associated with the use of preventive therapy in developing countries. The first one that I would like to mention is the selection of patients.

In North America individuals are selected for preventive therapy on the basis of a positive tuberculin test indicating previous exposure to tuberculosis and hence the danger of developing reactivation disease in the face of a declining immunity. I would emphasize, however, that in most developing countries, the routine use of BCG vaccination decreases the usefulness of the tuberculin test in identifying those at risk of reactivation of latent infection. In addition, it has been shown that tuberculin anergy is not uncommon in an HIV-positive patient. Furthermore, as has been pointed out by Dr O'Brien, anergic patients with HIV infection may be at increased risk of developing tuberculosis. Thus one problem with the implementation of preventive therapy in this setting would be to identify which patients require this intervention. This problem could be avoided by ignoring the tuberculin test as a screening measure and offering all HIV-positive individuals tuberculous preventive therapy on the assumption that due to the high prevalence of tuberculosis the vast majority of people would have been exposed to infection at some point.

This, however, begs another question. If there is a high rate of latent infection in the community, how does one ensure that the HIV-positive individual has not already developed reactivation disease? It is clear from studies on the impact of HIV on tuberculosis that there has been an increase in extrapulmonary disease in persons with dual HIV and tuberculosis infection. Clearly exclusion of these forms of tuberculosis is not easily achieved in the ordinary clinical situation that prevails in most areas.

With the current concern over the emergence of multidrug-resistant tuberculosis, monotherapy needs to be avoided at all cost. Routine chest X-rays to exclude active pulmonary tuberculosis, aside from being very costly, have associated problems with the interpretation of findings that are not obviously abnormal. It is not uncommon for an HIV-infected person without respiratory symptoms to have diffuse nodular shadows on chest radiograph. Hilar adenopathy also appears to be a relatively common finding and it is not clear whether these are due to primary tuberculosis or a part of HIV-associated adenopathy. In this setting too, with poor living conditions and overcrowding, what interpretation does one place on respiratory symptoms which would tend to be quite common? Adequate investigations to exclude tuberculosis in a patient presenting with the history of a cough of more than 3 weeks' duration requires, in my opinion, at least three negative sputum cultures, given the low sensitivity and specificity of sputum smear in the presence of HIV infection. This requires access to mycobacterial culture facilities which are not widely available. Mycobacteria, being slow growing organisms, need a minimum of 6 to 8 weeks for a culture result and the accuracy of the result is affected not only by the quality of the laboratory but also by the manner in which the sputum specimen is handled from collection by the patient to delivery to the laboratory for processing. It is interesting to note that in the Uganda study, almost 6% of PPD-positive patients were found to have active tuberculosis.

What is the optimum duration of preventive treatment for developing countries? For developed countries the duration of preventive treatment has been set at 6 to 12 months. This appears adequate in areas with a low prevalence of infection and hence a very low risk of reinfection. However, as Dr O'Brien has said, this may not be adequate for areas where there is a high prevalence of infection and continued risk of reinfection. Preventive therapy will sterilize tissues and prevent reactivation of infection. However, due to the poor socio-economic conditions that prevail in many developing countries the risk of reinfection after prophylaxis is still high. In this situation with a high prevalence of infection, preventive therapy for tuberculosis for a limited time will have less effect on the incidence of tuberculosis. Is lifelong therapy the answer? If lifelong therapy is required then possibly the long-acting preparations will have a bigger role to play.

In developing countries the emergence of the HIV epidemic has had the effect of increasing the numbers of tuberculosis cases. In Zambia there has been an increase in reported cases of tuberculosis of almost 20% per year since 1985. It is clear that in many of these countries the main objective of the NTPs should be case finding and adequate treatment, in order to reduce the infectious pool in the community. These countries, apart from being faced with increased numbers of tuberculosis cases, are also overburdened with other HIV and non-HIV related problems including depressed economies from drought, famine and the effects of a worldwide recession. I agree, then, that the implementation of tuberculous preventive therapy in developing countries cannot be considered solely in the framework of the national tuberculosis control programme due to limited resources available and logistical problems. Tuberculous preventive therapy will have little or no public health impact on the control of tuberculosis in these countries even in the HIV era.

It may appear from the discussion so far that preventive therapy for developing countries is neither feasible nor desirable due to some of the factors so far discussed. Another problem, discussed by Dr O'Brien is that of compliance to treatment. It is, indeed, my belief that under the present circumstances in most developing countries today, preventive therapy cannot be used as a control measure for tuberculosis and neither would it be possible to offer it on a nationwide scale to all HIV-infected individuals. I do, however, feel that if preventive therapy proves to be effective, as has been demonstrated by Wadhawan et al. (1992), it may be necessary to consider preventive therapy for certain well-defined groups in society. In addition there is an urgent need to strengthen national control programmes in their efforts to control tuberculosis.

The HIV epidemic has mainly affected the young economically active segment of society. In countries where the population pyramid is such that more than half of the population consists of children this has disastrous consequences on both the economy and social structure. Tuberculosis, being more virulent than other opportunistic infections, tends to present relatively early on in the course of immunosuppression. Whilst response to treatment has been found to be not too different in comparison to an HIV-negative individual, there is still considerable associated morbidity and mortality. In addition it is not inconceivable that tuberculosis will act as a cofactor in increasing the rate of progression of asymptomatic HIV infection into full blown AIDS.

Furthermore in a setting where currently available specific anti-HIV therapies like zidovudine are clearly out of reach, tuberculous preventive therapy may provide one means of prolonging the active disease-free life of the economically active population.

The final aspect that I would like to consider regarding the use of tuberculous preventive therapy in developing countries is who will pay the bill? The national tuberculosis control programmes cannot do this as they rely quite heavily on external funding for their treatment drugs. Preventive therapy would have to compete for funds from a limited source. Governments cannot do this as their limited resources are already fully stretched by other non-HIV-related problems. One possibility is to involve business concerns to provide the drugs for their workforce. They stand to benefit from an increased active working life of their employees. This would have the added advantage of possibly reducing the problem of non-compliance to treatment as administration of drugs could be done within the work environment or other stipulated place in order to preserve confidentiality. As has been mentioned, the national AIDS control programmes could be used to provide reliable HIV testing facilities and indeed tuberculous preventive therapy could be integrated into their activities. In this setting, the national tuberculosis control programmes could work together with the AIDS control programme to provide technical assistance by way of screening of patients to exclude active tuberculosis and to provide treatment for all cases of tuberculosis identified.

Last, but certainly not least, what possible role could the pharmaceutical industry have in this area? Would they be willing to provide funds to answer some of these questions in the form of grants for research? As a humanitarian gesture would they be willing to supply drugs at a reduced cost for use in specific groups of people?

Clearly, there are many questions still to be answered on the usefulness and feasibility of tuberculosis preventive therapy in developing countries. One important question that needs to be addressed is the cost of preventive therapy compared to the cost of treating a case of smear-negative tuberculosis. This will have important implications when considering the feasibility of preventive therapy in developing countries. The effect that preventive therapy may have on drug resistance is another important question in the face of the emergence of multidrug resistance in the United States.

In conclusion it may be worth reiterating that under the present circumstances preventive therapy for tuberculosis in developing countries cannot be considered as part of the tuberculosis control programme's efforts to control tuberculosis. This should be part of the national AIDS control programme and may possibly be offered in the context of voluntary testing centres as a point of identification of HIV-positive individuals. Clearly, this intervention cannot be offered on a nationwide scale and initially should be offered to selected groups of people.

These answers may provide the only chance that thousands of HIV-infected people in the poorer developing countries have of some hope amidst hopelessness.

8
Control strategies and programme management

Jaap F. Broekmans

Royal Netherlands Tuberculosis Association, The Hague, The Netherlands

Introduction

In the absence of effective treatment, case fatality of tuberculosis in developed and developing countries was extremely high, around 50% (National Tuberculosis Institute, Bangalore, 1974; Drolet, 1938). Lindhart in Denmark even reported a case fatality of patients with 'open' (smear-positive) tuberculosis of 44% within 1 year after diagnosis. This proportion increased to 61% after 3 years and to 66% after 5 years (Lindhart, 1939). An untreated smear-positive patient remains, on average, infectious for approximately 2 years and then dies or recovers (Holm, 1970). In those 2 years, a single patient infects on average 20 contacts (Styblo, 1978). Of these infected contacts, on average two persons eventually break down with active disease, of which one has smear-positive pulmonary tuberculosis (Styblo, 1991). In this way, the chain of transmission of tuberculosis essentially remains steady, reflecting, in itself, a well-adjusted host–parasite relationship of man and *Mycobacterium tuberculosis*. This host–parasite relationship can be seen as the end result of co-evolution of mankind and *M. tuberculosis* and presents us with a vivid illustration of Burnet's theory on the *Natural History of Infectious Disease* (Burnet and White, 1972).

From this insight into the natural history of the disease stems our understanding of why detection and isolation of infectious cases in the pre-chemotherapy era and, since the early 1950s, effective chemotherapy of infectious tuberculosis cases, tip the balance in favour of man and against *M. tuberculosis*. Effective treatment reduces the infectious period considerably and thus reduces transmission. Already in 1961, Crofton concluded that good chemotherapy, combined with good case finding, is one of the most important, if not *the* most important preventive measure against tuberculosis (Crofton, 1962). In retrospect, it is interesting to note that he also stated that it is a grave error to allow incorrect use of the drugs by inadequately

Tuberculosis: Back to the Future. Edited by J.D.H. Porter and K.P.W.J. McAdam
© 1994 John Wiley & Sons Ltd

qualified staff, because it compromises the future of the campaign against tuberculosis by encouraging the spread of resistant tubercle bacilli.

Compelling epidemiological evidence indicates that good treatment programmes are also the best tuberculosis prevention programmes by effectively reducing transmission.

Transmission of *M. tuberculosis* in a population is quantified by estimating the annual rate of infection in that population. The annual rate of infection expresses the proportion of a population that becomes infected or reinfected with *M. tuberculosis* in the course of 1 year (Styblo *et al.*, 1969). The acceleration in the decline of the annual rate of infection from 4–5% per year before, to 12–13% after, World War II in The Netherlands and other industrialized countries is well documented in this respect (Figure 8.1) (Styblo, 1991).

The simultaneous decline in the case rates in children and young adults in The Netherlands in the same period demonstrates the impact of the reduction of transmission on the incidence of disease (Figure 8.2) (Styblo and Meijer, 1976).

Estimates on the prevalence of infection in the total population of The

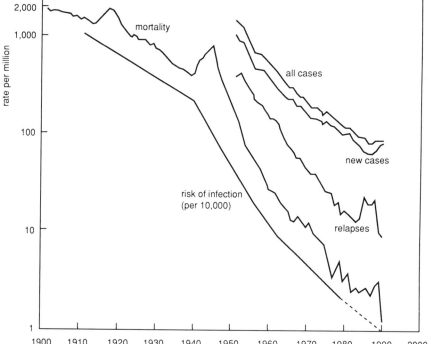

Figure 8.1 Tuberculosis mortality (1900–90), incidence (1951–90), reactivation (1951–90) rates (per million) and the annual risk of infection (1910–90) (per 10 000), The Netherlands. Source: Chief Medical Officer of Infectious Diseases. Ministry of Welfare, Health and Culture, Rijswijk, The Netherlands

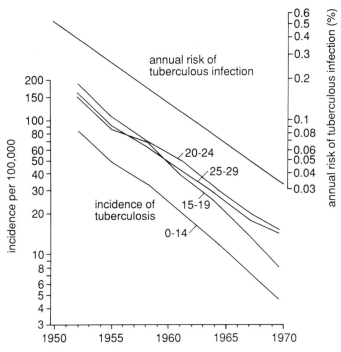

Figure 8.2 Annual risks of tuberculous infection and incidence of new active tuberculosis in subjects aged 0 to 14, 15 to 19, 20 to 24, and 25 to 29 years, The Netherlands, 1952–70. Source: Styblo and Meijer (1976) *Tubercle. 57*, 17–43. With permission of Churchill Livingstone.

Netherlands in 1945, 1975 and for 2005 (Figure 8.3) demonstrate that 'elimination' of infection is a preliminary to 'elimination' of disease (Bleiker, 1984). It illustrates the maximum that can be achieved with the application of current technologies, of which effective treatment delivery, which substantially reduces transmission from the sources of infection, is the most important. In 1990, approximately 15% (or more than 2 million) of the Dutch population of 15 million were still infected with *M. tuberculosis*, most of them in the higher age-groups, due to tuberculous infection before 1950 (Broekmans, 1993). Elimination of tuberculosis in The Netherlands is not foreseen before the year 2025 (Styblo, 1990). This fact underlines the need, even in low prevalence countries, for an uninterrupted continuation of control measures for at least 3 decades to come. From an ecological perspective, one cannot but admire the tenacity of *M. tuberculosis* to remain with such a firm foothold in the human population for such a long period of time under such adverse conditions against its existence.

The experience in the late 1980s and early 1990s in some of the metropolitan areas in the USA demonstrates that a premature breakdown of effective treatment delivery, among other factors, may have led to a resurgence of tuberculosis and an

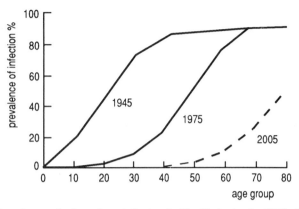

Figure 8.3   Prevalence of tuberculous infection in The Netherlands, 1945, 1975 and 2005.
Source: Bleiker (1984)

upsurge of multidrug-resistant tuberculosis (Brudney and Dobkin, 1991). Undoubtedly it will be demonstrated in these cities that it is possible to improve the situation, provided that new, bacteriologically confirmed cases are treated effectively.

Control strategies

The epidemiological model of transmission of infection and disease occurrence described above enables us to understand the current epidemiological situation in developing countries (Styblo, 1991).

The current level of the risk of infection in most developing countries is comparable to the size of the tuberculosis problem in industrialized countries in the late 1930s making tuberculosis in developing countries the most important public health problem caused by a single pathogen (Murray et al., 1990).

While the decrease in the risk of infection in most industrialized countries may still be in the order of 10% per year, the decline in the risk of infection in most developing countries was in the pre-HIV era in the order of 1–5% per year (Table 8.1), which was less than the decrease in industrialized countries in the pre-chemotherapy era (Murray et al., 1990). Moreover, the gap between developed and developing countries (Figure 8.4) with respect to tuberculosis has been widening year by year (Broekmans et al., 1990).

The current decline in the risk of infection of 1–5% in most developing countries is outweighed by population increases of 3%, creating a situation in which the *absolute* number of tuberculosis cases has not declined over the past 30–40 years worldwide. The only positive aspect of this trend in the epidemiological situation of tuberculosis was that, in the pre-HIV era, the incidence *rates* of the disease were slowly decreasing.

Table 8.1 Estimated risks of tuberculous infection and their trends in developing countries, 1985–90

Area	Estimated risk of tuberculous infection (%)		Estimated annual decrease in the risks of infection (%)
Sub-Saharan Africa	1.50	2.50	1–2
North Africa and western Asia	0.50	1.50	4–5
Asia	1.00	2.00	1–3
South America	0.50	1.50	2–5
Central America and Caribbean	0.50	1.50	1–3

Source: Murray *et al.* (1990) with permission of the International Union against Tuberculosis and Lung Disease.

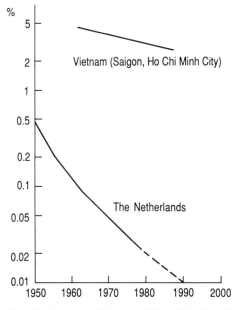

Figure 8.4 Annual risk of infection in Vietnam (Saigon/Ho Chi Minh City) 1961–87 and The Netherlands 1950–90. Source: Broekmans *et al.* (1990)

The failure to introduce effective treatment programmes in developing countries is the main reason why the chain of transmission continues unchanged in the developing world. Despite an international consensus on the overall control strategy (as expressed in the WHO Expert Reports on Tuberculosis in 1964 and 1974), the actual application of ambulatory treatment programmes using standard chemotherapy in the treatment of smear-positive tuberculosis in national programmes under routine programme conditions has been, by and large, a dismal failure.

The most important failure has been the failure to cure the sources of infection that were identified.

Grzybowski and Enarson were the first to review systematically the results of treatment of standard chemotherapy in developing countries under routine programme conditions (Grzybowski and Enarson, 1978). Their study showed that quiescence of the disease was achieved in about 60–65% of all patients under treatment (Table 8.2). The proportion of death from tuberculosis was about 10–16%.

Table 8.2   Fate of bacillary cases of tuberculosis when treated under mass chemotherapy programmes in certain developing countries

| Country | No. of cases | Year | Duration of follow-up | % died | Bacteriology | |
					% positive	% negative
Taiwan	237	1968	2 years	10.5	24.1	65.4
Korea	288	1968	1.5–2 years	11.1	26.0	62.9
Kenya	739	1968	> 1 year	15.6	21.5	62.9
India	292	1974	1 year	9.6	27.0	63.4

Source: Grzybowski and Enarson (1978) with permission of the International Union against Tuberculosis and Lung Disease.

The proportion of chronic bacillary excretors remained high (approximately 25%). The review of Grzybowski and Enarson concerned relatively small cohorts of patients. Styblo demonstrated that, even in well managed programmes covering a whole country in which drugs for all patients were available as in Tanzania, the overall success rate of standard chemotherapy evaluating all smear-positive patients diagnosed between 1979 and 1982 remained low. There was no improvement of the cure rate from 1979 to 1982, which at the end of treatment remained stable at a mere 50–55% (Table 8.3) (National Tuberculosis/Leprosy Program). Similar disappointing results have been reported from other programmes, supported by the International Union against Tuberculosis and Lung Disease (IUATLD).

Table 8.3   Results of treatment with standard chemotherapy under routine programme conditions, Tanzania, 1979–82

| Year | Number assessed | Results in percentages | | | | | |
		Cured	Treatment completed	Transferred out	Defaulted	Still on treatment	Died
1979	5418	31	13	10	23	18	5
1980	5867	39	16	13	15	10	7
1981	5527	39	14	12	18	10	7
1982	5498	37	15	15	14	13	6

Source: Ministry of Health, Dar es Salaam, Tanzania.

A cure rate of 50–60% of all sources of infection identified is insufficient to reduce transmission significantly. The main reasons are:

1. The proportion of undiscovered and untreated patients who continue to spread *M. tuberculosis*. Even in good programmes in developing countries, a certain proportion (35–40%) of the true incidence remains undiscovered and untreated.
2. The proportion of failure cases who continue to spread *M. tuberculosis*. The distinct advantage of inadequate chemotherapy is that it reduces case fatality to about 15% at the end of the first year after the onset of treatment. The most serious disadvantage is that it creates a high proportion (25–30%) of failure cases, often harbouring resistant bacilli, who may become chronic excretors and will continue to spread *M. tuberculosis*.

Styblo and Bumgarner (1991) recently summarized the net result of case finding and treatment under various programme conditions on the overall prevalence of smear-positive cases in the population. Their findings are summarized in Table 8.4, referring to a population in which the incidence of smear-positive tuberculosis is 100 per 100 000. From these calculations it can be inferred that from a cure rate of

Table 8.4 Prevalence of smear-positive cases assuming an incidence of 100 smear-positive cases per 100 000 under routine programme conditions with varying results of case finding and cure rates

Case finding rates (%)	Cure rates			
	35%	50%	75%	85%
35	215	197	173	161
50	218	196	159	146
65	223	193	145	125
70	223	192	140	119

Source: Styblo and Bumgarner (1991).

75% and higher one can expect a substantial reduction in the prevalence of sources of infection in the population compared to the situation in which no control measures are applied (Table 8.5). The other extreme (Table 8.6) is provided by the programme that applies optimal control measures (based on detailed epidemiological studies in The Netherlands) in which a 'maximum' reduction of 66% is reached in the prevalence of sources of infection at any given point in time.

Even with the onslaught of HIV transmission and its negative effect on the incidence of tuberculosis cases, Styblo demonstrated conclusively in the mid 1980s in the national programmes supported by IUATLD that with a result-oriented application of short-course chemotherapy under routine programme conditions, the

Table 8.5 Prevalence of smear-positive cases assuming an incidence of 100 per 100 000 population, if no control measures are applied

---

Prevalence of smear-positive cases = incidence × 2

Example Incidence of smear-positive cases = 100/100 000
Prevalence of smear-positive cases = 200/100 000

Number of infected contacts: 200 × 10 = 2000/year

Number of TB cases in 2000 infected contacts: 2000 × 0.10% = 200
of which 100 smear-positive and 100 smear-negative or extra-pulmonary tuberculosis

---

Source: Styblo and Bumgarner (1991).

Table 8.6 Prevalence of smear-positive cases assuming an incidence of 100 per 100 000 if optimal control measures are applied

---

Incidence of smear-positive cases: 100/100 000 Case finding rate: 90% Cure rate: 95%	Prevalence of smear-positive sources
Undiscovered: 10 × 2 (years)	20
Delay of 4 months in 90 discovered cases: (90 ÷ 3)	30
Delay of 4 months in 12 relapses: (12 ÷ 3)	4
5% of failure cases: 5 × 3 (years)	15
Total prevalence	69
Decrease in the prevalence: (200 – 69) ÷ 2	66%

Source: Styblo and Bumgarner (1991).

great majority of infectious cases can be effectively cured, and the failure rate reduced (Figure 8.5).

These results are being confirmed in other national programmes that followed the IUATLD methodology, for example Vietnam. Table 8.7 and Table 8.8 present the results of treatment with short-course chemotherapy under routine programme conditions in four countries. This remarkable achievement provided the basis for WHO's new Global Program against Tuberculosis aiming at a verifiable cure rate of 85% of all infectious cases identified in national programmes in developing countries.

Before the HIV epidemic, such high cure rates under routine programme conditions could have accelerated the then minimal decline in developing countries in the annual rate of infection with an estimated 5% per year, thus halving the rate of infection and the disease in children and young adults in about 15 years. Now, with a two-fold increase of sources of infection in countries where HIV infection becomes widespread, the most important target is to contain the present rate of

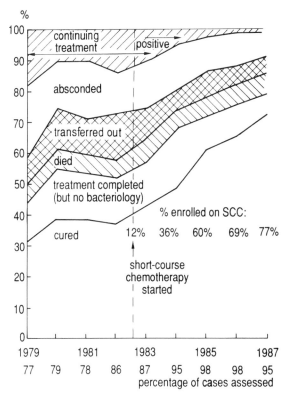

Figure 8.5 Results of treatment (%) with standard chemotherapy (1979–82) and with short-course or standard chemotherapy (1983–87). Tanzania 1979–87. Source: National Tuberculosis/Leprosy Program. Ministry of Health, Tanzania

Table 8.7 Results of treatment with short-course chemotherapy under routine programme conditions. Tanzania, Malawi, Benin, Vietnam

	Tanzania 1983–91	Malawi 1984–90	Benin 1984–90	Vietnam 1989–91
Number enrolled	55 330	12 593	5112	8953
Cured (negative) (%)	80	85	80	90
Failure (positive) (%)	2	1	2	2
Died (%)	7	8	6	2
Absconded (%)	8	2	11	4
Transferred out (%)	4	4	1	2
Total (%)	100	100	100	100

Source: National Tuberculosis Programmes of Tanzania, Malawi, Benin and Vietnam.

Table 8.8 Results of retreatment short-course chemotherapy under routine programme conditions. Tanzania, Malawi, Benin, Vietnam

	Tanzania 1983–91	Malawi 1984–90	Benin 1984–90	Vietnam 1989–91
Number enrolled	4922	1410	612	2620
Cured (negative) (%)	72	88	64	82
Failure (positive) (%)	4	2	5	10
Died (%)	9	6	8	4
Absconded (%)	11	3	18	2
Transferred out (%)	4	1	3	2
Total (%)	100	100	100	100

Source: National Tuberculosis Programmes of Tanzania, Malawi, Benin and Vietnam.

transmission by effective treatment delivery to all diagnosed new smear-positive cases and to keep the tuberculosis problem within manageable proportions until the rate of HIV transmission levels off. After levelling off of HIV infection, a decrease in the rate of tuberculous infection can then be expected which will be followed by a decrease in tuberculosis incidence. Till that time, we must prevent the situation that tuberculosis becomes managerially and epidemiologically out of control.

Conclusion on control strategies

In most industrialized countries, the application of effective chemotherapy tipped the balance in favour of man against *M. tuberculosis*. However, elimination is still decades away. This fact requires a maintenance of the existing tuberculosis surveillance network and specific diagnostic, therapeutic and surveillance expertise within the general health service of industrialized countries.

In high prevalence countries, HIV infection threatens to tip the balance in favour of *M. tuberculosis* against man. In these countries, there is an urgent need to develop effective national tuberculosis programmes in order to curtail transmission, reduce case fatality and prevent the emergence of multidrug resistance.

Programme management

Programme management in low prevalence countries

In low prevalence countries, the aim is to maintain the infrastructure of a tuberculosis service until elimination is achieved. In The Netherlands, with the relatively low notification rate of 9.2 (foreigners included) per 100 000 in 1990, for a population of 15 million people, 45 tuberculosis units within the national network

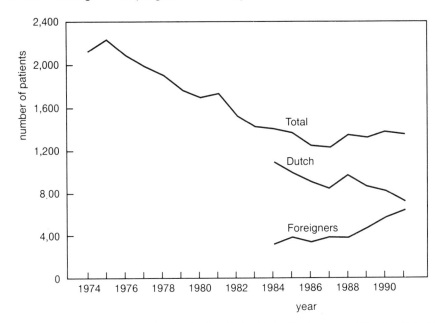

Figure 8.6 Tuberculosis notification in The Netherlands (foreigners and Dutch) 1971–91. Source: Chief Medical Officer of Infectious Diseases, Ministry of Health, Welfare and Culture, Rijswijk, The Netherlands, based on the registration of the Municipal Health Services

of Municipal Health Services are operational, with about 25 tuberculosis surveillance officers and 40 tuberculosis public health nurses in active service. In The Netherlands, tuberculosis is increasingly a disease imported from high prevalence countries (Figure 8.6). Specific policy measures include active case finding in foreigners and other risk groups (drug abusers, homeless people, prisoners, etc.), containment of micro-epidemics, and extensive tracing of contacts around newly detected cases and persons with (recent) infections.

Programme management in developing countries

The structure of a national tuberculosis programme and its key managerial and technical issues are discussed in this chapter. This description is based on the experience of the successful IUATLD-assisted programmes in developing countries, the national tuberculosis programme of Vietnam, and the World Bank/WHO supported national programme in China.

For a more detailed description the reader is referred to the chapter on 'National Tuberculosis Programmes' in the forthcoming publication of Reichman and Hershfield *Tuberculosis: a Comprehensive International Approach* (Styblo and Salomao, 1993).

Structure of a national tuberculosis programme. A national tuberculosis programme demands a continuous and long-term effort. In general, three levels are recognized.

- *National level.* At the Ministry of Health, there must be a single directing authority, e.g. a Central Tuberculosis Unit (CTU). The CTU is overall responsible for the planning, implementation and coordination of all programme activities. Its main tasks are surveillance, supervision, supplies, training and advocacy.
- *Intermediate (provincial or regional) level.* Under the Regional Director of Health, a specialized medical officer as Regional Tuberculosis Coordinator (RTC) is responsible for the implementation and coordination of the national programme in the area. The RTC's main task is the supervision of the staff involved in case finding and treatment, with special emphasis on the monitoring of treatment results.
- *District level.* Under the District Medical Officer, a specialized medical assistant as District Tuberculosis Coordinator (DTC) is responsible for the implementation of the national programme in the area. The DTC's main tasks are the day-to-day execution of the activities of the national programme with special emphasis on supervision of treatment delivery, case finding and recording and reporting.

Most national programmes function as an integral component of the primary health care system. Diagnosis (by smear examination in general hospital laboratories at district level) and treatment (supervised or self-administered) depend to a large extent on the general health staff at district and village level. The specialized staff at regional and district level function in most programmes much more as facilitators and advisers to the general health staff.

Key managerial and technical issues. The following key managerial and technical issues are recognized.

1. *Treatment issues.*
   (a) *Short-course chemotherapy for smear-positive patients.* The regimens are based on an initial intensive phase of 2 months of isoniazid, rifampicin, pyrazinamide and streptomycin (or ethambutol) and a continuation phase of isoniazid and rifampicin (for 4 months) or isoniazid and thiacetazone or ethambutol (for 6 months).
   (b) *Supervised intake of drugs during the intensive phase of treatment.* The success of short-course chemotherapy depends on a successful completion of the intensive phase of treatment. Sputum conversion at 8 weeks should be approximately 90%. If sputum is still positive at 8 weeks, the intensive phase should be prolonged with another 2 or 4 weeks.

Table 8.9 Examples of (supervised) treatment regimens in four countries

Country	Treatment regimen	Application of a supervised intensive phase	Continuation phase
Tanzania	2SHRZ/6TH	Rural areas: hospitalization Urban areas: supervised ambulatory treatment	Self-administered treatment Sputum examination at 5 and 8 months
Vietnam	2SHRZ/6HE	Urban areas: supervised ambulatory treatment Rural areas: self-care unit or hospitalization	Self-administered treatment Sputum examination at 5 and 8 months
China	$2S_3H_3R_3Z_3/4R_3H_3$	Supervised ambulatory treatment at village level	Supervised ambulatory treatment at village level Sputum examination at 4 and 6 months
Kenya (nomads)	4(S)HRZ/3TH	Self-care unit (manyatta) with extended intensive phase of treatment	Self-administered treatment No sputum examination at 7 months

Sputum conversion after the intensive phase of treatment is identified as the single most important parameter of the programme. After sputum conversion at 8 or 12 weeks after the onset of treatment, the patient switches to the continuation phase of treatment.

Alternative for the supervised treatment in the intensive phase are described in Table 8.9.

Streptomycin in the intensive phase acts as a "leash" to ensure fully supervised treatment in the intensive phase. Replacement of streptomycin (an injectable drug) by ethambutol (an oral drug) has not yet been demonstrated to be effective under routine programme conditions.

(c) *Retreatment regimen for failure and relapse cases.* The retreatment regimen for failure and relapse cases recommended by IUATLD and WHO has been shown to be effective under routine programme conditions and, besides reducing the number of (chronic) sources of infection, reduces substantially the risk of emergence of (multi)drug resistance. It should be applied fully supervised throughout.

2. *Monitoring of treatment results.*

(a) *Bacteriological examination on entry and monitoring of treatment results by bacteriology.* Each smear-positive patient has his or her treatment (after at least two positive smears on enrolment) closely monitored by bacteriology: at the end of the intensive phase (at 2 or 3 months), during treatment at 4 or 5 months and at the end of treatment (at 6 or 8 months).

Reliable bacteriology and monitoring of treatment results by bacteriology in individual patients constitute the basis of the quarterly cohort analysis of all smear-positive patients enrolled on treatment.

(b) *A standardized recording and reporting system at district level consisting of a district tuberculosis register, laboratory register and a patient card.* Recording of all patients diagnosed in one single district register establishes the cohort to be analysed, enables supervisory staff to check the entries with laboratory register and patient card, gives full information to trace individual patients, and forms the basis of the quarterly reports to provincial and national level.

(c) *Evaluation of treatment and case finding results by quarterly cohort analysis.* The results of treatment of each patient are evaluated at the end of treatment according to six categories: negative, treatment completed (but no bacteriology), positive (failure), died, absconded or transferred out (of the district). The cohort analysis uses as denominator all smear-positive cases enrolled. Continuous monitoring of treatment results by means of cohort analysis (reported every quarter by district level) is the key management tool in the delivery of the programme and enables provincial (and national) staff on the early improvement of treatment delivery in 'weak' districts. To what extent the treatment results achieved under routine programme conditions approximate the results obtained in control clinicial trials is the most important issue of the monitoring of treatment.

3. *Case detection and diagnosis.*

(a) *Passive case finding among suspects.* Case finding among suspects who attend health facilities on their own initiative with a productive cough lasting more than 3 weeks is the most important case finding activity of any tuberculosis programme in developing countries.

It is estimated that, in well-managed programmes in developing countries, about 60–70% of the true incidence is discovered by passive case finding.

(b) *Diagnosis by smear microscopy.* Diagnosis by smear microscopy examining at least three specimens of each suspect enables the programme to diagnose the most important sources of infection in the population. In large cities with many tuberculosis suspects, fluorescent microscopy should be introduced.

Smear-microscopy using the Ziehl–Neelsen staining technique can be considered as an intermediate technology that can be effectively and reliably applied at district level in any developing country. It is stressed that diagnosis of smear-negative tuberculosis, based on clinical and X-ray examinations, must be documented by at least three negative smear examinations, in particular in high HIV prevalence developing countries.

4. *Supportive activities.*

(a) *Supervision.* Regular and focused supervision from provincial to district and from national to provincial level is a key element in strengthening the national programme.

(b) *Regular supply of drugs.* The regular supply of drugs is a *sine qua non* for the effective delivery of short-course chemotherapy under routine programme conditions.

Although situations vary from country to country, the supply of isoniazid and streptomycin is often the responsibility of the Central Medical Stores. The regular supply of rifampicin, pyrazinamide and ethambutol should be closely supervised by the CTU and the RTC.

(c) *Tuberculosis manual.* A tuberculosis manual, delineating tasks and procedures for case finding, treatment and recording and reporting, is an important component of any programme, especially for paramedical staff and non-specialized medical officers.

Programme management in developing countries in the era of HIV transmission

At present, the most important tool available to curtail the impact of HIV infection on the epidemiological situation of tuberculosis is scrupulous maintenance of a high cure and detection rate of smear-positive cases of tuberculosis.

Tuberculosis patients who have been infected with HIV usually respond well to short-course chemotherapy and can be cured as quickly as HIV-negative patients. Their clinical improvement, however, is frequently a great deal less pronounced than that of HIV-negative tuberculosis patients.

HIV-infected tuberculosis patients are more likely to die while on treatment for tuberculosis than are patients without HIV. Thus, in countries with a high prevalence of dual infection, the fatality rate for tuberculosis is rising. In reviewing patients with the dual infection, it is frequently observed that those who die while on treatment do so after sputum conversion, when their tuberculosis has improved bacteriologically and clinically (Mohammed *et al.*, 1990).

Among patients who survive, treatment response to therapy does not appear to differ, whether the patient is infected with HIV or not. In IUATLD-assisted national programmes where HIV prevalence has been rapidly rising, rates of sputum conversion after the onset of treatment have not changed and appear to be the same in districts with a high prevalence of HIV infection as in districts where HIV infection is uncommon. Since the life expectancy after completion of treatment of patients with HIV infection is relatively short, the likelihood of relapse is necessarily reduced.

While on treatment for tuberculosis, adverse reactions to medications have been noted to be more common among those who are HIV-positive. This is especially true in developing countries where resources are limited and programmes must use thiacetazone. Diagnosis of tuberculosis in HIV-infected persons may be difficult in other than smear-positive cases. The principal presenting features of patients with AIDS are relatively non-specific. However, in the majority of cases there is pulmonary involvement, and in a high proportion of cases this is infectious (sputum smear-positive). Such cases can be diagnosed, by smear microscopy, and form the most important group of tuberculosis patients resulting from HIV infection, because of their infectious potential.

Since a proportion (as yet not reliably documented) smear-negative tuberculosis cases among HIV-infected persons are culture-positive, it is necessary, whenever possible, to improve case finding of smear-negative tuberculosis cases. At present, the most suitable method is screening patients suspected of having tuberculosis by chest X-ray, and to examine those with pathology on chest X-ray by microscopy and, if possible, by culture for the tubercle bacilli.

The safety of staff and of other patients is a matter of consideration where HIV infection is common. It is extremely important when injections (for example, streptomycin) are given, or when blood from such patients is handled, that proper sterilization and disposal procedures for hazardous materials be strictly practised.

In developing countries with a high prevalence of HIV infection, proper management of excess tuberculosis cases is very difficult in large cities. The personnel dealing with tuberculosis patients, and especially with those enrolled on outpatient chemotherapy, have become overstretched. Operational research is urgently needed to explore how to cope with the substantial and continuing increase in tuberculosis cases in large cities.

Although a steady increase in tuberculosis incidence has been observed in several developing countries with the prevalent dual infection, it is likely that the transmission of tuberculous infection will not increase accordingly due to a higher case fatality. However, if the current rate of tuberculous infection is high and the annual decrease in the risk is low, the extra infectious tuberculosis cases attributable to HIV may gradually increase the risk of infection. If a substantial decrease in the rate of infection is achieved by efficient case finding and by a high cure rate of smear-positive cases, the increase in the risk of infection caused by HIV infection might be contained.

In retrospect, it is a fortunate coincidence that, as part of the national tuberculosis programme of Tanzania, a National Tuberculin Survey was executed in the early years of the programme. A prevalence of infection of 11% was established in 1985 in schoolchildren aged on average 10 years. A survey carried out in the same schools established a prevalence of infection of 10% in 1990 (Styblo, 1992a, 1992b).

Despite a 4.5% annual increase in the case detection rate of smear-positive cases from 1985 until 1990, these preliminary results show no increase in the prevalence of infection in the same period.

Acknowledgement

The author would like to thank Dr K. Styblo, director of the Tuberculosis Surveillance Research Unit, for his suggestions in the preparation of this manuscript and his permission to quote from his publications.

References

Bleiker MA (1984) Tuberculine en tuberculine-onderzoek. In *Leerboek der Tuberculosebestrijding*. KNCV, The Hague, Chapter VI, pp. 1–19

Broekmans JF (1993) Evaluation of applied strategies in low prevalence countries. In Reichman LB, Hershfield ES (eds) *Tuberculosis: a Comprehensive International Approach*. Marcel Dekker, New York pp. 641–667

Broekmans JF, Planting KE, Nguyen Dinh Huong (1990) The extent of the tuberculosis problem in Vietnam and its trend. Poster presentation, 1990 World Conference of Lung Health, Boston

Brudney K, Dobkin J (1991) Resurgent tuberculosis in New York City. Human immunodeficiency virus, homelessness, and the decline of tuberculosis control programmes. *American Review of Respiratory Disease, 144*, 745–749

Burnet M, White DO (1972) Evolution and survival of host and parasite. In Burnet M (ed.) *Natural History of Infectious Disease*, 4th edition. Cambridge University Press, London, pp. 137–154

Crofton J (1962) The contribution of treatment to the prevention of tuberculosis. *Bulletin of the International Union Against Tuberculosis, 32*, 643–653

Drolet GJ (1938) Present trend of case fatality rates in tuberculosis. *American Review of Tuberculosis, 37*, 125–151

Grzybowski S, Enarson DA (1978) The fate of cases of pulmonary tuberculosis under various treatment programmes. *Bulletin of the International Union Against Tuberculosis, 53*, 70–75

Holm J (1970) Our enemy. The tubercle bacillus. *International Tuberculosis Digest*, no. 5. International Union against Tuberculosis

Lindhart M (1939) *The statistics of pulmonary tuberculosis in Denmark, 1925–1934. A statistical investigation on the occurrence of pulmonary tuberculosis in the period 1925–1934, worked out on the basis of the Danish National Health Service file of notified cases and of deaths*. E. Munksgaard, Copenhagen

Mohammed A, Lwechungura S, Chum HJ *et al.* (1990) Excess fatality rate after sputum conversion of new smear-positive patients enrolled on short-course chemotherapy in a country with prevalent HIV infection. Poster presentation at the 1990 World Conference on Lung Health, Boston

Murray CJL, Styblo K, Rouillon A (1990) Tuberculosis in developing countries: burden, intervention and cost. *Bulletin of the International Union Against Tuberculosis and Lung Disease, 65*, 6–24

National Tuberculosis/Leprosy Program, From *Annual Reports of the Program*, Ministry of Health, Tanzania

National Tuberculosis Institute, Bangalore (1974) Tuberculosis in a rural population of South India: a five-year epidemiological study. *Bulletin of the World Health Organization, 51*, 473–488

Styblo K (1978) State of the art. I. Epidemiology of tuberculosis. *Bulletin of the International Union Against Tuberculosis, 53*, 141–152

Styblo K (1990) The elimination of tuberculosis in the Netherlands. *Bulletin of the International Union Against Tuberculosis and Lung Disease, 65*, 49–55

Styblo K (1991) Epidemiology of tuberculosis. In Royal Netherlands Tuberculosis
Association, The Hague: Volume 24, Selected Papers

Styblo K (1992a) The first round of the National Tuberculin Survey in Tanzania, 1983–1987.
Tuberculosis Surveillance Research Unit Progress Report, 1, 127–164

Styblo K (1992b) A preliminary report on the second round of the National Tuberculin
Survey in Tanzania in the first 19 regions (1988–June 1992). *Tuberculosis Surveillance
Research Unit Progress Report, 2*, 113–161

Styblo K, Bumgarner JR (1991) Tuberculosis can be controlled with existing technologies:
evidence. *Tuberculosis Surveillance Research Unit Progress Report, 2*, 60–72

Styblo K, Meijer J (1976) Impact of BCG vaccination programmes in children and young
adults on the tuberculosis problem. *Tubercle, 57*, 17–43

Styblo K, Salomao MA (1993) National Tuberculosis Programmes. In Reichman LB,
Hershfield ES (eds.) *Tuberculosis: A Comprehensive International Approach.* Marcel
Dekker, New York, pp. 573–600

Styblo K, Meijer J, Sutherland I (1969) The transmission of tubercle bacilli. Its trend in a
human population. *Bulletin of the International Union Against Tuberculosis, 42*, 5–104

Discussion

Erik Glatthaar, *University of Pretoria, Republic of South Africa*

I will present my comments from a Southern, and in particular, South African
perspective.

In discussing the epidemiological model of transmission and disease occurrence
of tuberculosis no mention was made at all of the socio-economic, environmental
and other stress determinants controlling this formidable disease and of the
essential role community involvement/participation plays in the management and
control of tuberculosis. Expensive treatment regimens and sophisticated control
measures will not achieve the desired results without socio-economic upliftment,
multisectoral/disciplinary cooperation, and full community participation.

The plenary paper does not present a true reflection of the complexity
surrounding tuberculosis control in developing countries in Africa and of the many
and intricate problems facing these communities. Too much emphasis is placed on
the curative, epidemiological and research aspects of tuberculosis control instead of
addressing the basic, grassroots issues determining this disease. The tuberculosis
situation in many African countries is probably far worse than that reflected by
notification figures. In South Africa we are dealing with an annual case load of
134000 and incidence rates varying between 300 and 600 per 100000 (Küstner, 1993).

Urbanization is a serious problem in Africa and especially in South Africa where
approximately 80% of the population will be in and around cities by the year 2000.
The rural areas are being depopulated and the availability of health professionals in
rural areas is a luxury! In the urban squatter areas the demand for health care
services totally outstrips the resources available. Furthermore, violence seriously

disrupts and overloads the health services.

The discussion on control strategies presents a good overview of International Union against Tuberculosis and Lung Diseases (IUATLD)-supported strategies in developing countries with the focus on the curative aspects of standard chemotherapy. However, no critical evaluation of these strategies is made and essential elements such as disease surveillance, training of health workers, resource utilization and community awareness are not discussed.

A review of programme management for both developed and developing countries has been excellently presented. However, the following aspects must be discussed if we wish to progress to reasonable control of tuberculosis disease.

First, although the overview given of tuberculosis services in The Netherlands is not expected to differ widely from other regions of low prevalence, a summary of management principles used in other areas (e.g. the USA) would be useful for purposes of comparison.

Second, the comprehensive presentation on programme management in developing countries must unfortunately be challenged and debated on a number of issues:

1. *National tuberculosis programme.* The structure presented of a national tuberculosis programme for developing countries based on the experiences of the IUATLD-assisted programmes is excellent but must of course be adapted to the needs and circumstances of each country and region. Although the structure in South Africa is very similar to that discussed, a Tuberculosis Advisory Group was introduced some years ago to advise the Department of Health on the control and management of tuberculosis.

2. *Treatment issues.* The use of streptomycin as a standard drug in the treatment of smear-positive cases must be questioned, especially in the wake of HIV infection and the doubtful efficacy of the drug (Raviglione *et al.*, 1992). The argument that streptomycin serves as a 'leash' is unacceptable; other methods to improve compliance should be designed.

   Also, the routine use of thiacetazone is no longer recommended, due to severe adverse effects in HIV-positive individuals and very high initial resistance rates reported in Africa (e.g. Zaire 80%, Rwanda 59.5%, etc. (Institute for Tropical Medicine, Belgium)).

   South Africa discontinued the routine use of thiacetazone 15 years ago and that of streptomycin 5 years ago. Both the World Health Organization and the IUATLD have recommended discontinuation of streptomycin and thiacetazone (Raviglione, 1992; IUATLD, 1991).

   It is astounding that, in view of the intricate and very complex interrelationships in Africa and the serious tuberculosis situation, we still opt for complicated, impractical, ineffective, treatment programmes which are not cost-effective. In Africa programmes involving an initial intensive supervised treatment phase followed by a less effective unsupervised phase should be discontinued as these regimens present logistic problems, are morally unacceptable and do not achieve the cure rate we so desperately need. Treatment programmes in Africa should be cure-directed, manageable, innovative and should be tailored to meet local needs and situations. All therapy should be fully supervised and a standard regimen containing at least isoniazid, rifampicin and pyrazinamide should be administered for 6 months.

For several years South Africa has been using the following regimen: Rifater-80 administered Mondays to Fridays only under full supervision on an ambulatory basis for 6 months. The use of a combination tablet is also in line with the IUATLD recommendations (IUATLD, 1991).

The cure rate in South Africa is approximately 75% and this is achieved mainly by maximizing community participation. The majority of patients are attached to a treatment supervisor or buddy in the community. Supervisors are in turn managed by appointed monitors. A case holding programme is presently being developed in the Western Cape which involves a reward or incentive system for both patients and supervisors.

3. *Monitoring of treatment results.* Bacteriological examination on entry and monitoring of treatment results for quarterly cohort analysis is certainly the ideal. This will, however, be difficult to achieve in developing countries with large patient loads and a lack of a well-established infrastructure.

4. *Case detection and diagnosis.* While agreeing that passive finding among suspects 'is the most important case-finding activity of any tuberculosis programme in developing countries' it is equally important to establish passive case finding facilities to create community awareness and to ensure alert and motivated health personnel. The effectiveness of passive case finding can, therefore, be improved by a triple strategy of increasing programme accessibility (convenient location, ready availability of diagnostic and treatment facilities), improving acceptability (rapid sympathetic patient handling) and educating the public.

Diagnosis by sputum smear microscopy remains the cornerstone in a successful tuberculosis programme. However, with increasing demands on both financial and human resources the feasibility of examining 'at least three specimens' from each suspect has to be questioned. Also, laboratory technicians require refresher training, supervision and motivation, and ongoing reviews of workload and efficiency should be made.

My personal view is that the emphasis should be on culture examination and that small decentralized culture laboratories should be established. Not only is diagnosis by culture definitive and logistically simpler, but this method also discovers more excreters than does diagnosis by microscope.

The discussion on key managerial and technical issue ends with three supportive activities, that is supervision, regular supply of drugs and a tuberculosis manual. Further issues which need to be addressed as key components of a successful tuberculosis control programme in developing countries include:

- *Surveillance*: Surveillance is an important tool in planning, managing and evaluating the tuberculosis control strategy. Surveillance can be epidemiological (e.g. risk of tuberculosis infection, drug resistance trends, tuberculosis meningitis rates, prevalence of HIV seropositivity in tuberculosis-infected and diseased persons), operational (e.g. BCG vaccination coverage, adherence to chemotherapy, patient and health system delay) or sociological (e.g. improvement in public knowledge, patient satisfaction).
- *Training of health care and laboratory workers*: Training general health care workers in techniques of BCG vaccination, tuberculin testing, communication, case finding and case holding, and to enable them to perform these activities as part of their daily work, is the cornerstone of programme implementation.

Programme management: developing countries—The era of HIV transmission

The following statement in the plenary paper is endorsed as of extreme importance 'the most important tool available to curtail the impact of HIV infection on the epidemiological situation of tuberculosis is scrupulous maintenance of a high cure and detection rate of smear-positive cases of tuberculosis.'

The above statement emphasizes the importance of case holding as the cornerstone of tuberculosis control.

While agreeing wholeheartedly with the views expressed regarding the management of tuberculosis cases with HIV infection and AIDS cases with tuberculosis infection, it is regretted that no mention is made of the HIV-infected person with a dormant tuberculosis infection (that is tuberculin positive skin test). It is well known that HIV infection will accelerate the development of active tuberculosis disease and vice versa (Narain *et al.*, 1992). It follows, therefore, that if we are serious in curtailing the transmission of the tubercle bacillus, every possible step should be taken to achieve this. In South Africa it is now policy to monitor closely all HIV-infected persons with a positive tuberculin test and if supervised treatment is possible, to consider treatment with Rifater-80 for 6 months.

In conclusion I permit myself the following comments:

1. We urgently need global commitment and a uniform plan of action to control the transmission of tuberculosis disease.
2. We must establish regional cross-border task forces to manage and coordinate effective, disciplined control programmes.
3. We must, as a matter of priority, ensure maximum community involvement and participation.

4. We must encourage multisectoral/disciplinary cooperation.
5. Our aim should be practical, effective, needs-directed, and community-based control measures.

References

IUATLD (1991) Meeting, Paris

Küster HGV (1993) *Epidemiological comments, 20*(1) January

Narain JP, Raviglione MC, Kochi A (1992) HIV-associated tuberculosis in developing countries: epidemiology and strategies for prevention. *Tubercle and Lung Disease, 73,* 311–321

Raviglione MC, Narain JP, Kochi A (1992) HIV-associated tuberculosis in developing countries: clinical features, diagnosis, and treatment. *Bulletin of the World Health Organization, 70*(4), 515–526

9
Resource allocation priorities: value for money in tuberculosis control

Christopher J.L. Murray

Harvard University, Cambridge, MA, USA

Introduction

Often the most useful recommendations to decision-makers such as how health moneys should be precisely spent are the hardest to ground in rational analysis. This chapter examines the question of how much should be spent on tuberculosis control. With the work of the last decade, do we have sufficient understanding of the cost-effectiveness of different health interventions and tuberculosis control in particular to estimate the share of health sector resources that should be spent on tuberculosis? Can the available body of evidence provide useful guidance on how moneys for tuberculosis control can best be spent to decrease the burden of tuberculosis on the individual and society? Such recommendations require extensive information including knowledge of the burden of different disease, the cost-effectiveness of most major health interventions, a detailed analysis of the cost-effectiveness of different tuberculosis control options and the human and physical resources of the health system. For each of these clusters of information, we do not have empirical estimates for all the relevant parameters.

We should draw two mutually compatible conclusions from this longstanding dilemma. First, the policy process continues despite inadequate information. Decisions must be and indeed are made. Decision-makers allocate resources between competing sectors and within sectors between programmes every year. It would be short-sighted and counter-productive to refuse to use what information is available to inform decisions. The appropriate response to the need for conclusions in the face of uncertainty is to make our most plausible estimates. Care must also be taken to highlight the fragility of many of the conclusions and the continued need to revise assessments as new information becomes available. Second, in settings

Tuberculosis: Back to the Future. Edited by J.D.H. Porter and K.P.W.J. McAdam
© 1994 John Wiley & Sons Ltd

where important allocation decisions are founded on partial information collected in widely differing environments, a premium is placed on new information acquired through operational research. From the following discussion built in many cases on weak data, a clear agenda for operational research will also emerge. Making best estimates for missing data does not belittle the value of sound research; rather it heightens awareness of the importance of research results for policy-makers.

The analysis in this chapter is based on a specific framework for resource allocation decisions. Two key assumptions underlie this framework. First, health resources should be allocated in such a way that the most health gains are achieved for the budget devoted to health. Other considerations beyond maximizing gains in health are not explicitly considered. For example, the distribution of health gains amongst different groups in the society is not explicitly incorporated. A focus on equity would only heighten the importance of tuberculosis control in many regions, as it remains a disease of the poor and disadvantaged. Second, we claim that health benefits can at present best be measured using disability adjusted life years (DALYs). DALYs are a measure of years of life lost due to a premature mortality and years of life lived with a disability (Murray, 1993). This measure, which forms the basis of the cost-effectiveness and burden of disease work presented by the World Bank in the *World Development Report 1993* on health (World Bank, 1993), is further described below. Taken together these assumptions imply that available health sector resources should be allocated in such a way as to maximize the number of DALYs averted.

Distributing resources for health between competing programmes in order to maximize the number of DALYs saved requires detailed information on the number of DALYs caused by each major health problem, the cost-effectiveness of major health interventions and available human, financial and physical resources. A decade ago such a sectoral approach to cost-effectiveness could not be entertained because so few studies have been completed with comparable methods. In the late 1980s, the World Bank stimulated the collation, reanalysis and new analysis of cost-effectiveness of many major health interventions (Jamison and Mosley, 1993). For the first time, cost-effectiveness estimates of nearly 75 interventions became available using comparable methods and assumptions. This body of work provides a rational framework within which we can evaluate the cost-effectiveness of tuberculosis control strategies and the comparative cost-effectiveness of controlling tuberculosis versus other health interventions.

The rest of the paper is structured in five parts: the burden of different forms of tuberculosis in terms of DALYs by region, the major interventions available to control tuberculosis and the share of the total tuberculosis burden that can be addressed with each, the cost-effectiveness of different control options, limitations of generalizing results from one environment to another, and the priority of tuberculosis within the overall health sector. A final discussion provides a summary of the major conclusions and some observations on priority areas for operational research on resource allocation for tuberculosis.

The burden of tuberculosis

For the evaluation of different health interventions, a general measure of health outcomes must be used (Murray, 1990). Most cost-effectiveness studies are now based on the years of life lost family of outcome indicators (Jamison and Mosley, 1993). For the 1993 *World Development Report*, a study was commissioned on *The Global Burden of Disease* (Murray *et al.*, 1993a). This study used a specific form of a years of life lost health indicator: disability adjusted life years (DALYs). This indicator captures years of life lost due to premature mortality and years of life lived with a disability, adjusted for the severity of the disability. The technical details of the indicator and the basis for the estimates for each disease are discussed in full in Murray *et al.* (1993a). The *Global Burden of Disease* (GBD) study provides estimates of DALYs for eight regions and over 100 health problems by age and sex including tuberculosis. Table 9.1 illustrates that tuberculosis accounts for 46.5 million DALYs lost each year. More than 3% of the total global burden of disease is due to tuberculosis. These figures confirm the tremendous importance of tuberculosis as a cause of both mortality and disability found in previous analyses (Murray *et al.*, 1990; Styblo, 1989).

Table 9.1 Disability adjusted life years from all forms of tuberculosis, 1990 (thousands)

Region	Male	Female	Total
Established market economies	106	46	152
Former socialist economies of Europe	308	53	361
Middle East, North Africa and south-west Asia	2 165	1 880	4 045
India	6 282	4 518	10 800
China	3 469	2 445	5 914
Other Asia and Pacific	5 165	3 771	8 936
Latin America and the Caribbean	1 508	1 061	2 569
Sub-Saharan Africa	7 464	6 209	13 673
Total	26 468	19 982	46 450

As the cost-effectiveness of interventions targeted to different forms of tuberculosis in HIV-positive and HIV-negative individuals will be different, we need to distinguish the burden of tuberculosis for these different forms. Table 9.2 provides estimates of the burden of tuberculosis disaggregated into pulmonary smear-positive, pulmonary smear-negative and extrapulmonary tuberculosis. The burden is also disaggregated into HIV-positive and HIV-negative tuberculosis. The estimates of HIV attributable tuberculosis burden, based on the calculations of Murray *et al.* (1993b), are crude, being derived from estimates of the TB/HIV coinfections. WHO estimates of the seroprevalence of HIV and prevalence of tuberculosis infection are used to estimate likely coinfections to which breakdown rates for TB/HIV coinfections observed in New York City intravenous drug users (Selwyn *et al.*, 1989, 1992) have then been applied. Some observations from sub-

Table 9.2   Disability adjusted life years from tuberculosis by type and HIV status, 1990

HIV status	Smear-positive	Smear-negative	Extrapulmonary	Total
HIV-negative	22 528	18 248	4 280	45 057
	48.5%	39.3%	9.2%	97.0%
HIV-positive	697	543	154	1 394
	1.5%	1.2%	0.3%	3.0%
Total	23 225	18 790	4 435	46 450

Saharan Africa suggest that these annual coinfection breakdown rates may be too high and the resulting estimates of HIV-positive cases exaggerated. Table 9.2 shows that in 1990, only 3% of the total burden of tuberculosis is in HIV-positives. This will undoubtedly increase by the end of the decade but will still be less than 10% of the total burden of tuberculosis.

The potential burden averted through different interventions

As addressed in several other chapters, many options are available for tuberculosis control programmes. Interventions fall into three large categories based on the technology involved: BCG, case treatment and chemoprophylaxis. For each intervention we need to understand its potential role in terms of the share of the total tuberculosis burden that can be addressed in the short and long terms.

BCG

BCG warrants little discussion in this context. First, it is already the most used immunization in the world with an estimated global coverage over 80% (UNICEF, 1992). Second, despite being the most popular immunization, its effectiveness in different environments remains uncertain (Rodrigues and Smith, 1990; Clemens *et al.*, 1983). Third, because BCG is given at birth and there is little or no evidence of an effect after 15 years, BCG has had little effect on the epidemiological trend of tuberculosis (Styblo and Meijer, 1976). There is no serious discussion of retrenching the coverage of BCG already achieved. Likewise, for the tuberculosis community to devote significant energy to increasing the coverage of BCG would appear to be unwarranted. Conveniently, BCG is administratively the province of the Expanded Programme of Immunization so that policy debate on tuberculosis need not focus on the ongoing BCG controversy. An open issue, however, is school age BCG revaccination. Several countries in eastern Europe and Latin America have at various times had BCG revaccination programmes. The efficacy of BCG revaccination has not been studied and should best be considered in the category of potential interventions that may warrant further operational research.

Case treatment

The second category of intervention, case treatment, can be divided into many sub-categories, four of which are emphasized here: chemotherapy of HIV-negative smear-positive pulmonary tuberculosis, chemotherapy of HIV-negative smear-negative pulmonary tuberculosis, chemotherapy of HIV-positive smear-positive pulmonary tuberculosis and chemotherapy for HIV-positive smear-negative pulmonary tuberculosis.

1. *Case treatment with short-course chemotherapy of HIV-negative smear-positive pulmonary tuberculosis cases passively detected by the health system.* This category of patients has long been the focus of tuberculosis control programmes. In 1990, it accounted for about 48% of the total burden of tuberculosis. WHO has established targets for developing countries to detect 70% of smear-positive cases and treat effectively 80% of those detected. While the majority of countries are far from achieving these targets, meeting these goals would avert only 56% of the current burden of smear-positive tuberculosis, slightly more than a quarter of the total burden of tuberculosis in the community. It is conceivable that a passive case detection system with heightened awareness of health care workers for the diagnosis of tuberculosis could increase case detection to greater than 80%, so that two-thirds of the current burden of smear-positive tuberculosis could be averted with this intervention.

These rough calculations of the current burden that can be addressed through the detection and treatment of smear-positive patients do not take into consideration that treating smear-positive tuberculosis patients will probably decrease the transmission of tuberculosis and the burden of tuberculosis in future years. Chemotherapy for smear-positives today may avert much more than a quarter of the burden of tuberculosis in 10 years. The cost-effectiveness studies on treating smear-positives indicate that for every DALY averted at the time of treatment, four will be averted over the next two decades (Murray *et al.*, 1991). Judging the desirability of investments in tuberculosis control as compared to other health interventions will be complicated by the multi-time period benefits of treatment.

We will not devote significant attention to the choice of two-drug 'standard' long chemotherapy regimens versus short-course regimens in the treatment of smear-positives. Cost-effectiveness studies have demonstrated that over a wide range of conditions, short-course regimens are more cost-effective (Barnum, 1986; Murray *et al.*, 1991; DeJonghe *et al.*, 1993). As most governments have indicated a desire to change to short-course regimens and WHO now recommends short-course regimens, it should no longer be a major tuberculosis policy debate.

2. *Case treatment with short-course chemotherapy of HIV-negative smear-negative pulmonary tuberculosis cases passively detected by the health system.* As with smear-positive tuberculosis, we will only discuss short-course regimens. The

rationale for using short-course regimens for smear-negatives is the same as for smear-positives. There is a clear relationship between the probability of default and the duration of treatment (Murray *et al.*, 1991b). Shortening regimens will increase the case completion rate and thus the cure rate. This is addressed further in the section on cost-effectiveness. With 80% case detection and 80% case cure, 64% of smear-negative burden could be averted or 25% of total tuberculosis burden. Eighty per cent case detection in countries with X-ray widely available in the periphery may not be unrealistic; many Asian countries with extensive access to chest radiography may have a problem of over-diagnosis rather than under-diagnosis.

3. *Case treatment with short-course chemotherapy of HIV-positive smear-positive pulmonary tuberculosis cases passively detected by the health system.* The total burden in 1990 is small, although relatively large in sub-Saharan Africa. By the year 2000, this category may account for nearly 4–5% of the burden of tuberculosis. The proportion of HIV-positive smear-positive tuberculosis cases that can be detected may not be substantially different from HIV-negatives judging by the large volume of HIV-positives diagnosed in Tanzania and Malawi. The impact of treatment has not been sufficiently studied. Evidence from Kenya suggests more than half of those completing treatment may relapse by 18 months (Nunn *et al.*, 1992). The attributed burden includes the stream of life lost due to death as a young adult. Treatment will not avert all the lost stream of life as the individual will probably succumb to some other opportunistic infection. If treating HIV-positives with tuberculosis adds 2–3 years of disability adjusted life (an optimistic assumption), treatment will alleviate only 10% of the current burden. As with treating HIV-negative smear-positives treatment may substantially reduce the future burden of tuberculosis through decreased transmission.

4. *Case treatment with short-course chemotherapy of HIV-positive smear-negative pulmonary tuberculosis cases passively detected by the health system.* The information on the feasibility of detection and treatment of HIV-positive smear-negatives is the least developed. One can observe that a relatively small proportion of the attributable burden can be directly averted through case treatment.

For each of these intervention categories, there is a complex array of detailed strategies. Different supervision strategies, drug regimens and health workers can be utilized. Supervision can differ in intensity, location and the health worker involved. Some, usually unsuccessful, programmes such as the government services in India may use largely self-administered regimens with no real supervision of chemotherapy. At the other extreme, a number of successful programmes will supervise all of the intensive phase of treatment (e.g. Tanzania, Malawi, Mozambique, Nicaragua) or even the entire continuation phase as well (e.g. China and Botswana). Fully supervised intensive or continuation phases can be delivered in hospitals, clinics, health posts or even on home visits. In Botswana, patients are often hospitalized for as long as is necessary to assure supervised chemotherapy. In the new programme in China, village doctors supervise chemotherapy at the village level on an ambulatory basis. Even the cadre of health worker used to supervise chemotherapy differs widely, from doctors in China, to nurses in Tanzania to family welfare educators in Botswana or community health volunteers in some parts of Bolivia. One general formula for success cannot be detailed. All the successful programmes, however, do have an emphasis on heavy supervision to ensure a high treatment completion rate. Failures such as the programme in New York City are characterized by virtually no supervision (Brudney and Dobkin, 1991; Bloom and Murray, 1992). The most appropriate method depends on the available infrastructure and cadres of health workers; in all settings, it forms a major cost of delivering short-course chemotherapy.

A wide array of drugs and regimen durations are in use in different programmes. The regimen used in a number of programmes supported by the International Union against Tuberculosis and Lung Disease (IUATLD), 2SHRZ/6HT, is an example of widely used short-course regimen. A number of programmes use shorter continuation phase regimens that include rifampicin such as 2SHRZ/4RH. The advantage of a four drug regimen in the intensive phase is not entirely captured in the cost-effectiveness analyses. The probability of secondary resistance and subsequent primary resistance in contacts is much lower. The clear relationship between the probability of default and the duration of treatment argues strongly for investing in the shorter regimens including shorter continuation phases.

Chemoprophylaxis

The third major category of tuberculosis interventions is chemoprophylaxis. This is the mainstay of control policy in the United States. The IUAT trial of chemoprophylaxis demonstrated that it can be up to 90% effective in preventing the breakdown of infection to disease (IUAT, 1982). The share of total tuberculosis burden that can be addressed with this intervention is difficult to assess. In most developing country settings where half or more of adults are infected, it is probably unfeasible to use chemoprophylaxis on all PPD-positives. Even if the decision analyses that suggest the risk of isoniazid hepatitis outweighs the benefits of decreased breakdown were applicable (Colice, 1990; Comstock and Edwards, 1975; Tsevat *et al.*, 1988; Taylor *et al.*, 1981; Rose *et al.*, 1986), the number eligible for chemoprophylaxis would be unfeasible. There are many reasons to question whether the US decision analyses are relevant to developing countries, particularly the assumed case fatality rate from tuberculosis.

Chemoprophylaxis of high risk groups is a more viable option. Candidate high risk groups must include PPD-positive children detected through contact tracing and HIV-positives. An extremely small share of the total current burden of tuberculosis could be addressed with contact tracing. For HIV-positives, feasibility studies are underway. Preliminary results from a trial in Uganda suggest that less than 10% of HIV/TB coinfected patients could be reached (WHO, unpublished). Within this group the total attributable burden that can be averted is restricted by the fact that HIV-positives will eventually die from other causes. If only 10% of the burden from HIV/TB can be averted with treatment, chemoprophylaxis will probably avert a tenth of that or 1%. While further data are urgently required on efficacy and feasibility, this is not an intervention that will avert a significant burden of tuberculosis. As with case treatment, it could decrease future burden through decreased caseloads and reductions in transmission.

Cost-effectiveness

Over the last 6 years, evaluation of short-course chemotherapy programmes in Malawi, Mozambique, Tanzania, China and Botswana have demonstrated that short-course chemotherapy for pulmonary smear-positives is extremely cost-effective (Murray et al., 1990, 1991, 1991b, DeJonghe et al., 1993; World Bank, 1991). Table 9.3 summarizes the average programme costs in four programmes when patients are hospitalized during the intensive phase of treatment. For the

Table 9.3 Summary of average programme cost per DALY averted with short-course chemotherapy with hospitalization during the intensive phase of treatment for pulmonary smear-positive tuberculosis (prices in US$ 1990)

Country	Cost per case treated	Cost per DALY averted
Botswana	367	6.2
Malawi	103	1.8
Mozambique	161	2.7
Tanzania	132	2.2

health sector resource allocation model discussed below, these are the most important unit costs as opposed to the average costs which include an arbitrary component of the infrastructure costs attributed to the tuberculosis programme. The use made of general health system resources by a particular programme is better captured directly in terms of the number of bed-days or clinic personnel hours consumed. The cost in dollars per patient treated and the cost per DALY averted through these interventions are provided. While the figures based on hospitalizing patients are substantially higher than ambulatory treatment, it is conservative to generalize the cost-effectiveness of chemotherapy for smear-positives on these numbers.

Few other health interventions except the package of childhood immunizations have been as extensively evaluated. The basic cost-effectiveness of short-course chemotherapy for smear positives appears to be a robust conclusion supported by

Table 9.4   The top ten most cost-effective health interventions

	Disease	Intervention	Cost per DALY
1.	Leprosy	Targeted screening	$0.5
2.	Tuberculosis	Short-course chemotherapy	$3
3.	Micronutrient deficiency	Fortification of sugar with vitamin A	$5
4.	Tetanus	Immunization	$6
5.	Tuberculosis	BCG added to DPT programme	$7
6.	Leprosy	Multidrug therapy clinic	$7
7.	Micronutrient deficiency	Iodization of salt or water	$8
8.	Measles	Immunization	$9
9.	Micronutrient deficiency	Semiannual vitamin A for children 0–5	$9
10.	Diarrhoeal diseases	Measles vaccine	$10

Note: Where cost per DALY is a range of values, calculations are based on the midpoint of that range.

results from countries with widely differing incomes per capita and health systems. With the World Bank Health Sector Priorities Review, it has emerged that chemotherapy for smear-positive tuberculosis is one of the five most cost-effective health interventions available (Table 9.4) (Jamison and Mosley, 1993).

Few programmes have cohort results of treatment for smear-negatives. In Botswana, where cohort results are available for all forms of tuberculosis, the results of treating smear-negatives are as good as for smear-positives (Murray *et al.*, 1993c). Not surprisingly, it is much more difficult to estimate formally the cost-effectiveness of treating smear-negatives. The direct benefits to the individual treated are easily calculated (Murray *et al.*, 1993b). As the case fatality rate for smear-negatives is lower than for smear-positives, the cost per DALY will be slightly higher. Cost-effectiveness for smear-negatives turns on two key issues: specificity of diagnosis and the transmission benefits. In regions where smear-negative diagnosis is largely based on chest radiographs, there is a major potential for false positive diagnosis. Second, the traditional viewpoint is that treating smear-negatives will have a minimal effect on decreasing transmission and the future incidence of tuberculosis. This may be incorrect. A proportion of smear-negatives progress to become smear-positive. Estimates range from approximately 5% to 50% over 5 years (Olakowski *et al.* 1972, Hong Kong Chest Service, 1984). Treating a smear-negative that may become a smear-positive will also have the extra bonus of preventing the significant component of pre-diagnosis transmission. Murray *et al.* (1991b) estimate that the cost per DALY of treating smear-negatives will be 3.5 to 8 times greater than treating smear-positives. Despite the higher cost, treating smear-negative tuberculosis would be one of the more cost-effective interventions available.

Cost-effectiveness of short-course chemotherapy for HIV-positive smear-positives has not been clearly defined. The direct benefit in terms of DALY averted in the individual treated is much reduced. Relative cost-effectiveness depends on the transmission potential for HIV-positive smear-positives. Are they more likely to transmit or at least transmit to groups at higher risk of subsequent breakdown? Or do they die sooner and thus have a lower transmission potential? Murray *et al.* (1991a) argued that if they transmit at the same rate as HIV-negatives, then the cost per DALY averted is only slightly more than for treating HIV-negatives, because transmission accounts for nearly four-fifths of the benefit. Recent studies suggest that the benefits may be overestimated as a high proportion of patients apparently relapse within a short period of time (Nunn *et al.*, 1993).

Cost-effectiveness of HIV-positive smear-negatives is extremely hard to assess. No hard evidence is available on either the direct benefits of treatment or the putative transmission benefits. In the absence of any information, one can only speculate that, as with HIV-negative smear-negatives, a proportion may progress to become smear-positive. Preventing this progression would be a worthwhile investment.

Chemoprophylaxis for HIV-positives is now a widely discussed intervention. Formal studies of the cost-effectiveness have awaited further clarification of the feasibility, costs and effectiveness of chemoprophylaxis. Pending real data, we can speculate on the cost-effectiveness of chemoprophylaxis. If the only benefits of chemoprophylaxis were averting the costs of treatment of future cases of clinical tuberculosis, would chemoprophylaxis be a good investment? With coinfection breakdown rates of 7% per year and assumed duration of HIV coinfection of 5 years, one would treat three to four patients to prevent one case, assuming 80% effectiveness. Is the true cost of chemoprophylaxis less than one-quarter of treatment? Counting costs of screening, drugs and delivery, chemoprophylaxis may not be cheaper than waiting for cases to develop. This speculation ignores the pre-diagnosis transmission that would be averted through chemoprophylaxis. If this were large, it could make chemoprophylaxis a desirable and cost-effective intervention.

Generalizing cost-effectiveness results

Each cost-effectiveness analysis is conducted for a specific programme in a particular social, economic, political and epidemiological environment. How confidently can we generalize the results of cost-effectiveness studies in one environment to another? There are two major factors that must be taken into consideration when using cost-effectiveness results from one setting and applying them to another: the cost of non-traded goods and differences in infrastructure.

Programme costs can be divided into traded goods and services and non-traded goods and services. The price of traded goods and services follows international markets closely so that they are relatively constant across different countries. For example, ignoring shipping costs, the cost of rifampicin is similar in Paraguay, Tanzania and the Philippines. The cost of non-traded goods and services, most notably labour, varies markedly from country to country in rough proportion to the gross domestic product (GDP) per capita. For example, generalizing costs from

Tanzania with an income per capita under $300 to a country in Latin America with an income 5 to 10 times higher would be inappropriate because the cost of labour will be much higher. A more recent study on the cost-effectiveness of chemotherapy in Botswana demonstrates that the cost of labour is nearly proportional to GDP per capita. In Table 9.3, the cost per DALY averted through chemotherapy is, not surprisingly, higher in Botswana.

Tuberculosis control strategies depend substantially on the infrastructure available. In rural sub-Saharan Africa, the network of clinics is often not accessible on a daily basis for many patients. Supervised chemotherapy must be delivered in some other setting such as a hospital or an intermediary facility. In China, the health system is extensive such that nearly every villager has easy access to a village doctor. Chemotherapy can be delivered to nearly all patients on an outpatient basis. Heavy investments in a deeper infrastructure mean that programme specific costs may be lower since hospitalization can be avoided. Tradeoffs between the development of infrastructure and the unit costs for a specific programme are not unusual. Similar results would be found for a wide range of programmes.

Chemotherapy for tuberculosis is so cost-effective that even if the studies are all underestimating the cost per DALY by a factor of ten, it still remains extremely cost-effective. This leeway allows generalization of cost-effectiveness results from one country to another with some confidence.

Tuberculosis as a health sector priority

Too much of the discussion of tuberculosis control emphasizes competing priorities within tuberculosis control. Should the focus of programmes be smear-positive or smear-negatives, HIV-negatives or HIV-positives etc.? Perhaps more important is establishing the relative importance of tuberculosis control as compared to other available health sector interventions. The cost-effectiveness principles can be applied to the health sector as a whole as well as to alternative disease control strategies. The information requirements for a sectoral approach to cost-effectiveness are heavy. We must know or estimate the cost-effectiveness of the major health interventions under consideration, the available infrastructure and its service capacity, the physical and social access of the population to different components of the health system, and the burden of disease. With this approach one can attempt to allocate health sector resources in such a way as to maximize the total number of DALYs averted throughout the health sector.

Two years ago such an ambitious approach to health sector priority setting could only be discussed not undertaken. With the codification of cost-effectiveness data by the World Bank and the elaboration of the *Global Burden of Disease* study, this approach is feasible. Using the algorithm developed by Murray *et al.* (1993d), we have estimated how resources should be allocated across interventions. Two aspects deserve note. Marginal costs of programmes are assumed to rise within districts and to be higher on average in more peripheral districts. The results make these estimates of total expenditure for tuberculosis conservative. Second, this framework includes improving infrastructure as an option so that the common criticism that the cost-effectiveness approach does not address the need for improvements in the health system does not apply.

The system that should be spent on tuberculosis depends critically on the total resources available for the health sector. As case treatment for smear-positive and smear-negative tuberculosis is relatively cheap when compared with many health interventions, even at low levels of health expenditure countries should invest to avert nearly all feasible cases of tuberculosis. In percentage of total budget terms, tuberculosis expenditure should be a very high percentage in a low budget environment and a declining percentage but increasing absolute amount as more resources for health are available.

The model predictions for sub-Saharan Africa illustrate that for a country that spends $10 per capita for all health services, $0.86 should be spent on tuberculosis control. This is an extraordinarily large share of the health budget reflecting the large existing burden and the potential to address more than half of the current burden and a larger share of the future burden with interventions that are cost-effective. Given the current level of expenditure in developing countries on health by the public sector, Table 9.5 shows the percentage of the entire annual health budget that should be spent on the tuberculosis control programme in two different regions. The shares differ by region for three reasons. First, labour costs are different in different regions. Second, the available infrastructure varies and finally, the burden of tuberculosis is also different. Tuberculosis case treatment is such a relatively attractive investment that in some environments the construction of new district hospitals may be warranted by the potential to expand tuberculosis treatment alone.

The logic of cost-effectiveness leads one to the conclusion that tuberculosis

Table 9.5 The optimal budget allocation for controlling tuberculosis. Estimates for average countries in different regions, based on a cost-effectiveness approach to health sector resource allocation

Region	Percentage of GDP spent by public sector on health	Percentage of public sector health budget that should be spent on tuberculosis	Optimal tuberculosis expenditure per capita (US dollars)
Sub-Saharan Africa	3.0	8.4	0.86
Latin America and the Caribbean	5.0	1.7	1.65
India	2.4%	4.5%	0.60
Other Asia and islands	4.0%	2.4%	0.94

control is heavily under-funded in nearly all countries. Exact information on the current expenditure for tuberculosis is hard to obtain. Budget data disaggregated by programme activity is not available for most governments. Based on estimates of the number of cases treated and the likely average cost per case treated, one can crudely estimate that currently only 300–500 million is spent on tuberculosis control. The model results suggest that the global total should be closer to 1.75 billion dollars per year. The shortfall of nearly one and quarter billion dollars must be filled.

Conclusions

Priorities within tuberculosis control given our current state of knowledge are: (1) case treatment with short-course chemotherapy of HIV-negative pulmonary smear-positives; (2) case treatment with short-course chemotherapy of HIV-positive pulmonary smear-positives; (3) case treatment with short-course chemotherapy of HIV-negative pulmonary smear-negatives; (4) case treatment with short-course chemotherapy of HIV-positive pulmonary smear-negatives; (5) chemoprophylaxis of PPD-positive close contacts; and (6) chemoprophylaxis of other high risk groups such as HIV-positives. This ranking is not based on hard evidence of the costs and effectiveness of each of these interventions. Rather, it is based on reasonable inference from past studies. Operational research is needed to confirm both the ordinal rank of these interventions but also the specific cost-effectiveness of each.

Several operational research priorities emerge from this uncertain ranking. First, studies on the natural history of smear-negatives are needed in order to establish the real transmission benefits of treating smear-negatives. I would argue there is already sufficient evidence to warrant investment in treating smear-negatives with short-course chemotherapy as cost-effective intervention. Second, countries with good cohort results of treatment for smear-positives should be encouraged to collect and collate similar data for the treatment of smear-negatives. Third, if treatment of smear-negatives becomes a more important priority, studies defining the most cost-effective drug combination and duration will be needed. Fourth, increased treatment of smear-negatives will require studies to defined diagnostic protocols that will minimize costly false positive diagnosis. Fifth, ongoing and further studies will help define the real direct and transmission benefits of treating HIV-positive smear-positives. While such studies will be informative, they are unlikely to alter the decision to treat HIV-positives. It is likely that few governments will choose to exclude tuberculosis patients who are found to be HIV-positive from treatment even if that treatment has a high cost per DALY. If this supposition is true, then operational research on the topic will not contribute substantially to the policy debate. Sixth, studies on the progression of HIV-positive smear-negatives as with HIV-negatives could substantially alter the perceived cost-effectiveness of treating smear-negatives.

From the health sector point of view, the first four interventions just listed are clearly good investments. Even low income countries, should invest in treating both smear-positives and smear-negatives with short-course chemotherapy. This is a radical departure from the traditional tuberculosis control message which emphasized the relative priority within tuberculosis of smear-positives. Major gains in averting the burden of tuberculosis remain to be achieved with improving and expanding short-course chemotherapy programmes for smear-positives. But, major gains can also be made in virtually every developing country by increasing resources for tuberculosis control to the point where short-course chemotherapy can be provided for smear-negatives as well. An urgent priority for WHO and other advocacy groups is to persuade governments that tuberculosis control is so attractive that major budgetary shifts are needed.

The extraordinary cost-effectiveness of most tuberculosis control efforts leads to a different set of operational research priorities than the traditional approach of looking for the best way to spread scarce tuberculosis control resources. The dictum that case treatment should be improved to the point where 80% of cases complete treatment before considering expanding case detection remains essentially true. Strategies to increase case detection once case treatment has been improved become options. More active methods of case detection may need to be re-evaluated. If the cost-effectiveness of virtually all forms of case treatment is widely appreciated, upgrading rural facilities to facilitate X-ray diagnosis of smear-negatives would be an immediate priority in a number of regions.

The HIV epidemic is a small component of the tuberculosis problem in 1990. Using the results of the estimates of HIV seroprevalence by age and sex for 2000 calculated by the WHO Global Programme on AIDS as part of the *Global Burden of Disease* study, we can calculate coinfection and likely numbers of HIV-positive tuberculosis cases. This is shown in Table 9.6 for the eight World Bank regions. By the end of the decade, there will be an extra 600 000 cases of tuberculosis. This assumes no increase in the annual risk of infection brought about by the extra HIV-

Table 9.6 Estimated HIV/TB coinfections and HIV-positive tuberculosis cases, in the year 2000 (figures in thousands)

Region	HIV-infected population	TB/HIV coinfections	HIV-positive tuberculosis cases
Established market economies	960	11	0.7
Former socialist economies of Europe	70	1	0.1
Middle East, North Africa and south-west Asia	170	48	3.4
India	6 211	2 560	179.2
China	72	26	1.8
Other Asia and Pacific	3 079	1 279	89.5
Latin America and the Caribbean	2 262	574	40.2
Sub-Saharan Africa	10 481	4 102	287.0
Total	23 305	8 601	602

positive cases, a conservative assumption. With an increased case load by the end of the century, the desirable level of expenditure on tuberculosis control in a cost-effectiveness framework will only be higher.

The message from cost-effectiveness studies is clear. Tuberculosis control is a highly attractive health intervention that is currently under-funded in nearly all regions of the world. Cogent advocacy is needed to convince donor agencies and governments that tuberculosis needs more resources. WHO, the World Bank and other agencies must provide the technical guidance and marginal resources required to improve case treatment programmes. Operational research should be pursued to provide answers to a range of questions on how to adapt successful programme strategies to differing environments and types of cases.

References

Barnum HN (1986) Cost savings from alternative treatments for tuberculosis. *Social Science and Medicine, 23*, 847–850

Bloom B, Murray CJL (1992) Tuberculosis: Commentary on a reemergent killer. *Science, 257*, 1055–1064

Brudney K, Dobkin J (1991) Resurgent tuberculosis in New York City: human immunodeficiency virus, homelessness, and the decline of tuberculosis control programs. *American Review of Respiratory Disease, 144*, 745–749

Clemens JD, Chuong JJH, Feinstein AR (1983) The BCG controversy: a methodological and statistical reappraisal. *Journal of the American Medical Association, 249*, 2362–2369

Colice GL (1990) Decision analysis, public health policy, and isoniazid chemoprophylaxis for young adult tuberculin skin reactors. *Archives of Internal Medicine, 150*, 2517–2522

Comstock GW, Edwards PQ (1975) The competing risks of tuberculosis and hepatitis for adult tuberculin reactors. *American Review of Respiratory Disease, 111*, 573–577

DeJonghe E, Murray CJL, Chum HG, Nyangulu DS, Salamao A, Styblo K (1993) *International Journal of Health Policy and Management* (In press)

Hong Kong Chest Service/Tuberculosis Research Centre, Madras/British Medical Research Council (1984) A controlled trial of 2-month, 3-month, and 12-month regimens of chemotherapy for sputum smear-negative pulmonary tuberculosis. *American Review of Respiratory Diseases, 130*, 23–28

International Union Against Tuberculosis Committee on Prophylaxis (1992) Efficacy of various durations of isoniazid preventive therapy for tuberculosis: five years of follow-up in the IUAT trial. *Bulletin of the World Health Organization, 60*, 555–564

Jamison DT, Mosley H (eds) (1993) *Disease Control Priorities in Developing Countries.* Oxford University Press for the World Bank, New York

Murray CJL (1990) Rational approaches to priority setting in international health. *Journal of Hygiene and Tropical Medicine, 93*, 303–311

Murray CJL (1993) Disability adjusted life years. In submission

Murray CJL, Styblo K, Rouillon A (1990) Tuberculosis in developing countries: burden, intervention and cost. *Bulletin of the International Union Against Tuberculosis and Lung Disease, 65*, 2–20

Murray CJL, DeJonghe E, Chum JH, Nyangulu DS, Salamao A, Styblo K (1991a) Cost effectiveness of chemotherapy for pulmonary tuberculosis in three sub-Saharan African countries. *Lancet, 338*, 1305–1308

Murray CJL, Lopez A, Jamison DT (1993a) *The Global Burden of Disease.* World Bank, Washington DC

Murray CJL, Styblo K, Rouillon A (1991b) Tuberculosis. In, Jamison DT, Mosley H (eds.) *Disease Control Priorities in Developing Countries*. Oxford University Press for the World Bank, New York

Murray CJL, Hamers F, Kumaresan J, Maganu E (1993c) Cost-effectiveness of short-course chemotherapy for tuberculosis in Botswana. In submission

Murray CJL, Kreuser J, Whang W (1993d) A cost-effectiveness model for allocating health sector resources. In preparation

Nunn P, Brindle R, Carpenter L et al. (1992) Cohort study of human immunodeficiency virus infection in patients with tuberculosis in Nairobi, Kenya: analysis of early (6 month) mortality. *American Review of Respiratory Diseases, 146*, 849–854

Nunn P, Gathua S, Kibuga D, Binge R, Brindle R, Odhiambo J, McAdam K (1993) The impact of HIV on resource utilization by patients with tuberculosis in a tertiary referral hospital in Nairobi, Kenya. *Tubercle and Lung Disease, 74*, 273–279

Olakowski T, et al. (1972) Controlled trials on BCG vaccine: vaccination of new born infants with BCG vaccine prepared from the French BCG substrain in Warsaw. *Gruzlica Chor, Pluc, 40*, 403–409

Rodrigues LC, Smith PG (1990) Tuberculosis in developing countries and methods for its control. *Transactions of the Royal Society of Tropical Medicine and Hygiene, 84*, 739–744

Rose DN, Schechter DB, Silver AL (1986) The age threshold for isoniazid chemoprophylaxis: a decision analysis for low-risk tuberculin reactors. *Journal of the American Medical Association, 256*, 2709–2713

Selwyn PA, Hartel D, Lewis VA et al. (1989) A prospective study of the risk of tuberculosis among intravenous drug users with human immunodeficiency virus infection. *New England Journal of Medicine, 320*, 545–550

Selwyn PA, Sckell Bm, Alcabes P (1992) High risk of active tuberculosis in HIV-infected drug users with cutaneous anergy. *Journal of the American Medical Association, 268*, 504–509

Styblo K (1989) Overview and epidemiological assessment of the current global tuberculosis situation with an emphasis on control in developing countries. *Reviews of Infectious Diseases, 11* (supplement 2), S339–S345

Styblo K, Meijer J (1976) Impact of BCG vaccination programmes in children and young adults on the tuberculosis problem. *Tubercle, 57*, 17–43

Taylor WC, Aronson MD, Delbanco TL (1981) Should young adults with a positive tuberculin test take isoniazid? *Annals of Internal Medicine, 94*, 808–813

Tsevat J, Taylor WC, Wong JB, Pauker SG (1988) Isoniazid for the tuberculin reactor: take it or leave it. *American Review of Respiratory Disease, 137*, 215–220

UNICEF (1992) *State of the World's Children*. Oxford University Press for UNICEF, New York

World Bank (1991) *China Infectious and Endemic Disease Project*. World Bank, Washington DC

World Bank (1993) *World Development Report 1993*. Oxford University Press for the World Bank, New York

Discussion

D.K. Kibuga, *Ministry of Health, Nairobi, Kenya*

Tuberculosis has been one of the top ten causes of morbidity and mortality in most of the developing world. Just as many countries were beginning to come up with well organized tuberculosis control programmes, the HIV pandemic has struck a devastating blow to control activities. This has resulted in a sharp rise in tuberculosis cases especially in the 15–35 year age group who are the most economically productive members of the society.

Any control activity resulting in an increase in the disability adjusted life years (DALY) saved is of benefit to the population in affected countries. We should, however, note that while in the developed world many governments have welfare packages for their citizens and feel financially responsible for the welfare of their citizens, in poorer countries many of the people affected with tuberculosis are the poor and self-employed individuals who are totally responsible for their own economic welfare. No welfare monies are paid to the unemployed in most of these countries. When we therefore sell the concept of DALY to the policy-makers, who are already economically strained and overburdened by too many requests for very little funds available, they are unlikely to buy it, since it implies that governments are taking total responsibility for the economic welfare of citizens who are supposed to look after themselves.

The association of tuberculosis with HIV and the unacceptability of the HIV pandemic as a disease like any other is also causing strains in some sectors of the administration when it comes to allocation of resources. Although short-course chemotherapy has been accepted as the most effective method of treatment worldwide, this means that a country has to spend more now to save in the future. Do many countries have enough resources to loan to the future?

The treatment of smear-negative tuberculosis with short-course chemotherapy is an even bigger economic burden because in the developing world diagnosis of smear-negative pulmonary tuberculosis has its handicaps in that x-ray facilities are expensive and therefore scarce and even where they exist, the shortage of radiologists is another handicap. Pathologists are also few. The clinical acumen of primary health care staff is also low and in many developing countries the doctor to population ratio is between $1:10000$ and $1:20000$ population.

When it comes to the treatment of HIV-associated diseases including tuberculosis, there has been considerable laxity in spending by administrators simply because of the stigma associated with HIV. When the issue of chemoprophylaxis is taken into account it is even more difficult to convince the treasuries that substantial amounts of money should be used to prevent a disease we are not sure is likely to occur, especially since the survival period with HIV is substantially lower in the Third World than in the Western World. Testing for HIV is quite expensive too and there is a marked shortage of counsellors.

Although short-course chemotherapy is more cost-effective than standard chemotherapy, the poorer countries need much support from richer countries to sustain such programmes. Are the richer countries always ready to assist?

A very high priority is health education to general health staff and the public to reduce the delay in diagnosis which sometimes extends several months in many countries.

Attention should also be drawn to countries where health facilities are highly inaccessible due to long distances and sparse population like the arid and semiarid parts of Africa. In these parts, modified forms of treatment like the manyatta programme of Kenya should be emphasized.

Tuberculosis control has to compete with other health problems and within tuberculosis control itself, allocation of funds should be based on priorities determined by cost-effectiveness of the intervention.

I will provide an example to illustrate the political implications of basing resource allocation on DALY. The example is a model Third World country named the Maskini Republic.

Example

Vital data of Maskini Republic

Population of 25 million
GNP per capita US$ 400
Health budget US$ 1000 million
Registered doctors 3000 (1 : 10 000)
Registered nurses 20 000 (1 : 1000)
Doctor's salary $100–300 per month
Nurse's salary $50–100 per month

Outpatient morbidity

Disease	No. of cases per year	Cost of one course of treatment
Malaria	5 000 000	$1
Diarrhoeal disease	700 000	$3
Acute respiratory infections	4 000 000	$2–5
Skin diseases	1 000 000	$5–10
Hypertension	150 000	$1000 per year
Diabetes	40 000	$700 per year
Tuberculosis	15 000	$150

From the above data it is apparent that the number of individuals who suffer from malaria and acute respiratory infections far outweights the number with tuberculosis, even if the DALY is not proportional. This has political implications in that the population will not support increased spending on tuberculosis, if it means reducing the expenditure on the other diseases. This is unrealistic in that some diseases like malaria and acute respiratory diseases are cheap to treat per patient compared to tuberculosis.

The budget allocation remains 20% of the requirement. The population therefore has to be convinced that allocation should not be uniformly distributed at 20% of requirements for each disease.

The low staff salaries have caused a low morale among staff with many resignations resulting in very poor staff performance. I feel the following order of priority should be followed:

1. Adequate funds for staff training, salaries and incentives.
2. Short-course chemotherapy for smear-positive tuberculosis.
3. Standard treatment for all other forms of tuberculosis.
4. Operational research
5. Chemoprophylaxis

Conclusions

1. While tuberculosis control is definitely a priority for governments worldwide, the allocation of resources is usually not proportional to the DALY saved by proper tuberculosis control.
2. While short-course chemotherapy for all forms of tuberculosis would be the ideal, many governments are not in a position to spend more now as an investment for the future. Non-governmental organizations (NGOs) and other donor organizations should be encouraged to assist the less rich governments.
3. Chemoprophylaxis is logistically different in areas where the prevalence of both tuberculosis and HIV is high.
4. The international professional community, especially tuberculosis control experts and organizations such as WHO and IUATLD, should direct their efforts to disseminating the knowledge already available on the need for adequate resource allocation for tuberculosis control by all governments.

10
Future research needs

Douglas B. Young

RPMS, Hammersmith Hospital, London, UK

Research perspectives

There are two general perspectives from which one can view research needs in tuberculosis. One line of reasoning is to suggest that, since tuberculosis is a disease for which (in most cases) an effective treatment is available, the role of research should be to provide tools which facilitate delivery of that treatment. Alternatively, one can reason that, despite the availability of effective treatment for more than 30 years, there has been a failure to control tuberculosis in most of the developing world, and research should therefore be set the broader goal of identifying radical new approaches to disease control. It is essential that both of these perspectives are included in designing a tuberculosis research programme. The need for development of tools to assist current control strategies is self-evident, but it is important that the dynamic of basic scientific research is also harnessed in pursuit of these goals. In envisaging a 'future' to which we might aspire to go back, tuberculosis research in the early 1950s provides an attractive model. The first antituberculosis drugs emerged from a research environment in which the best scientists of the day were dedicated to detailed and imaginative investigation of every possible aspect of the microbiology and pathogenesis of tuberculosis. In renewing our attempts to control the 'white plague', we must try and regenerate the scientific impetus and breadth of vision characteristic of that period of tuberculosis research.

Long-term goals

To motivate basic scientists, and to obtain the maximum benefit from scientific progress, tuberculosis research must stir the imagination as well as the social conscience. This can be achieved by setting demanding—'blue skies'—research goals which can in themselves be seen as providing a significant advance in the human condition. The goal of developing a tuberculosis vaccine provides just such

Tuberculosis: Back to the Future. Edited by J.D.H. Porter and K.P.W.J. McAdam
© 1994 John Wiley & Sons Ltd

a motivation. Undoubtedly, an effective vaccine could radically alter worldwide prospects for tuberculosis control; and, undoubtedly, vaccine development presents a major scientific challenge.

In search of protective immunity

Tuberculosis is not an inevitable consequence of infection with *M. tuberculosis*, and the concept of reinforcing the body's natural ability to cope with infection has obvious attraction as a means of tuberculosis control. At the dawn of the chemotherapy era in the 1950s, Dubos outlined the dramatic effect of changing social conditions on the incidence of tuberculosis and predicted that 'Tuberculosis will be conquered only when man has learned to function according to a physiological way of living that renders him more resistant to tubercle bacilli' (Dubos and Dubos, 1952). While nutritional and other factors associated with a 'physiological way of living' should not be forgotten, advances in scientific understanding—and, more acutely, the dramatic link between HIV-associated immunosuppression and tuberculosis—focus attention on strategies for direct stimulation of the immune system. To go back even further in search of a brave new future: at the start of the century we find Sir Ralph Bloomfield Bonington expostulating 'There is at bottom only one genuinely scientific treatment for all diseases, and that is to stimulate the phagocytes' (Shaw, 1906). While appreciating the scientific principle, we should bear in mind that, having killed his patient by its application, Sir Ralph later laments that 'if I didn't know as a matter of scientific fact that I'd been stimulating the phagocytes, I should say I'd been stimulating other things'. To understand protective immunity to *M. tuberculosis* at a cellular and molecular level is perhaps the most important research goal for the 1990s, with direct implications not only for vaccine development, but also for diagnosis, treatment, and epidemiology as described below.

From animal models of infection, and from the HIV epidemic, we know that T lymphocytes play a central role in protection against tuberculosis. Crude measurements of T cell activation—the PPD skin test response, or *in vitro* proliferation of peripheral blood lymphocytes—are capable of detecting exposure to *M. tuberculosis*, but are unreliable in distinguishing protected individuals from tuberculosis patients. Identification of immunological parameters which correlate wtih protective immunity would represent a crucial step towards vaccine development. Attempts to characterize the immune response have focused on analysis of T cell responses to individual antigenic components of the tubercle bacilli and, more recently, on analysis of the profile of cytokines released by activated immune cells. A broad spectrum of mycobacterial antigens has now been defined, with recombinant DNA techniques providing detailed structural information in many instances (reviewed by Young *et al.*, 1992). For the most part, it has not been possible to distinguish the response of tuberculosis patients from that of BCG vaccinees on the basis of antigen repertoire. A notable exception has been a recent report documenting a lack of response to one particular peptide-defined determinant in patients with active disease (Vordermeier *et al.*, 1992). Activation of different subsets of T cells—TH1 and TH2—resulting in release of different sets of soluble mediators, or cytokines, is an important factor in determining the outcome of infection (Sher and Coffman, 1992). The distinction between the different polar forms of leprosy is reflected in the particular pattern of cytokines seen within lesions (Yamamura *et al.*, 1991), for example, and there is considerable interest in the possibility that differences in cytokine profile may provide a measure of immune status in relation to *M. tuberculosis* infection. It is likely that protective immunity will come to be understood as a balance achieved by networks of locally interacting cells, rather than as the action of a single subset of specifically 'protective' cells. Cytokines represent one mechanism utilized by the immune system to coordinate such multicellular interactions.

Unravelling the tubercle bacillus

While protective immunity remains an elusive goal, the last few years have seen distinct progress in the microbiology of tuberculosis, with the introduction of modern molecular genetics (reviewed by Young and Cole, 1993). The goal of such research is to understand virulence; to identify at a molecular level the properties of *M. tuberculosis* which are responsible for causing disease. At present we have no idea why BCG, or the H37Ra isolate of *M. tuberculosis*, differ from virulent strains in their ability to cause disease, but the availability of detailed information on the structure of mycobacterial genomes (Eiglmeier *et al.*, 1993), along with the ability to transfer genes between mycobacterial strains (Snapper *et al.*, 1988), will undoubtedly provide new insights into such questions within the next few years. Bacterial pathogens must generally adapt their patterns of gene expression in order to assume an appropriate phenotype for optimal survival within the environment of the infected host (Miller *et al.*, 1989), and it seems most probable that adaptation will similarly hold the key to understanding the virulence of *M. tuberculosis*. In terms of disease control, an understanding of virulence will contribute to development of rationally attenuated variants of *M. tuberculosis* perhaps surpassing BCG in vaccine efficacy, and may also lead to the identification of novel immune targets. While T cell stimulation will obviously represent the primary target for immune intervention, the possibility that antibodies directed to specific surface structures might be used to modulate certain stages of *M. tuberculosis* infection cannot be discounted. The lack of efficient methods for generation of defined *M. tuberculosis* mutants remains an important technical limitation for these studies. Another major microbiological goal is to understand the phenomenon of mycobacterial persistence. The nature of tuberculosis as a reactivation disease, and the requirement for extended chemotherapy, both suggest an ability of *M. tuberculosis* to persist in some 'dormant' form in infected tissues. Understanding of the molecular basis of persistance could have a profound impact on disease control.

Interventions designed to 'activate' dormant *M. tuberculosis* could contribute to shortening of treatment schedules; while the reverse strategy might be used to prevent reactivation disease.

HIV and M. tuberculosis

Characterization of the deadly synergy between HIV and *M. tuberculosis* represents another key area for basic research. Enhanced susceptibility to tuberculosis occurs at a relatively early stage in the course of HIV infection—prior to development of susceptibility to *Mycobacterium avium-intracellulare*, for example—and detailed analysis of the immune status of individuals at this stage of disease might provide insights relevant both to HIV-associated tuberculosis, and to the more 'conventional' reactivation disease. Identification of the mechanisms by which tuberculosis potentiates progression of HIV also represents an important basic research goal with obvious relevance to development of improved treatments for dually infected populations.

Short-term goals

While the grand goals of protective immunity and virulence will provide the impetus for fundamental research in tuberculosis, it is important that the energy and ideas from such research are used to drive progress in development of tools of immediate use in current disease control programmes.

Diagnostic tools

Improvements in the diagnosis of tuberculosis have been based on improved understanding of clinical features of disease and, over the last century, on refinement of techniques for detection of *M. tuberculosis*. Molecular biology has provided important new possibilities for detection of bacteria. Techniques based on the polymerase chain reaction (PCR) present the potential for detecting very small numbers of bacteria in a matter of hours, and clearly this goal is being achieved in many laboratories (e.g. Brisson-Noel *et al.*, 1991; Eisenach *et al.*, 1991). Inherent in the exquisite sensitivity of PCR, however, are problems of laboratory contamination, and it can be questioned whether the technique in its present form is sufficiently robust to be suitable for widespread clinical application. Such problems are not specific to tuberculosis and it is probable that the considerable financial market available for such tests will stimulate development of improved PCR—or related DNA amplification techniques—during the next few years. An alternative application of molecular biological techniques has been pioneered by Dr Jacobs and his colleagues at the Albert Einstein College of Medicine in New York. Applying the principle of constructing a bioluminescent reporter phage, they have developed an approach which has the attraction of reflecting not only the presence, but also the viability, of mycobacteria. Development of such innovative approaches into clinically useful protocols represents a major research goal.

Recent excitement in relation to implementation of molecular biology techniques has diverted attention from development of diagnostic techniques based on detection of the disease process. Characterization of defined mycobacterial antigens, and advances in understanding of the immune response, offer the potential for development of novel immunodiagnostic tests. Tests based on measurement of circulating antibodies have been evaluated in many laboratories using crude antigen extracts, or purified defined antigens (reviewed by Ivanyi *et al.*, 1988). Antibody levels reflect the antigen load and, under optimal conditions, such serological tests have a sensitivity comparable to that of bacterial smear analysis. Large numbers of serological assays can be conducted in centralized facilities and, in some circumstances, this may be seen as providing a technical advantage over smear analysis. The nature of the immune response to tuberculosis makes it attractive to think in terms of development of improved immunodiagnostic tests based on measurement of T cell reactivities. Three types of improvement on the present PPD skin test could be envisaged. Firstly, the PPD reagent is difficult to standardize from batch to batch, and it would be advantageous if it could be replaced by one or more defined antigens eliciting a response with similar sensitivity. Secondly, it would be useful to generate a skin test reagent—based on a species-specific antigen, for example—which would discriminate between BCG vaccination and exposure to *M. tuberculosis*. Finally, it is attractive to envisage a reagent which could discriminate between the immune response resulting from exposure, or subclinical infection with *M. tuberculosis*, from the response associated with onset of clinical disease. In order of increasing complexity, these represent three important practical goals driven by the basic studies of *M. tuberculosis* antigens described above.

Drugs and drug resistance

The emergence of multidrug-resistant tuberculosis in the United States has had a dramatic effect on prospects for new drug development. A number of pharmaceutical companies are interested at least in screening available compounds for reactivity against *M. tuberculosis*. There is a particular interest in developing screens based on defined *M. tuberculosis* enzymes, or metabolic pathways, since such systems would provide a feasible starting point for future drug development programmes. This initiative from pharmaceutical companies will provide a stimulus for further biochemical and genetic characterization of biosynthetic pathways in *M. tuberculosis*. Enzymes which are specific to the mycobacteria—for example, those involved in cell wall biosynthesis—are seen as being especially interesting in this regard.

There has been a corresponding revival of interest in elucidating the mechanisms involved in action of established drugs and in determining the genetic basis of drug resistance. A key role for the catalase-peroxidase enzyme in the action of isoniazid has recently been demonstrated, with deletion of the corresponding gene accounting for drug resistance in some clinical isolates of *M. tuberculosis* (Zhang *et al.*, 1992). Point mutations in genes encoding RNA polymerase are associated with development of resistance to rifampicin (Honore and Cole, 1993). Development of techniques for genetic manipulation of mycobacteria opens a range of new research possibilities in this area, and it is likely that mechanisms for susceptibility and resistance to all of the major antituberculosis drugs will be elucidated within the next few years. Development of rapid tests for drug resistance will also have a high priority. It can be envisaged that these may be based either on tests specific for individual drugs, or perhaps single tests which, like the bioluminescent reporter phage, can be used to screen for resistance to a panel of drugs.

Contingent on progress in fundamental research, it is worthwhile considering the possible development of drugs targeted, not at the bacteria, but at specific host functions. Agonists, or antagonists, related to immune activation and cytokine networks would be obvious candidates, although at present it is difficult to envisage how such treatments could be administered to elicit local responses against infection, without triggering potentially damaging systemic effects.

Epidemiological tools

Progress in research on the genome structure of mycobacteria has provided a new epidemiological tool in the technique of DNA fingerprinting (Van Embden *et al.*, 1993). Typing methods based on the IS*6110* repetitive element have been used to demonstrate transmission of individual strains in local outbreaks—including those involving multiple drug resistance (Daley *et al.*, 1992)—and will be useful in establishing the relative contributions of reactivation and reinfection in onset of clinical disease. The availability of efficient strain typing methods, along with improved immunological tools for monitoring infection and disease as discussed above, will promote increased research on the epidemiology of tuberculosis. Insights into the role of genetic and environmental factors in determining variations in tuberculosis incidence and vaccine efficacy amongst different populations will be of fundamental importance in designing improved strategies for disease control.

Priorities and resources

Assessment of priorities will always have a strong subjective element. At the top of my own list would be the need to maintain a close link between the ambitious 'blue skies' research and the more applied practical goals outlined above. Different funding agencies will obviously highlight different areas. Research on elucidation of the basic mechanisms of protective immunity and virulence is likely to be funded by national agencies—the Medical Research Council in the UK, for example, and more recently, the National Institutes of Health in the USA—and clearly must be able to compete with other disciplines in terms purely of scientific merit. Funding agencies with closer links to tuberculosis control programmes are likely to favour funding of research with more immediate clinical connection. Research funding by the private sector will be an increasingly important factor. Renewed public concern about tuberculosis in developed countries, and the emergence of multidrug-resistant strains, provides an important market for new drugs and diagnostic kits. The involvement of pharmaceutical companies was an essential factor in development of the first generation of drugs against *M. tuberculosis*, and as we proceed 'back to the future', the pharmaceutical industry and smaller biotechnology companies will again have a key role in translating research efforts into new tools for disease control.

References

Brisson-Noel A, Aznar C, Churea C *et al.* (1991) Diagnosis of tuberculosis by DNA amplification in clinical practice evaluation. *Lancet, 338*, 364–366

Daley CL, Small PM, Schechter GF *et al.* (1992) An outbreak of tuberculosis with accelerated progression among persons infected with the human immunodeficiency virus. An analysis using restriction-fragment-length-polymorphism. *New England Journal of Medicine, 326*, 231–235

Dubos R, Dubos J (1952) *The White Plague. Tuberculosis, Man, and Society*. Rutgers University Press, New Jersey

Eiglmeier K, Honore N, Woods SA, Caudron B, Cole ST (1993) Use of an ordered cosmid library to deduce genomic organisation of *Mycobacterium leprae*. *Molecular Microbiology, 7*, 197–206

Eisenach KD, Siffird MD, Cave MD, Bates JH, Crawford JT (1991) Detection of *Mycobacterium tuberculosis* in sputum samples using a polymerase chain reaction. *American Review of Respiratory Disease, 144*, 1160–1163

Honore N, Cole ST (1993) The molecular basis of rifampicin resistance in *Mycobacterium leprae*. *Antimicrobial Agents and Chemotherapy, 37*, 414–418

Ivanyi J, Bothamley GH, Jackett PS (1988) Immunodiagnostic assays for tuberculosis and leprosy. *British Medical Bulletin, 44*, 635–649

Miller JF, Mekalanos JJ, Falkow S (1989) Coordinate regulation and sensory transduction in the control of bacterial virulence. *Science, 243*, 916–922

Shaw GB (1906) *The Doctor's Dilemma*. Penguin, Harmondsworth (1975 edition)

Sher A, Coffman RL (1992) Regulation of immunity to parasites by T cells and T cell-derived cytokines. *Annual Review of Immunology, 10*, 385–409

Snapper SB, Lugosi L, Jekkel A, Melton RE, Kieser T, Jacobs WR (1988) Lysogeny and transformation in mycobacteria: Stable expression of foreign genes. *Proceedings of the National Academy of Science of the USA, 85*, 6987–6991

Van Embden JDA, Cave MD, Crawford JT *et al.* (1993) Strain identification of *Mycobacterium tuberculosis* by DNA fingerprinting: Recommendations for a standardized methodology. *Journal of Clinical Microbiology, 31*, 406–409

Vordermeier HM, Harris DP, Friscia G *et al.* (1992) T cell repertoire in tuberculosis: selective anergy to an immunodominant epitope of the 38-kDa antigen in patients with active disease. *European Journal of Immunology, 22*, 631–2637

Yamamura M, Uyemura K, Deans RJ *et al.* (1991) Defining protective responses to pathogens: Cytokine profiles in leprosy lesions. *Science, 254*, 277–279

Young DB, Cole ST (1993) Leprosy, tuberculosis, and the new genetics. *Journal of Bacteriology, 175,* 1–6

Young DB, Kaufmann SHE, Hermans PWM, Thole JER (1992) Mycobacterial protein antigens: a compilation. *Molecular Microbiology, 6,* 133–145

Zhang Y, Heym B, Allen B, Young D, Cole S (1992) The catalase-peroxidase gene and isoniazid resistance of *Mycobacterium tuberculosis. Nature, 358,* 591–593

Discussion

Barry R. Bloom, *Albert Einstein College of Medicine, New York, USA*

I cannot forgo noting the fact that the session on Future Research Needs follows that on Resource Allocation. I am afraid that may be significant, and may imply that research is something to consider if there are any funds left over after allocations have been made for other important things. In fact, why do we need research? Let me suggest three reasons: (i) The obvious one is when we need to know something more or gain greater understanding. (ii) I believe we also need research when we think we know something important. Let me remind you that there are few fields that have promised more and disappointed expectations more than TB. In 1890 Robert Koch reported the 'cure' for tuberculosis; In the 1920s Calmette promised us the vaccine; and in the 1940s Waksman had the drug for TB. (iii) I will argue that we also need research to mobilize resources as well.

Studies on the burden of disease have a history that begins in London. The first epidemiological work ever published in English was that of John Graunt, Citizen of London, in 1662, who carried out the first assessment of the burden of disease by looking at Bills of Mortality in London. Graunt found TB to be responsible for 19% of the deaths in London, and regrettably it has remained worldwide the largest cause of death from a single infectious agent ever since.

Dr Young did a wonderful job of reviewing the biomedical research challenges, and I can add little but some of my enthusiasms. Basic molecular genetic systems have been developed over the past 5 years that now allow scientists to move genes in and out of the genome of the tubercle bacillus or BCG and to uncover the precise molecular basis for drug action and resistance in tuberculosis. In just the past year the target molecules for isoniazid, rifampicin, streptomycin and ethambutol resistance have been molecularly characterized. Several gene amplification techniques offer the possibility of more rapid diagnosis, but are technically demanding and costly, and it remains unclear whether they are optimal for clinical use in industrialized countries, let alone in developing countries at present. We can study pathogenesis by putting genes from virulent strains into avirulent ones. By screening libraries of H37Rv made in H37Ra, it has been possible, for example, to isolate certain cosmid clones from mice containing specific DNA sequences associated with more rapid growth in lungs and spleen of mice, possibly relating to virulence. The TB Genome Project will define every gene, every antigen, every enzyme, every drug target over the next 4–5 years. The principle genetic tool ultimately limiting our understanding of the molecular basis of drug resistance of pathogenesis remains the peculiar inability to obtain homologous recombination that would enable gene replacement to be carried out in slow growing mycobacteria.

Together with Bill Jacobs we have tried to develop a very simple and hopefully inexpensive test for rapidly assessing drug sensitivities. It is based on luciferase, the enzyme that makes fireflies glow and which represents the most sensitive known biological reporter molecule. Firefly luciferase depends on ATP levels, perhaps the best measure of cell viability we have, to produce quanta of light in cells possessing ATP. We deliver luciferase by a recombinant mycobacteriophage which, if the cells are drug resistant, produces light, but if susceptible, produce no or reduced signals. We have now applied that assay successfully to multidrug-resistant (MDR) strains in New York City in our laboratory with some success, but it remains now to adapt the assay to early detection of a small number of organisms in clinical specimens.

There is lots about the pathogenesis of TB we do not understand. We do not know how the bacillus gets into the body from the outside world, how it attaches to cells, how it is taken into cells, how it survives the cytocidal mechanisms of the macrophages, how it is transported from the initial site to distant sites, how it causes disease or even why it kills. One of the areas we thought we did understand is that *M. tuberculosis* entered macrophages and grew only in the phagocytic vacuoles by inhibiting the fusion of lysosomes containing the killing armamentarium. We have recently found that they can escape from the phago-lysosome into the cytoplasms, so that we probably have to rethink how and where we need to target drugs, and whether bacilli in the cytoplasm of infected cells are responsible for killing them.

The overarching problem in immunology is to understand the mechanisms of protection and proceed logically from there to identify the antigens that engender them. As the epidemiologists have been happy to remind us, the correlation between skin test positivity and protection in BCG trials is imperfect. Our hypothesis was that there might be another immunological mechanism involved in protection that is not reflected in a positive skin test. The availability of transgenic 'knockout' mice with disruptions in genes associated with specific immune functions offers an extraordinary opportunity to analyse *in vivo* immunological mechanisms necessary and sufficient for protection. For example, mice whose β_2-microglobulin gene has been disrupted cannot make or express MHC Class I antigens on any cell of the body. Since cytotoxic T lymphocytes (CTL) are dependent on MHC Class I antigen presentation, these mice lack the ability to generate or use CD8 CTL. Our results indicated that while control mice survive 10^6 *M. tuberculosis* for 20 weeks, 75% of the β_2M-mice (mice whose β_2 microglobulin has been disrupted) are dead in 3 weeks. Most gratifying was the finding that they had developed pathology, including breakdown of granulomas into the bronchioles and beginnings of cavity formation, resembling human pathology. Ian Orme and our group have similarly challenged mice that have a disruption in the gene for IFNγ and then found them to be equally susceptible. We have used monoclonal neutralizing antibodies to tumour necrosis factor (TNF) and found that such mice also become highly susceptible to *M. tuberculosis*. Finally, although it is widely believed that TNF is responsible for production of granulomas and for tissue damage associated with TB, we find using a monoclonal neutralizing antibody to TNF that infected animals die rapidly, but do form granulomas and tissue necrosis. Thus TNF is also needed for protection and necrosis can occur in the absence of TNF. My point here is that we still do not have an adequate understanding of the immune components required for generating pathology or protection. Since BCG does not kill in the β_2M-'knockout' mice, these results suggest that one reason that BCG is not an ideally effective vaccine is that it neither needs, nor perhaps generates, appropriate killer T cells required for protection. Another inference would be that, from the point of view of immunology, the proper study of tuberculosis is *M. tuberculosis*.

There is much about epidemiological and operational field research that is just as important as laboratory-based research in learning how to apply the currently existing drugs and tools more effectively, and which I have not time to discuss. Let me only say that no research in the last 30 years has had greater impact on TB than the operational research of Styblo that enabled control programmes to succeed in developing countries. One final reason for my excitement is that molecular tools have been developed that may make a real contribution to the epidemiology of tuberculosis. DNA fingerprinting or restriction fragment length polymorphisms (RFLPs) permit us, albeit in a crude way, to mark individual strains. While most studies have been used to show that outbreaks in nosocomial settings are caused by a limited number of strains, the real power of technology is to apply it out of the hospital, to find out the life and dynamics of the individual strains, particularly MDR strains, and follow their transmission within the community, or even between countries.

In many respects, as Dr Nabarro of the Overseas Development Administration pointed out, TB is a problem of resource allocation. Resources for overseas development, and particularly health, have been flat or declining for many years. If we care about TB we must make the best case we can to obtain resources to address the problem. The burden of TB is an important, but not sufficient argument, since TB has been a major burden since the 17th century. If the only strategies we can conceive of developing are better 'case finding' and 'case holding', I do not believe we can attract the support we need. There is an undercurrent in the TB community that control and research activities are separate, and that research represents a diversion of resources from the important priorities. My belief is that everyone has something to contribute to the problem of TB. We must realize that TB keeps changing and that we constantly need better tools; otherwise, if our tools are so terrific, an agency could legitimately enquire why there is a problem? Finally it is my fervent hope that we can all recognize a shared and common interest between control and research activities, if we are to bring new people, new approaches and new resources to the problem of tuberculosis.

11
Multidrug resistance

The New York Experience

Dale L. Morse, *PHLS Communicable Disease Surveillance Centre, London, UK and Bureau of Communicable Disease Control, Albany, New York, USA*

> Darkling I listen; and, for many a time
> I have been half in love with easeful Death,
> Call'd him soft names in many a mused rhyme,
> To take into the air my quiet breath;
> Now more than ever seems it rich to die,
> To cease upon the midnight with no pain,
>
> 'Ode to a Nightingale', John Keats (1795–1821)

Introduction

In the 18th century of Keats, tuberculosis (TB) was not only common in England, but was one of the leading causes of death in the United States and New York State (Dubos and Dubos, 1987). In the early 1990s sanatoria were built to isolate infectious patients from society and provide supportive care. In the absence of effective drugs, TB mortality approached 50% (Bloom and Murray, 1992).

The introduction of effective chemotherapy in the 1950s made tuberculosis a curable disease and contributed to average declines in TB incidence rates of 6% per year until the 1980s. This decline was halted by the HIV epidemic which has contributed to an estimated excess of up to 50 000 TB cases in the USA since 1980.

In New York State (population approximately 18 million) the resurgence of TB has been even more dramatic with a doubling of cases since 1978 (Figure 11.1). This increase was most dramatic in New York City (NYC) where case rates have exceeded 50 per 100 000 and are approximately five times those for the United States (Table 11.1). This increase was associated primarily with the HIV epidemic, but was also linked to homelessness, immigration, intravenous drug use,

Tuberculosis: Back to the Future. Edited by J.D.H. Porter and K.P.W.J. McAdam
© 1994 John Wiley & Sons Ltd

poverty and poor access to primary health care (Snider and Roper 1992). Indeed, the geographic distribution of TB cases in NYC (Figure 11.2) has been very similar to that seen for HIV and for a number of socio-economic factors (Morse *et al.*, 1991).

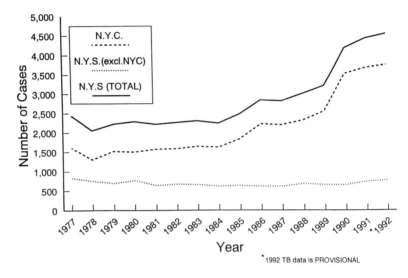

Figure 11.1 Reported tuberculosis cases in New York State 1977–92. Source: TB Control Program, BCDC. NYS Department of Health

Table 11.1 Tuberculosis case rates per 100 000, NYC, NYS (excluding NYC) and the USA, 1982–1992[a]

Year	New York City	New York State (excl. NYC)	United States
1982	22.7	6.5	11.0
1983	23.3	6.3	10.2
1984	22.9	5.9	9.4
1985	25.7	6.1	9.3
1986	30.7	5.8	9.4
1987	30.0	5.8	9.3
1988	31.7	6.5	9.1
1989	34.5	6.2	9.5
1990	48.1	6.1	10.0
1991	50.2	7.0	10.4
1992[a]	51.1[a]	7.3[a]	[b]

Source: TB Control Program, BCDC NYS Department of Health.
[a] 1992 TB data for New York is provisional.
[b] 1992 TB data for USA is not yet available.

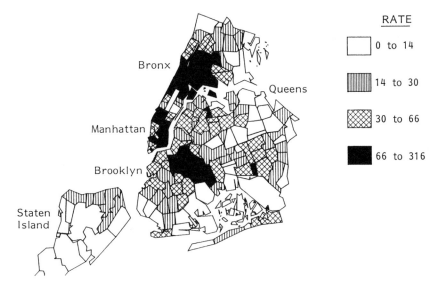

Figure 11.2   New York City TB incidence, rate per 100 000, 1991

Emergence of multidrug resistant tuberculosis (MDR-TB)

NYC nosocomial MDR-TB outbreaks

While drug-resistant TB had long been recognized as a treatment issue for individual patients (e.g. TB patients who were foreign born, homeless, recalcitrant or had reactivated TB) MDR-TB only surfaced as a major public health issue in the 1990s. On 30 August 1991 the Morbidity and Mortality Weekly Report reported on four outbreaks of nosocomial transmission of MDR-TB, three of which occurred in NYC (Centers for Disease Control, 1991). These outbreaks were noteworthy because of widespread transmission of MDR-TB to patients and staff (Pearson *et al.*, 1992; Edlin *et al.*, 1992; Busillo *et al.*, 1992). Cases were predominantly HIV infected and had high mortality rates (70–90%) and extremely short survival (median of 4–16 weeks from diagnosis until death) (Centers for Disease Control, 1991). The MDR-TB strain at one hospital (Hospital C) was resistant to seven of the most common TB drugs with the potential of taking us back to the TB era of the 18th century when TB was virtually untreatable. The potential implications of these findings were staggering. While the federal, state and city health officials began to take action and prepare for the onslaught of expected publicity and public reactions, surprisingly little happened when the article was published. The phones were relatively silent, perhaps because of the perception that what happened in the '4th World County' of NYC was not relevant to the rest of the world.

The Syracuse MDR-TB hospital outbreak

In September 1991, the New York State Department of Health learned about a cluster of PPD skin test conversions in health care workers (HCWs) in an Upstate New York hospital. An epidemiological investigation identified 46 HCWs with new TB infections and showed an association with exposure to an HIV-infected prisoner who had been admitted for treatment (Ikeda *et al.*, 1992). He had 7-MDR-TB with the same antibiotic and restriction fragment length polymorphism (RFLP) pattern as that seen in NYC Hospital C. Subsequent epidemiological, environmental and laboratory evidence also supported nosocomial transmission of the same strain of 7-MDR-TB resulting in tuberculosis disease in three patients and the inmate's guard (three of whom died), a pathologist (needlestick granuloma), and two HCWs along with evidence for PPD conversions in two autopsy department staff. Unlike the outbreaks in NYC, this outbreak resulted in widespread publicity; in threatened industrial action by prison officers, health care workers and their unions; and in a general awakening of the public at large who finally became cognizant of the implications of what was happening in New York City.

MDR-TB in New York State prisons

The Syracuse hospital outbreak identified the same 7-MDR-TB strain in six inmates; four from the same prison. An investigation at that prison identified eight inmates with epidemiological links to each other and TB isolates indistinguishable by RFLP (Centers for Disease Control, 1992). In addition, 30% of inmates at the prison had converted their PPD skin tests since beginning incarceration. A subsequent review of MDR-TB isolates from the entire 68 000 inmate New York State Correctional System demonstrated that the 7-MDR-TB strain had been introduced into as many as 23 prisons with at least 26 inmates with MDR-TB having been previously hospitalized at NYC Hospital C (Valway *et al.*, 1992). As inmates are moved frequently from prison to prison for security reasons and are released after an average incarceration time of 2 years, there is ample opportunity for transmission of this strain within prisons and to the general community.

Additional evidence for MDR-TB spread

Since 1991, additional hospital outbreaks of MDR-TB have been identified and are under investigation in NYC. A retrospective study of TB cases at one NYC hospital has showed 21% of homeless individuals to have drug resistance compared to 8% in non-homeless persons (Pablos-Mendez *et al.*, 1990). A 1 month laboratory survey of all TB isolates in NYC in April 1991 showed resistance to one or more drugs in 33% of patients and to isoniazid (INH) and rifampicin in 19% of patients (Frieden *et al.*, 1992). For new TB patients, resistance to one or more anti-TB medications had increased from 10% in 1982–1984 to 23% in 1991: combined resistance to INH and rifampicin had increased from 3% to 7% of patients. Preliminary results from isolates in Upstate New York have shown that multiple drug resistance has not been limited to NYC.

Assessment and public health response

The emergence of MDR-TB in NYS and elsewhere has made it one of the leading health issues of the 1990s. The federal tuberculosis programme which had been in mothballs has been recommissioned with increases in CDC TB funding from $8 million to greater than $100 million within a few years. In New York the NYC and NYS Departments of Health have committed millions of dollars in resources and staff to a multifaceted approach to dealing with tuberculosis as well as some of its contributing factors. A wide spectrum of TB surveillance, epidemiological study, prevention and control, regulatory, laboratory, educational and special population activities are planned or underway (Table 11.2).

Table 11.2 Spectrum of some NYS MDR-TB prevention and control efforts

I Surveillance and outbreak investigations
   A. Development of Statewide TB and MDR-TB case reporting and management registries
   B. Creation of an occupational TB registry
   C. Laboratory surveillance of TB susceptibility
   D. Formation of MDR-TB outbreak investigation teams

II Epidemiological studies
   A. Matching of multiple registries
   B. Case-control study of MDR-TB and drug-susceptible TB cases
   C. Environmental surveys of AFB isolation in prisons and health care facilities
   D. Evaluation of Directly Observed Therapy (DOT) Programmes
   E. Health care utilization studies

III Local prevention and control
   A. State grants for DOT, case management and jail TB control
   B. Utilization of TB outreach workers
   C. Coordination of TB and HIV supportive housing services
   D. Construction of special TB units with adequate acid-fast bacillus (AFB) isolation

IV Regulatory activities
   A. Monitoring of local TB programmes
   B. Inspections of health care facilities
   C. Surveys of provider TB control practices
   D. Oversight of mandatory TB skin testing programmes

V Prison initiatives
   A. PPD and chest X-ray screening of inmates at entry
   B. Annual PPD testing of employees and inmates
   C. Implementation of DOT for all TB treatments
   D. Construction of AFB isolation facilities

VI Miscellaneous
   A. Establishment of TB homeless shelters for men and women
   B. Spectrum of patient and provider education programmes
   C. Upgrading of laboratory service and research (e.g. RFLP) capabilities
   D. Mobilization of collaborative activities of multiple agencies
   E. Etc.

Postscript

> Where youth grows pale, and spectre-thin, and dies;
> Where but to think is to be full of sorrow
> And leaden-eyed despairs;

'Ode to a Nightingale', John Keats (1795–1821)

Keats may have written some of his best poetry while dying of tuberculosis, but let us not forget it is a horrible way to enhance one's creativity and a tragic loss of human potential. MDR-TB, if not controlled, has the potential to take us back to an era of untreatable tuberculosis to which we do not want to return.

References

Bloom BR, Murray CJL (1992) Tuberculosis: commentary on a re-emergent killer. *Science, 257*, 1055–1064

Busillo CP, Lessnau KD, Sanjana V *et al.* (1992) Multidrug resistant *Mycobacterium tuberculosis* in patients with human immunodeficiency virus infection. *Chest, 102*, 797–801

Centers for Disease Control (1991) Nosocomial transmission of multidrug-resistant tuberculosis among HIV-infected persons—Florida and New York, 1988–1991. *Morbidity and Mortality Weekly Report, 40*, 585–591

Centers for Disease Control (1992) Transmission of multidrug-resistant tuberculosis among immunocompromised persons in a correctional system—New York 1991. *Morbidity and Mortality Weekly Report, 41*, 507–509

Dubos R, Dubos J (1987) *The White Plague*. Rutgers University Press, New Brunswick, NJ. pp. 1–277

Edlin BR, Tokars JI, Greico MH *et al.* (1992) An outbreak of multidrug-resistant tuberculosis among hospitalised patients with the acquired immunodeficiency syndrome. *New England Journal of Medicine, 326*, 1514–1521

Frieden TR, Sterling T, Kilburn J, Crawford J, Gunn R, Dooley S (1992) Abstract and Presentation, 41st Annual EIS Conference, Centers for Disease Control, Atlanta, Georgia

Ikeda RM, Birkhead GS, Di Ferdinando CT, Bornstein D, Morse DL (1992) Nosocomial transmission of multidrug-resistant tuberculosis, New York. Abstract and presentation, 41st Annual EIS Conference, Centers for Disease Control, Atlanta, Georgia

Morse DL, Lessner L, Medvesky MG, Glebitis DM, Novick LF (1991) Geographic distribution of newborne HIV seroprevalence in relation to four sociodemographic variables. *American Journal of Public Health, 815*, 25–29

Pearson ML, Jereb JA, Frieden TR *et al.* (1992) Nosocomial transmission of multidrug-resistant *Mycobacterium tuberculosis. Annals of Internal Medicine, 117*, 191–196

Pablos-Mendez A, Raviglione MC, Battan R, Ramos-Zuniga R (1990) Drug resistant tuberculosis among the homeless in New York City. *New York State Journal of Medicine, 90*, 351–355

Snider DE, Roper WL (1992) The new tuberculosis. *New England Journal of Medicine, 326*, 703–705

Valway S, Greifinger R, DiFerdinando G *et al.* (1992) Multidrug-resistant tuberculosis in the New York State Correctional System. Late-breaker presentation, 41st Annual EIS Conference, Centers for Disease Control, Atlanta, Georgia

Danger for the Third World

Sir John Crofton, *University of Edinburgh, UK*

With the incipient HIV explosion in Asia, widespread drug resistance could make tuberculosis uncontrollable. At the Coordination, Advisory and Review Group (CARG) meeting of WHO's TB unit in November 1991 some of us thought that there had been too little attention given to the resistance problem. Accordingly, Knut Ovreberg, of Norway, and I submitted a memorandum (Crofton and Ovreberg, 1992) on the subject to WHO in January 1992. Following this, WHO is working to develop a practical, cost-effective sample survey technique (Felten, in preparation) and is collecting what data on national resistance prevalences are available in the literature (Vareldzis, in preparation) (see also a brief review in the paper by Weyer and Kleeberg, 1992). The present paper is based on our memorandum and to some extent on a previous publication (Crofton, 1987) covering preventive and treatment aspects. It will deal briefly, in a Third World context, with determining drug resistance prevalence, potential causes of resistance and possible ways of preventing or reducing the problem.

Problems in determining resistance prevalence

These include: (1) absent or unreliable laboratory facilities (Stewart and Crofton, 1964; Rist and Crofton, 1960); (2) lack of systematic sample surveys; (3) possible exaggeration of resistance prevalence because laboratory data derive mainly from 'chronics'; (4) difficulty in differentiating 'primary' from 'initial' resistance, because of unreliable treatment histories from patients.

Potential causes of drug resistance

These include:

1. Use of a single drug: this can be due to ignorance (e.g. over-the-counter therapy or alternative medicine practitioners); to residual (or transmitted) isoniazid resistance from the period when WHO recommended single isoniazid therapy for the Third World; to past use of isoniazid in cough mixtures; to use of penicillin/streptomycin combinations, or of rifampicin, for other diseases.
2. Use of unreliable combinations, e.g. ethambutol/isoniazid or thioacetazone/ isoniazid as initial treatment, with an appreciable failure rate; or of initial rifampicin/isoniazid in areas with high primary isoniazid resistance.
3. The 'addition syndrome' (Crofton, 1987), in which another drug is added when the patient appears to deteriorate clinically: if resistance has developed to the

drugs in use, this amounts to using the additional drug alone. There is temporary improvement until resistance to the added drug emerges. The process may then be repeated with a further drug. This is probably the commonest cause of multiple drug resistance.

4. Use of unreliable drugs due to unscrupulous dilution or to poor bioavailability (particularly rifampicin/isoniazid/pyrazinamide combinations): an important problem in India and perhaps elsewhere.
5. Irregular drug supply: if only one drug is available, should you give the patient this or let him deteriorate with no treatment?
6. Ignorant or unscrupulous treatment by doctors, alternative medicine practitioners or even over-the-counter. This includes patient ignorance. He may only be able to afford a week or two of rifampicin but continue to take another drug or drugs unprotected.

Prevention and remedies

To tackle the problem in any one country one has to have a baseline sample survey to determine the prevalence of resistance in (presumptively) new patients ('initial' resistance) and in those presenting for retreatment ('acquired' resistance). Progress can be monitored by regular surveys. Surveys need not be too elaborate. One needs only to know whether resistance is a small, large or medium problem, and to what drugs. Standard initial and retreatment regimens can then be planned.

Experience has shown that where there is an effective national tuberculosis control programme (Crofton *et al.*, 1992), giving good treatment with kindness and consideration and convenience, patients use it rather than chaotic private services. In consequence resistance prevalence is low. Where resistance has been high, it diminishes when a good service is established. I understand that this is now happening in South Korea.

To prevent ignorant or unscrupulous treatment, the ideal is to establish government legislation to confine the availability of antituberculosis drugs to those trained to use them. This has been done at least in Norway and Libya. In Libya the policy resulted in a dramatic decrease in resistance prevalence (Khalil and Sathianathan, 1978).

Where legislation is politically impossible there must be intensive and ongoing undergraduate and postgraduate education. This should include regular updating newsletters to doctors, and also to alternative medicine practitioners if these are allowed access to the drugs. If over-the-counter prescribing cannot be prevented by law, as it should be, there must be intensive education of shopkeepers, who in many countries are quite untrained. A possible sanction is to advertise to the public that misuse of chemotherapy amounts to malpractice. Patients deteriorating owing to misuse could resort to litigation against the practitioner or shopkeeper responsible. This might frighten them into conformity with good treatment.

Conclusions

A high prevalence of drug resistance could make tuberculosis uncontrollable. This is a particular threat as the HIV epidemic explodes in Asia. The problem is entirely preventable. It is essential, in all threatened countries, to have an effective national tuberculosis control programme in place before the HIV epidemic sweeps in. Governments must be prepared to take firm action to prevent disaster from this global emergency.

References

Crofton J (1987) The prevention and management of drug-resistant tuberculosis. *Bulletin of the International Union Against Tuberculosis and Lung Disease, 62*, 6–11
Crofton J, Ovreberg K (1992) *Drug resistance and national tuberculosis control programmes.* Memorandum to WHO, January
Crofton J, Horne N, Miller F (1992) *Clinical Tuberculosis.* Macmillan, TALC, International Union Against Tuberculosis and Lung Disease, London and Basingstoke
Felten M. *Surveillance of Drug Resistance in Tuberculosis. A Sample Survey of Initial and Acquired Resistance.* WHO, Geneva. In preparation
Khalil H, Sathianathan S (1978) Impact of antituberculosis legislative actions in Libya on the prevalence of primary and acquired resistance to the three main drugs at a major tuberculosis centre. *Tubercle, 59*, 1–12
Rist N, Crofton J (1960) Drug resistance in hospitals and sanatoria. A report to the Committee on Laboratory Methods and to the Committee on Antibiotics and Chemotherapy of the International Union Against Tuberculosis. *Bulletin of the International Union Against Tuberculosis, 30*, 2–41
Stewart SM, Crofton JW (1964) The clinical significance of low degrees of drug resistance in tuberculosis. *American Review of Respiratory Disease, 89*, 811–829
Vareldzis B. *Review Paper of Drug Resistance in Tuberculosis.* WHO, Geneva. In preparation
Weyer K, Kleeberg HH (1992) Primary and acquired drug resistance in adult black patients with tuberculosis in South Africa: results of a continuous national resistance surveillance programme involvement. *Tubercle and Lung Disease, 73*, 106–112

The molecular basis of drug resistance in *Mycobacterium tuberculosis*

Stewart T. Cole, *Institut Pasteur, Paris, France*

Although chemotherapy has been used for over forty years to treat tuberculosis, it is only recently that our understanding of the mode and site of action of antituberculosis drugs has improved significantly. *Mycobacterium tuberculosis* is naturally resistant to most antimicrobial agents, probably as a result of its highly lipophilic cell envelope acting as an effective permeability barrier. In the late

1940s, streptomycin was first used in the treatment of the disease while isonicotinic acid hydrazide or isoniazid (INH), which is exquisitely potent against *M. tuberculosis*, was introduced shortly afterwards. Problems of resistance, leading to therapeutic failure, were often encountered when these compounds were employed singly. This led to the implementation of multidrug therapy, in which patients are given suitable drug combinations, as this is an efficient means of preventing the emergence of mutants resistant to individual components. The five main drugs currently available for the treatment of tuberculosis are streptomycin, rifampicin, pyrazinamide, ethambutol and INH.

By analogy with other bacteria, streptomycin probably provokes translational defects by interacting with the ribosomes of *M. tuberculosis* whereas rifampicin is believed to block transcription by inactivating RNA polymerase. Experimental support for the mode of action of these drugs in mycobacteria was lacking until very recently. Pyrazinamide is tuberculostatic but its precise action is unknown and this is also the case for ethambutol which is believed to perturb cell wall synthesis. INH appears to have pleiotropic effects and has been reported to disrupt intermediary metabolism, to affect nucleic acid synthesis, and to inhibit the production of mycolic acids.

In recent years, an important sequel of the AIDS epidemic in industrialized countries has been the re-emergence of tuberculosis as a public health problem, after several decades of steadily declining incidence. One of the more alarming features of the disease in HIV-infected individuals is the increasingly common isolation of strains of *M. tuberculosis* resistant to two or more antituberculosis drugs. Although the emergence of such strains probably reflects poor compliance of the patients, the potential of the threat posed to tuberculosis chemotherapy should not be underestimated given the limited number of active compounds available. It was thus both timely and appropriate to reappraise the problem of drug resistance in order to learn more about the mechanisms involved and to develop tests for rapidly identifying resistant strains.

A surrogate genetic approach was employed, using the fast-growing *Mycobacterium smegmatis* as host, to identify genes involved in the INH-resistance of *M. tuberculosis*. INH-resistant mutants of *M. smegmatis* have the same phenotypes as their *M. tuberculosis* counterparts namely greatly increased MICs (minimum inhibitory concentrations) for the drug, normal mycolate production, slower growth rate and reduced catalase-peroxidase activity. On screening a shuttle cosmid library, a clone was isolated that could restore INH sensitivity to such mutants and on subsequent characterization this was shown to carry the *katG* gene of *M. tuberculosis*. Several independent studies show that the toxic effect of INH is mediated via the *katG* gene product, the haeme-containing enzyme, catalase-peroxidase. It is conceivable that INH is converted into an activated form, by peroxidation, catalysed by the KatG protein. On examination of INH-resistant clinical isolates of *M. tuberculosis*, it was found that in some cases the *katG* gene had been deleted from the chromosome whereas in the majority it had been inactivated by point mutations.

Rifampicin has a strong bactericidal effect and, in *Escherichia coli* and

Mycobacterium leprae, rifampicin resistance is associated with missense mutations in the *rpoB* gene encoding the β-subunit of RNA polymerase. To determine whether this mechanism was also responsible for the rifampicin resistance of *M. tuberculosis*, the polymerase chain reaction (PCR) was employed to selectively amplify the corresponding segments of the *rpoB* gene from sensitive and resistant strains. A solid phase sequencing approach was then used to locate the mutations. No deviations from the wild-type *rpoB* sequence were found in drug-sensitive strains whereas, in virtually all of the resistant isolates, point mutations or in-frame deletions were located in a short stretch of the gene. In approximately 80% of the cases, resistance is due to missense mutations affecting only two amino acid residues: either His-420 or Ser-425. These mutations have also been described in *E. coli* and *M. leprae*.

A similar approach was employed to assess streptomycin resistance in *M. tuberculosis* for it was reasoned that this should stem from alterations in the drug target, the ribosome. As the nucleotide sequence of the *rpsL* gene of *M. leprae*, encoding ribosomal protein S12—a potential site of streptomycin action, had been determined recently it was a simple matter to adapt PCR to examine the *rpsL* genes from streptomycin-sensitive and -resistant strains of *M. tuberculosis*. After DNA sequence analysis of the wild-type and mutant alleles, it was found that in 50% of the resistant strains the codon corresponding to Lys-42 had been mutated. The sequences of the *rpsL* genes from the other resistant mutants were identical to that of the wild-type gene suggesting that there may be another mechanism of resistance.

Single-stranded conformation polymorphism (SSCP) analysis is a potent means of screening for mutations in a target gene. It is both simple and rapid and, in conjunction with PCR, provides a powerful tool for determining the drug susceptibility profile of *M. tuberculosis* isolates. SSCP-PCR tests for INH, rifampicin and streptomycin isolates. SSCP-PCR tests for INH, rifampicin and streptomycin resistance have been developed and these should find application in the fight against multidrug-resistant tuberculosis. As the procedure can be performed directly on clinical samples and requires less than 2 days it represents a potentially useful alternative to the slower antibiogram method which can take up to 10 weeks. Finally, from the findings described here it appears that multidrug resistance in *M. tuberculosis* results from the accumulation of mutations in chromosomal genes and not from a novel resistance mechanism.

The clinical management of multidrug-resistant (MDR) tuberculosis

Jerrold J. Ellner, *Case Western Reserve University, Cleveland, Ohio, USA*

The proper treatment of MDR-TB is not yet known and may require development of new drugs and other therapeutic modalities (cytokines, surgery). It must be emphasized that at the time of initial presentation the drug sensitivity of the isolate is not known. Therefore, the rising prevalence of drug resistance in certain geographic areas dictates a new approach to initial therapy as well as to definitive regimens that can be applied once drug sensitivity patterns have been established. Because of the seriousness of MDR-TB and the potential for nosocomial transmission, management of TB requires attention to basic principles that have been sadly ignored recently. These include: a high index of suspicion of TB, early diagnosis, rapid institution of isolation procedures in functioning, monitored facilities, selection of empirical regimen based on geography and setting, rapid determination of drug susceptibility, and continued isolation until there is a clear clinical and microbiological response (Edlin 1992, Fischl *et al.*, 1992a,b).

The increasing prevalence of resistant isolates of *M. tuberculosis* in the community reflects a failure of TB control programmes (Frieden 1993). Review of recent cases of isoniazid (INH) and MDR-resistant TB shows that 57% had neither of the traditional risk factors for resistant disease (foreign-born, prior treatment). Additional risk factors for resistance includes AIDS, HIV infection, and intravenous drug users. The prevalence of resistant TB in the community may be a useful guide to initial treatment of TB. If the prevalence of drug resistance is <4%, a standard three drug regimen is appropriate; at higher prevailing levels of resistance, initial therapy should consist of four drugs (isoniazid, rifampicin, pyrazinamide, ethambutol or streptomycin). If the level of resistance is >10%, addition of a quinolone should be considered. If a patient has been exposed to a known case of MDR-TB (or has demonstrated MDR-TB), the regimen should be tailored based on sensitivity tests. The goal is to include at least three drugs (and as many first-line drugs) to which the isolate is sensitive. The basic regimen should include an injectable (amikacin, kanamycin, capreomycin), a quinolone (ofloxacin), and (depending on sensitivities), ethambutol, pyrazinamide, rifabutin, paraminosalicylate, ethionamide, or cycloserine. The optimal duration of therapy is unknown. Even with optimal regimens in HIV-negative patients, response rates were only 65% in a recently reported series, and cure rates 56% (Goble, 1993). In the presence of HIV infection, few patients respond to therapy by sterilizing sputum, and mortality has been 70–80%. These dismal results have prompted initiatives to develop new drugs and renewed interest in cytokine therapy. As these approaches are unlikely to achieve fruition soon, attempts at basic principles of TB and infection control are key.

Assuring compliance with therapy is essential to prevent further emergence of drug resistance. Directly observed therapy has been advocated as a remedy but evokes logistic issues and some added expense. Contact tracing of patients exposed to MDR-TB is another vital issue although the approach to management of the documented tuberculin skin test converter is unknown. Decisions concerning preventive therapy depend on the likelihood that the infecting strain is MDR, and the likelihood that the individual if infected will progress to disease. If one or both of these issues suggest that preventive therapy is warranted, combination therapy with pyrazinamide plus ethambutol or ofloxacillin has been advocated.

References

Edlin BR, Tokars JI, Grieco MH, Crawford JT *et al*. (1992) An outbreak of multidrug-resistant tuberculosis among hospitalized patients with the acquired immunodeficiency syndrome. *New England Journal of Medicine, 326*(23), 1514–1521

Fischl MA, Daikos GL, Uttamchandani RB *et al*. (1992b) Clinical presentation and outcome of patients with HIV infection and tuberculosis caused by multiple-drug-resistant bacilli. *Annals of Internal Medicine, 117*, 184–190

Fischl MA, Uttamchandani RB, Daikos GL (1992a) An outbreak of tuberculosis caused by multiple-drug-resistant tubercle bacillii among patients with HIV infection. *Annals of Internal Medicine, 117*(3), 177–183

Frieden TR, Sterling, T, Pablo-Mendez A *et al*. (1993) The emerging of drug-resistant tuberculosis in New York City. *New England Journal of Medicine, 328*, 521–526

Goble M, Iseman MD, Madsen LA, Waite D *et al*. (1993) Treatment of 1712 patients with pulmonary tuberculosis resistant to isoniazid and rifampicin. *New England Journal of Medicine, 328*, 527–532

Pearson ML, Jereb, JA, Frieden, Crawford JT *et al*. (1992) Nosocomial transmission of multidrug-resistant *Mycobacterium tuberculosis*. *Annals of Internal Medicine, 117*, 191–196

WORKSHOP REPORTS

Workshop 1: Immunology and vaccines

Hazel M. Dockrell and M. Joseph Colston*

*London School of Hygiene and Tropical Medicine and *MRC National Institute of Medical Research, London, UK*

Major advances are occurring in our ability to dissect and manipulate host–parasite interactions. Targeted genetic changes in both the host and the infectious agent will enable us to understand the basis of immunity and virulence, and lead to novel approaches to manipulate the balance between them. It is essential that these advances in medical biotechnology should be applied to the study of tuberculosis so that, in the long-term, improved tools for disease control can be developed.

Which tests best reflect immunity to tuberculosis, and what does our experience on HIV, BCG and immunopathogenesis tell us about immunity to tuberculosis?

In order to develop new tests to measure immunity, we need to better understand the mechanism of protection against *M. tuberculosis*. Protective immunity against tuberculosis may include an innate or genetic mechanism of resistance, and an acquired immune response, which would protect an individual from developing clinical tuberculosis. More work is needed to understand how such long-lasting T cell memory is maintained.

The ideal test would measure the acquired or memory immune response against *M. tuberculosis*, and would be sufficiently simple for field use. Skin tests have been widely used but batch variation in antigens, age and sex variations in response, and a decline in response over time all complicate their analysis. There is evidence that those individuals with moderate rather than strong responses have the greatest degree of protection. It should now be possible to develop more specific skin tests using some of the recently identified antigens from *M. tuberculosis*. Antibody tests may indicate whether an individual is infected but do not seem useful as measures of immunity. The best *in vitro* cellular test would measure the killing of *M. tuberculosis* by macrophages, but such assays are technically very complex to perform.

Tuberculosis: Back to the Future. Edited by J.D.H. Porter and K.P.W.J. McAdam
© 1994 John Wiley & Sons Ltd

The development of TB infection early during an HIV infection indicates that CD4+ T cell function is required for immunity (although the final effector mechanisms may involve other cells including CD8+ T cells and macrophages). Mouse experiments have detailed complex kinetic responses in the different T cell subsets, involving CD4+ T cells, $\gamma\delta$T cells, CD8+ T cells and CD4+ CTL (cytotoxic T lymphocytes).

Priority points of action

1. We need to better understand the mechanism of protection against TB in order to develop new tests.
2. Experimental infections are providing new insights into immunological interactions. This is an important research area.
3. Work in mice suggests that the balance between TH1 and TH2 subsets, and Class I/II presentation is important. Correlations in man should be investigated.
4. Work on secreted antigens should be a priority; these could be tested as skin test reagents in man.

How should we approach the development of a new TB vaccine?

The search for a single protective antigen is continuing, although it may be that the type of immunity induced is more important. However, experiments using synthetic peptides can help to assess how many epitopes are required to give protection. A minimalist vaccine is therefore a long-term goal. To date, good protection against tuberculosis in animal models has only been induced by live organisms, although work with other delivery systems may reveal that the route of presentation of antigens is crucial for the induction of immunity. The ability to delete virulence genes from *M. tuberculosis*, or to introduce selected *M. tuberculosis* genes into *M. bovis* BCG or other fast growing mycobacteria is a new development which has great promise for vaccine development.

Priority points of action

1. We need to apply the rapid developments in immunology to understanding protective immunity to tuberculosis.
2. Developments in genetic manipulation will provide new attenuated/live vaccines. These are important in their own right for evaluation as vaccines and offer a completely new approach to investigating protective immune mechanisms.
3. The minimalist vaccine approach may also produce new vaccines or identify genes for expression in live/attenuated vaccines.
4. Any new vaccine showing promise in experimental systems will ultimately have to be tested in well-controlled double-blind trials before general use.

Workshop 2: Diagnosis and molecular epidemiology

Neil G. Stoker and Jan D.A. van Embden*

London School of Hygiene & Tropical Medicine, UK and *National Institute of Public Health and Protection, Bilthoven, The Netherlands

What is the role of the polymerase chain reaction (PCR) in developing countries?

Priority points of action

1. *The use of the polymerase chain reaction (PCR) in diagnosis.* The polymerase chain reaction (PCR) allows the specific detection of single bacterial cells in clinical material in a matter of hours. Therefore, it could potentially revolutionize the laboratory diagnosis of tuberculosis. Competing methods which are already well established are culture and microscopy, and PCR will have to show that it provides advantages over these methods if it is to be useful. The advantage of the rapidity of the PCR is most obvious for cases in which detection by microscopy fails. It was strongly felt that diagnosis of smear-negative TB cases is a priority, as many of these people become smear-positive, and hence more infectious, later. Furthermore, the workshop participants felt that a PCR test could in particular play a critical role in diagnosing suspected cases of meningitis and also of TB in HIV-infected patients, because of the difficulties of diagnosing TB in dually infected patients.

2. *The practicality of using PCR in developing countries.* Some optimism was expressed that although it is clearly not appropriate in all settings, in other centres it will be quite feasible. However, external quality control was felt to be critical. New isothermal methods which are being developed may be even more appropriate, as a thermal cycler would not be required.

3. *Diagnosis of drug resistance.* More rapid methods to test the susceptibility of *M. tuberculosis* to currently used antimycobacterial drugs are badly needed. Preliminary studies on rapid sensitivity testing, using molecular biological tools, were considered to be extremely promising. One method is based on the characterization of the genes that encode the target proteins for antimycobacterial drugs. Small differences in these genes between drug-sensitive and drug-resistant bacteria can be assayed after *in vitro* amplification by PCR-SSCP (single-stranded conformation polymorphism) within a day. It was reported that this methodology could currently detect 99% of rifampicin-resistant, 70% of isoniazid-resistant and 60% of streptomycin-resistant strains. Another approach is to assay the inhibitory effect of antimycobacterial agents by detecting light emitted by genes carried on genetically

engineered bacteriophages. This method takes 3 days, but it has the advantage that no knowledge is needed about the drug targets of which only a few have been characterized until now. It was suggested that clinical microbiologists would prefer a phenotypic test rather than a genotypic test. Further research to develop these methods for use in the bacteriological laboratory was considered of high priority.

What questions can be asked from DNA fingerprinting?

Priority points of action

Recently, various genetic markers have been identified that allow differentiation of *M. tuberculosis* strains from epidemiologically unrelated patients. The most frequently used marker for DNA fingerprinting is a genetic element, IS*6110*, which can move within the *M. tuberculosis* genome and which is usually present in multiple copies. Due to the great variability in fingerprint types, transmission of strains with a given DNA type can be detected. In this way the route of transmission and the spread of multiresistant strains within and among hospitals and penitentiary facilities in the USA has been established. DNA typing is potentially useful for outbreak investigations, hospital-acquired infections (for instance by bronchoscopes), and strain identification (e.g. of BCG). Furthermore, fingerprinting of *M. tuberculosis* has shown that cross-contamination may occur even in well equipped laboratories, leading to overdiagnosis. The panel felt that DNA typing of *M. tuberculosis* is ready for immediate use in reference laboratories to support the epidemiology and for quality control in the bacteriological laboratory. More sophisticated epidemiological studies are required to answer other questions, such as the relative importance of reactivation and reinfection. The use of different markers which evolve at different rates might allow different questions to be addressed. This may also overcome the problem that in some parts of the world, significant numbers of strains do not possess a copy of IS*6110*, a fact which is also relevant for diagnosis, as many PCR methods make use of this marker.

Workshop 3: Case finding and clinical management

Paul Nunn and Reginald C. Boulos*

*World Health Organization, Geneva, Switzerland and *Centres pour le Développement et la Santé, Port-au-Prince, Haiti*

The goals of the new WHO Tuberculosis Programme are to detect 75% of all smear-positive TB cases and to treat 85% of all identified cases. Case finding, case holding and clinical management are essential elements of a successful tuberculosis control programme.

What chemotherapeutic regimens should we be using in developing countries and what studies do we need to answer this question?

To better understand the importance of the first question, it is essential to remember that, at best, the treatment rate, in developing countries, has been around 55–65%. The failure to introduce effective chemotherapy in the developing countries is the main reason for the *persistence of the disease*. In general, in the Third World, treating identified cases has been a great disaster. In selecting the best regimens, several elements were reviewed: type of drugs, duration of treatment, type of supervision, frequency of treatment, loss to follow-up and organization of treatment.

Priority points of action

1. A good chemotherapeutic regimen is one that achieves successful treatment without creating resistance. In this context, resistance should be viewed as a major side effect and we should use the regimen that offers the safest choice.

2. Several regimens are available to programme managers. These include the 6 month short course, including four drugs, to the 8 month course with thiacetazone as well as the traditional 12 month course with streptomycin and thiacetazone. The choice of any of these regimens should rest entirely on resources available to each country. While there is agreement that the shorter courses are more likely to achieve a better treatment rate, individual countries should choose a regimen according to their resources and the capacity of the health system to implement a specific regimen. Regardless of the regimen chosen, two factors are essential for the success of the programme:

    (a) Good operation of the TB programme: resources are not only necessary to finance the drugs, but are important to pay for and support a working network. It is as important to provide for the human resources, the laboratory supplies and to establish proper supervision. Better drug procurement and distribution should be established.

    (b) Donor and government commitment to allocating the necessary resources should be sustained on a long-term basis. Programme and means need to be established for at least a five year period. A tuberculosis programme is a long-term action.

3. Treatment supervision is essential to good success. Direct observation therapy (DOT) is by far the best. When DOT is possible, intermittent therapy should be

used. There is no reason for supervised daily treatment. Daily treatment can be offered unsupervised.

4. Regarding thiacetazone and the risk of severe skin reactions, it is recommended that:

   (a) In places where resources are available and HIV infection is prevalent, thiacetazone should be replaced by another drug (ethambutol or rifampicin).

   (b) In areas where HIV testing is available, thiacetazone should be given only to HIV-negative patients.

   (c) When resources are not available and HIV testing is not a standard procedure, thiacetazone use should be supported by a strong health education programme and proper training of health workers.

5. Compliance with the drug regimen is considered a key element to the success of therapy. Compliance can be obtained through: good management of operations, including counselling at onset of treatment, capacity to follow up on patients and track down loss to follow-up. The attitude of health workers, primarily physicians, is considered an important factor for good compliance. Compliance would be the responsibility of the programme.

There is still room for research in the area of case finding and clinical management. The causes of failure and drug resistance should be investigated; we need to know why resistance occurs, and the effect of the exclusion of streptomycin from the treatment regimen should be evaluated. We know little about the cost-effectiveness of thiacetazone; the use of solutions excluding thiacetazone needs to be studied and research studies should look at the providers and the patient causes for poor adherence. The attitude of health workers needs to be evaluated. The possibility of using rewards and incentives to improve compliance should be the subject of operational research.

What is the role of the community in case finding and case holding?

Priority points of action

1. Community involvement from the start of the programme is *a must*. Tuberculosis control should be fully integrated within the development of the primary health care system. Community participation in the design and implementation of TB control activities will greatly increase the effectiveness of the programme and compliance.

2. Good quality of services will lead to successful case finding.

3. The role of community financing of case holding needs to be explored and investigated. Their application on a national level should be studied.

Workshop 4: Chemoprophylaxis and drug therapy

Alison Elliott and Denis A. Mitchison*

*University of Colorado, Denver, USA and *Hammersmith Hospital, London, UK*

How should we approach the development of new tuberculosis drugs?

Priority points of action

1. The need for new drugs. The introduction of the last major antituberculosis drug, rifampicin, took place 30 years ago. New drugs are needed for the following reasons:

- To shorten the duration of chemotherapy.
- To widen spacing of drug doses to make full supervision of dosage easier and to decrease drug costs.
- For cost-effective chemoprophylaxis.
- For treatment of drug-resistant tubercle bacilli.
- To avoid the appreciable toxicity of current second-line drugs.

The need is urgent because of the likely large increase of tuberculosis, in association with HIV infections, throughout the world during the next decade and because of the difficulty of treating patients with drug-resistant tuberculosis.

2. Collaboration with industry. The development of a new drug typically costs about 100 million pounds which a commercial firm cannot easily recoup when most sales are to developing countries. Public health and academic bodies should be encouraged to collaborate with industry since they carry out much of the initial drug screening and studies on pharmacokinetics, some of the animal experimentation and much of the clinical development, thereby reducing costs. Screening of old molecules might be cost-effective. While welcoming collaboration, the workshop regretted the failure of some commercial firms to license potentially valuable new wide-spectrum drugs, such as quinolones, for use in tuberculosis on the grounds that it might reduce profitability. There is also a very real need for independent bodies to compare the relative merits of competing drugs. Thus the tendency of funding bodies to refuse support if there is any possibility of obtaining it from commercial firms is regrettable since it encourages poor quality commercially-orientated protocols and bias in the eventual assessment.

3. Speeding up clinical development. Examples were given of the use of an assessment of early bactericidal activity to obtain a rapid, accurate and economical assessment of drug activity. This technique has been used to compare the potencies of rifabutin and rifampicin in a study in Hong Kong (Chan *et al.*, 1992) and later in South Africa (Sirgel *et al.*, 1993). In the South African study, the dose of rifabutin to give the same activity as rifampicin was 2.73 times higher with 95% confidence limits of 1.96 and 3.78. The comparison was done on only 50 patients. Examination of the amount of variation between patients suggests that the method can only be used in the acute disease found in African populations.

Early bactericidal activity is not the same as the sterilizing activity of a drug. Sterilizing activity is measured by the relapse rates during a follow-up period of about 2 years after the end of chemotherapy. A good indication of the relapse rates can be obtained from the proportion of patients who have negative sputum cultures at 2 months after the start of chemotherapy (Mitchison, 1993). Provisional FDA licensing of a new rifamycin is likely to be obtainable from the results of a study of early bactericidal activity and of 2 months' bacteriology, thus saving as much as 3.5 years of development time.

Given scarce resources, is chemoprophylaxis logistically feasible? If so, how can these programmes be targeted?

The use of preventive treatment for tuberculosis in people infected with HIV has been proposed with the following aims:

1. The prevention of active tuberculosis in people with HIV. It is believed that active tuberculosis may develop in at least 30% of dually infected individuals.
2. A possible reduction in the rate of progression of HIV infection to AIDS. Theoretically, activation of the immune system in response to active tuberculosis may promote viral replication and increase the rate of progression of HIV-disease, but this is not proven.
3. Prevention of spread of tuberculosis in the community.

The workshop was asked, primarily, to discuss whether preventative treatment of tuberculosis would be feasible in countries with limited resources for health care. Current studies in developing countries have identified several problems.

1. Identification of the population to receive prophylaxis. It was recognized that, at least initially, prophylaxis would be directed at selected groups, such as those identified as HIV-positive at voluntary testing centres, or company employees. It was agreed that preventative treatment for tuberculosis could not, currently,

be envisaged as a major component of national tuberculosis control programmes.

2. Exclusion of active tuberculosis. Experience reported by delegates from Uganda and Zambia indicated that the main risk of inducing drug resistance lay in the difficulty in excluding active tuberculosis in symptomatic HIV-positive individuals. The simplest test for tuberculosis remains the sputum smear. The risk of a sputum smear-negative patient, accidentally given monotherapy as 'prophylaxis,' proceeding to smear-positive (infectious) drug-resistant disease was not yet known.

3. Compliance. Difficulties observed in promoting compliance with therapy in people offered prophylactic treatment are similar to those well recognized in treatment of active disease.

Priority points of action

Participants agreed that, although some data are available regarding the efficacy of preventive treatment and its effect on survival in HIV-positive individuals, these are still inadequate. Studies which address these questions are, however, in progress in Zambia, Uganda, the United States and elsewhere. Research was also called for regarding type and duration of regimen to be used and, in particular, the implications of using single-drug prophylactic treatment for induction of drug-resistant disease in HIV-positive people.

In many developing countries tuberculosis control programmes are severely stretched by the current epidemic and would be quite unable to undertake a concurrent prophylaxis programme. It was suggested that tuberculosis prophylaxis might rather be approached as part of the AIDS control programme, with facilities for sputum smear examination made available at centres where HIV testing and counselling are performed. The support of the tuberculosis service would be required, especially for the management of new, active cases identified.

References

Chan SL, Yew WW, Ma WK *et al.* (1992) The early bactericidal activity of rifabutin measured by sputum viable counts in Hong Kong patients with pulmonary tuberculosis. *Tubercle and Lung Disease, 73*, 33–38

Mitchison DA (1993) Assessment of new sterilizing drugs for treating pulmonary tuberculosis by culture at 2 months. *American Review of Respiratory Disease, 147*, 1062–1063

Sirgel FA, Botha FJH, Parkin DP *et al.* The early bactericidal activity of rifabutin in patients with pulmonary tuberculosis measured by sputum viable counts. A new method of drug assessment. *Journal of Antimicrobial Chemotherapy*, in press

Workshop 5: Control strategies and resource allocation

Susan Foster and M. Angelica Salomão*

*London School of Hygiene & Tropical Medicine, UK and *Ministry of Health, Maputo, Mozambique*

The workshop focused on the contributing factors to the generally poor level of effectiveness of existing TB control programmes, and considered whether the problem was *lack* of funds, or rather whether other factors were equally important. On balance, with the major exception of funds for drugs, workshop participants did not feel that lack of resources per se was the main problem in failure to do better in TB control.

Given scarce resources, how can we best organize case finding, diagnosis, treatment, case holding, and eventually prophylaxis? How can we improve the effectiveness of the TB services?

Priority points of action

The target of 85% of patients completing treatment was far away; the workshop concluded that the main problem in attaining this goal was poor case holding; much of the expenditure on case detection and on treatment was wasted due to the failure to keep patients in treatment until the end. There were two sources of failure in this process; often the patient was blamed as 'non-compliant' when in fact it was the system which had failed the patient and not the reverse. Accordingly, it was felt that emphasis, and additional resources, should be devoted mainly to ensuring an adequate, secure, uninterrupted supply of drugs; without this no control programme could hope to attain the 85% target. Other factors which required attention included investigation of the behavioural factors influencing both patients and staff, and the quality or lack of quality of their interaction, and the role of poor patient/staff interaction in poor compliance. It is important to identify and if possible mitigate the economic barriers which patients experience in seeking and in complying with TB treatment, which is more difficult than virtually any other course of treatment.

What novel methods are there for improving compliance?

Priority points of action

In many countries various schemes have been introduced to provide financial support or encouragement of patients to continue treatment, such as offsetting their transport costs or providing a bonus at the successful completion of treatment; in Sierra Leone, patients were asked to pay a deposit on commencement of treatment which was returned to them at the end of the inpatient treatment phase. One participant stressed the need to move from an 'administrative culture' towards a 'management culture' wherein staff performance and commitment was taken seriously, and this suggestion was widely approved by the workshop. This management role will require better surveillance, recording and reporting of data, and evaluation and supervision should be given a more prominent role as well. Opportunities to link TB control with other control programmes in terms of vehicles, staff, etc., existed which needed to be made use of; this would not automatically lead to a weakening of the TB control effort but rather the contrary.

Finally, the workshop participants noted that not all countries actually have a TB control programme or strategy, yet this was essential. A successful TB control programme must also have strong leadership and political support; in countries without such a programme little improvement could be expected.

CLOSING SESSION
ADDRESSES

Tuberculosis

Ralph H. Henderson

Assistant Director-General, World Health Organization, Geneva, Switzerland

Professor John Kenneth Galbraith warned one of his audiences that, at the conclusion of his talk, they might not be a great deal wiser, but they certainly would be older. I do not promise wisdom here, but I hope at least to limit the ageing process. I would like to direct my remarks to three themes. They relate to thanks, to the role of WHO in the fight against tuberculosis and to the future of world health.

My thanks come from the World Health Organization to the London School of Hygiene and Tropical Medicine and to Dean Richard Feachem's team who have organized this Third Annual Public Health Forum on Tuberculosis as well as to the presenters, the discussants and the participants who have made this such a productive event. This has been a most stimulating set of reports from the workshops, and they reflect the energy and innovative thinking which has permeated this Forum.

This event illustrates for me the complementary roles which should be played between academic institutions and governmental or intergovernmental institutions. These roles are very often *not* played, however, for organizational inertia and differences in agendas frequently overwhelm the vision and good intentions of individuals found within the different bodies. The London School has not only overcome these difficulties in continuing to organize these Fora, but has used these events themselves to promote this vision of collaboration which extends beyond the academic–government axis to encompass all who have contributions to make in addressing public health problems. This is evident from the background of the participants, who represent a rich mixture of those from Ministries of Health, those from universities and research institutions, and those from non-governmental institutions, the private sector and from national and international development organizations. Please keep up the good work in organizing such Fora.

The role of WHO in the fight against tuberculosis is also one of promoting and catalysing collaboration between the many organizations and individuals who can contribute. We have, in addition, a special responsibility to the over 180 member

Tuberculosis: Back to the Future. Edited by J.D.H. Porter and K.P.W.J. McAdam
© 1994 John Wiley & Sons Ltd

states of WHO who have charged us with providing technical leadership and co-ordination in the international health field. WHO itself has few resources compared with the World Bank-estimated 1.9 trillion international dollars[1] being spent annually on health services in the world, or compared with the 360 billion international dollars being spent in developing countries. The WHO annual budget of approximately 0.9 billion US dollars does compare more favourably with the 4 billion international dollars being invested annually in developing countries by donors, but this is more a cause for concern about this level of donor investment than a cause for celebration by WHO.

How WHO uses its resources in promoting world health is the critical question. Is the organization providing 'value for money?' I think most would give us a mixed rating. Perhaps it is not surprising that we do better in circumstances in which we can provide a sound 'technological fix' rather than in circumstances which require more of a 'social fix.' I think our ratings are good, for example, in the field of standard setting for biologicals and pharmaceuticals, and in the coordination of research and development with respect to specific problems, including human reproduction, tropical diseases and tuberculosis. I also think we get good marks concerning leadership in promoting activities related to the control or eradication of certain infectious diseases, including acute respiratory infections, diarrhoeal diseases, leprosy, onchocerciasis, tuberculosis and vaccine-preventable diseases. We do less well with the problems related to chronic diseases, HIV and other sexually transmitted infections, malaria, nutrition, and substance abuse or those related to the basic development of the health infrastructure, all of which provide examples where the elements of broader 'social fixes' increase in importance relative to those of narrower 'technological fixes.'

We are now in a period of rather profound introspection and transition in WHO. We need to see how best to evolve within an environment which is also changing profoundly and rapidly. But I, at least, am convinced, that WHO does provide exceptional value for money in a number of its activities, and I am convinced that these include its leadership in the global fight against tuberculosis.

What is the future of world health, leaving aside the future of the World Health Organization? I doubt any of you need convincing that it is a *world* future which is at stake and no longer the isolated concern for its own well-being of a household, a community, or a country. There is no question in my mind that this reality will be increasingly shared by the world's population as the effects of world economy, environmental pollution, infectious disease, refugee movements and substance abuse pierce the barriers which have defended many, particularly the affluent, in the past. The question which does trouble me is whether public policy, in developing as well as industrialized countries, will reflect these realities quickly enough so that

---

[1]International dollars are derived from national currencies not by use of exchange rates but by assessment of purchasing power.

the human and financial resources needed are put in place to promote healthy sustainable development on planet earth. Tuberculosis illustrates this issue very well indeed. Let us use the global control of this disease as an example of how to do things right, both for ourselves and for future generations.

Lessons from the past

William H. Foege

The Carter Center Inc, Atlanta, Georgia, USA

Introduction

Public health continues to grow in complexity. Last week one of the Pulitzer Prizes was given for a series of articles written by Mike Toner, on 'When Bugs Fight Back.' At one time we could classify public health into programmes where people were getting the advantage and those that were a standoff. Now we have problems that have been solved (such as smallpox), problems that are improving (such as measles and polio), problems that are a standoff (such as cholera and malaria), and problems where public health is losing (such as AIDS and tobacco addiction).

My plan is to cover three topics:

1. What went on in the mind of an outsider to the tuberculosis problem during the last three days?
2. What are the signs of hope?
3. Based on experiences in other areas of public health, where might we go in tuberculosis?

My thoughts

First, I was struck by how the theme, *back to the future*, allowed us to emphasize one of the barriers to good public health decisions.

The first barrier to good global public health decisions concerns the distance between the places of decision-making and the effects of those decisions. It is very hard to make good decisions in London, Geneva or Atlanta when the effects will be felt in Zaire. Nonetheless, in recent years we have put great emphasis on our interdependence, the need for global decisions and the interrelationships of people around the world. This School has been particularly good at fostering that understanding.

But a second barrier has been the time between a decision and its effect. On a personal level that is why we have such a hard time making the right decisions on smoking, diet and exercise. The effects are years in the future. Collectively that is why we have trouble making good decisions on the disposal of toxic wastes or radioactive wastes. The effects are seen long after the decisions are made.

Tuberculosis: Back to the Future. Edited by J.D.H. Porter and K.P.W.J. McAdam
© 1994 John Wiley & Sons Ltd

A good reason for studying history is to become convinced that this is a cause and effect world. Every idea or product that we have today has a history. Likewise what we do today will have an impact 10, 100 and a thousand years from now. As we see ourselves dependent on the past, so is the future dependent on us.

A 4 year old girl asked me, several years ago, whether doctors had bosses. Having assured her that the patients are the bosses of doctors, I then asked the same question of public health workers. It is easy for them to see that their patients logically include all people, even in other countries. It is more difficult to see that their patients include all who will ever live. With that perspective, the decisions made in tuberculosis control today must make sense to those who live in the future.

Secondly I was also struck by the classic public health problems raised by the discussions of tuberculosis. The questions of social justice and the epidemiological puzzles.

On social justice, we heard in the introduction that the burden of tuberculosis is not equally shared. Repeatedly we heard that it is a disease of poverty. What does this tell us about approaching control plans? What responsibility do health people have for poverty? Mencius, the great Chinese scholar once said, 'The good ruler wars not against other countries but against the common enemy . . . poverty.' The good public health worker wars not only against disease but also poverty. Our research must encompass basic biology, application, but also how to alter the social problems that result in inequity. When you consider that our lifestyles are subsidized by the low wages of the poor, the correction of poverty can be seen as simple fairness.

A major public health lesson of the past few years is our need for other disciplines. While our basic science always seems to be lacking in answers, the fact is our science is always ahead of our ethics, our law, our sociology, our religion or our understanding. Whether dealing with AIDS, smoking, diet, injuries, tuberculosis or cancer, we are awakening to the need for social science expertise, not as step sciences but as full participants.

The epidemiological issues were no less intriguing. As a non-expert, the papers were full of surprises. I was surprised, for example, to hear of the exquisite research, the wonderful field trials, the state-of-the-art diagnostic and treatment abilities, and then find that the global populations of *Mycobacterium tuberculosis* bacilli in 1993 is about what it was in 1950. While rates have decreased in many places, the population has increased. The entire force of 20th century science, medicine and public health has resulted in a standoff and no decrease in organisms.

I was also surprised at the difficulties in characterizing the problem. Dr Dixie Snider in commenting on the global problem said that we simply do not know because we lack good surveillance. Knowledge is power and if we cannot characterize the problem with accuracy, it will be difficult to make the case for resources.

I will not dwell on the many problems of diagnosis, treatment and chemoprophylaxis other than to say that Dr Chris Murray is right when he says that we make decisions based on whatever information we have. We do the best we can. Whatever the problems, the bottom line is that you, the world's experts on tuberculosis, are expected to provide your best judgement on what should be done about the disease. I found, in the discussion, great hope rather than great despair.

Why the hope?

Admittedly, this is a difficult time in international health because many of the donor agencies have flat or declining budgets, the new possibilities for interventions must compete for those resources and international health has been mired in politics. But there are signs of real hope.

First, social interest in tuberculosis is again increasing. This is due to people like Dr Barry Bloom who have put tuberculosis on the media agenda but it is also due to the problems of AIDS, the startling resistance to drug therapy and the increase in cases. All of these problems bind us together to make the point that this is a shared problem. It makes it easier for us to show that if society invests, the benefits accrue to society. This is not a welfare programme for someone else. This is an investment for all of us.

Second, we benefit from the political interest in health that has developed very recently. Heads of state have discovered it is important to be interested in health. In September 1990, 71 heads of state met at the UN to discuss and make commitments to child health. To give only two examples, Mexico now reviews where they stand on those commitments every 6 months and the review is chaired by the head of state, President Salinas. Mrs Mubarek has continued to work with the Ministry of Health in Egypt to make sure that targets are being reached. In addition, President Clinton has not only shown his interest in health care reform but in public health with increased funding for immunization.

Third, there is a new scientific momentum in tuberculosis. Dr Paul Fine talks in his paper about 'immunologists with the courage to study this disease.' We are seeing increased interest and courage from the scientific community.

Fourth, the World Bank's World Development Report 1993, 'Investing in Health,' will be a watershed report. Keeping in mind the questions raised yesterday by Paul Fine, this report will now allow us to present a case not available before. We will be able to combine the impact of morbidity and mortality into a single number. We will be able to compare low mortality problems, such as Guinea worm, with high mortality problems such as meningitis. We will be able to compare traditional health problems with problems that have not been viewed in the domain of health. For example, the report shows that the impact of war in Africa exceeds the impact of cancer. And it allows us to do reasonable cost-effectiveness calculations and comparisons.

This report will become a powerful force in resource allocation decisions. This is important because the major medical–ethical battlefield of today is not in debate over the beginning of life or when to end life. The major battleground is in resource allocation. Ethicists often lack interest in the budget process and budget planners fail to see themselves as ethicists. This report could provide us with new tools.

If this meeting is successful, it could be similar to the 1984 Bellagio meeting on immunization sponsored by the Rockefeller Foundation. At that time less than 20% of children in the world had received their indicated immunizations. The principals at WHO, UNICEF, the World Bank and UNDP agreed to follow a single global plan on immunization, to meet every 3 months to share plans and experiences and to collaborate on providing compatible advice to countries. By 1990 immunization rates had increased from less than 20% to 80%.

So I end up with great hope that the same type of collaboration could develop for tuberculosis.

Public health lessons from other programmes

The basics of public health are applicable to a wide variety of problems. One must be careful not to claim greater lessons from experiences than they actually contain. However, there are five areas where lessons seem possible.

1. *Defining the problem.* This meeting has helped us to know what is known and what is needed. Nothing is more basic to epidemiology and to public health than adequate surveillance. What are the facts? Whatever the disease, accurate information is more likely to inspire political leaders to move. One example. guinea worm in Nigeria was reported only a few thousand times per year. A single survey demonstrated over 650 000 cases at one time and the President of Nigeria was so impressed that he pledged $1 million which in turn attracted outside resources. Nigeria is well on the way to eradicating guinea worm at this time.

With tuberculosis it is hard to overstate the problem. A few years ago, measles was the single most lethal agent known to the world with some 3 million deaths a year. Global immunization has changed that to the point that the most lethal agents now known to the world are tuberculosis and tobacco, with tuberculosis the most lethal microorganism. This must be conveyed to the world.

2. *Defining the best interventions.* It is important that you provide a vision of what could be done, based on the best science available, including an analysis of costs and effectiveness and a demonstration of what could be done at different resource levels.

It is also important that there be some agreement on that vision. Fragmenting the field may be great intellectual sport but the price is certainly paid in illness and death. We should ask:

- What can be done with what we have?
- What could be done with more resources?
- What could be done with better tools?
- What are reasonable targets?

When there is agreement of the experts, money will follow the plan. In 1984, Robert MacNamara suggested that the agreements on immunization should lead us to seek $100 million in external funds each year for the global programme. Most people argued that such funds were unrealistic and if found would have to be taken from other health programmes. MacNamara was correct and within 3 years no one would have settled any longer with $100 million per year.

Advocacy is also easier if scientists have reached an agreement. In 1985, President Reagan proposed a decrease in child survival funds for USAID. Instead, Congress voted a $100 million increase in the appropriation. An article in the *American Journal of Public Health* has traced that decision to the work of Bread For The World, an organization that alerted members to the possibilities in child survival, which in turn led to a flow of letters to members of Congress and an increase in funds.

There are two kinds of futurists: those who predict what will happen and those who actually change what happens. We need, collectively, to change what happens to the future of tuberculosis.

A vision, a plan, and good use of the World Bank analysis will be a very powerful argument.

3. *Improving the implementation strategy.* There is a great deal of experience in the Expanded Programme of Immunization (EPI), Diarrhoeal Disease Control, Acute Respiratory Infections and the UNICEF programme to draw on regarding surveillance, management, training, and evaluation. Continuous inspection is a mainstay. In the India smallpox programme we would use the motto that 'You get what you inspect, not what you expect.' The work is tedious but necessary. As William Blake has said, 'If we are to do good it must be in minute particulars. General good is the plea of the scoundrel. Art and science cannot exist but in minutely organized particulars.

4. *Outcomes.* Put a heavy emphasis on outcomes and provide rewards or recognition based on outcomes. Ambulatory care, diagnostic approaches, therapeutic approaches are all obviously important, but if the reward system is based on outcomes it makes the provider responsible for compliance, rather than the patient, it makes the provider responsible for stains for laboratory work, it makes the provider ultimately responsible for everything.

5. *Research.* We must provide a vision for research as part of the implementation plan. It is not something separate. We have heard repeatedly in the last two days that we have the tools. We have had the tools for smallpox eradication since 1796. Countries actually eliminated smallpox with liquid vaccine and straight pins. But freeze-dried vaccine and bifurcated needles made it much easier. When EPI added a research and development programme to their operations it quickly became one of the most exciting and effective parts of the programme

with over 200 research projects on everything from cold chain improvements and vaccine trials to better motor-cycle maintenance.

We heard yesterday that field needs should drive our research. The best field workers ultimately are those who are seeking better answers, and the best researchers are those who see their ideas implemented. Keep research and implementation intimately tied.

In research it is also important to have a vision of what you would like. In 1985, at an immunization meeting in Colombia, a hope was expressed for vaccine changes which would allow children to have lifetime protection with a single visit that combined vaccines, required no boosters, eliminated adverse reactions and used heat stable vaccines. Since then the Children's Vaccine Initiative has developed to seek that vision.

The same could be done for tuberculosis by using the ideas expressed in the last two days and putting them into a bold summary even if it appears impractical. We would like, for example, a vaccine that is protective against all forms of tuberculosis for life, usable in both skin test positive and negative persons, at any time after birth.

We would also like diagnostic tests that are inexpensive, non-invasive, easy to interpret and can be read without delay. It would be nice to combine what we heard yesterday into tests that differentiate active disease from exposure, BCG from disease, all with a single urine test that uses luciferase, or something similar, to activate different colours on a dipstick. You see how easy it is to develop an approach if you have no idea what you are talking about!

The research vision should include sustained release therapeutics to get away from the horrendous logistics problems that we are accepting as normal.

As part of the research agenda, until we have a better vaccine, we should revisit BCG. We do not know the relative value of BCG vaccines or in which geographic areas they might work. We do not have basic cost-effectiveness calculations to compare with other interventions. We ignore these knowledge gaps by saying that BCG is so inexpensive that it is not a major issue. But for every dollar spent on BCG we tie up an additional 10 dollars in storage, transportation and administration. We owe the world a more responsible approach. You heard Dr George Comstock of the Johns Hopkins School of Hygiene and Public Health suggest, this morning, a study that could give some answers in a few years, if a number of countries were willing to switch the type of BCG they were using on 1 January. With a few vaccines, changed in a few countries, following the cohorts of children over a few years, it should be possible to place relative values on the different vaccines used. Will it surprise you to know that Dr Comstock made that same proposal to WHO 20 years ago? Think where we might be if there had been action at that time.

Finally, yesterday, Dr Barry Bloom reminded us that it requires cooperation of the entire immune system to provide protection to the individual. Likewise, it requires cooperation of the entire social response system (and that means everyone in this room) to provide protection to society. We started on Monday with a prediction that we would end up saying we need 'more commitment, collaboration and generosity.' That was not a bad prediction.

There are many lessons we could take from other programmes. Lessons on surveillance, collaboration, interventions, simplification, inspection and evaluation. But certainly the most important lesson is the need for global collaboration. And there is great urgency. Tuberculosis is going ahead with its own implementation plan whether or not we put a better control plan in motion.

The question is not whether we will determine the future. We are writing that this very moment. The question is whether we will make the future better.

Back to the future: 'the ten commitments'

Keith P.W.J. McAdam

London School of Hygiene & Tropical Medicine, UK

In looking to the future we have to be careful to learn from the lessons of the past so beautifully illustrated for us by Bill Foege. However, we should pause for the thoughts of Sir Theodore Fox, a previous editor of *The Lancet*, who wrote

> We shall have to learn to refrain from doing things, merely because we know how to do them.

I have an illustration which might appeal to some of you who have been swimming or surfing in the sea. Perhaps you have felt the irresistible force of an undertow which makes some beaches so dangerous. Try as you might to fight against the current it merely exhausts you in your attempts to swim back to shore. This is an alarming situation even for strong swimmers who have a surf board. The temptation is to swim harder and exhaust yourself against the current, while nearby others seem to be catching waves which take them to the shore. Paradoxically the secret is to swim sideways or even to relax and allow the current to carry you round to another wave which can take you to shore.

At present the tuberculosis problem seems insuperable in some situations and it requires lateral thought and perhaps unlikely solutions for us to achieve the goal of TB control. We must be prepared even to challenge current dogma and to test alternative hypotheses, but only to be convinced by the best objective and scientific criteria.

It may sound trite but *the tuberculosis solution lies in identifying the key problems*, both as they exist today and as we can predict them in the future.

We have heard about the great changes in the global picture of tuberculosis that have emerged over the last 7 years: the incidence is rising, drug resistance of alarming proportions is being reported and the AIDS epidemic is like a tidal wave bringing in new susceptible immunocompromised people. They not only reactivate their latent *Mycobacterium tuberculosis* infection but also they are at higher risk of being infected.

This meeting has certainly helped to identify many problems and if we accept George Bernard Shaw's challenge in the preface to his book *The Doctor's Dilemma*, then 'All problems are *finally* scientific problems.'

Tuberculosis: Back to the Future. Edited by J.D.H. Porter and K.P.W.J. McAdam
© 1994 John Wiley & Sons Ltd

The secret for the scientist therefore is to ask the right questions. Sir Peter Medawar in his book *The Art of the Soluble* put it a slightly different way.

Let me quote: 'If politics is the art of the possible, research is surely the art of the soluble. Both are immensely practical-minded affairs. Good scientists study the most important problems they think they can solve. It is, after all, their professional business to *solve* problems, not merely to grapple with them.'

My thesis is therefore that the problems facing us in tuberculosis require urgent solution. They are not only *urgent* and therefore timely, but also *important*, so merit scientific investment. This may be self-evident to those scientists attending this Forum but that is not enough. We need *commitment* from many different sectors of society if tuberculosis is going to be controlled and not allowed to escalate out of control.

One key to the future is illustrated by the mix of disciplines attending this Forum: we need a multidisciplinary approach to the problems facing us. No longer can the social scientist ignore the advances of the basic sciences. Similarly, the basic scientists who pride themselves on objectivity will fail to make an impact on tuberculosis if they do not collaborate with their colleagues in the increasingly less subjective disciplines of social sciences.

The biotechnology revolution, of which we are currently an integral part, is a movement of heroic dimensions. We have heard about molecular genetics, gene transfer, cytokines, molecular modelling, polymerase chain reaction and molecular epidemiology but let us not be fooled into thinking that these are merely techniques. These are dependable ways to seek the solutions to critical problems in tuberculosis, to make the diagnosis quickly and identify drug-resistant organisms, to produce a new vaccine and design new drugs.

In parallel the social science disciplines need to be drawn increasingly into finding solutions to the critical problems of how to improve compliance, how to provide effective health education, how to lobby for political partnership and national resources.

Perhaps it is helpful to imagine a giant walking with a dwarf in that tall grass which I grew up to call 'elephant grass.' Neither can see anything but grass, even on tiptoes, they are being cut by the sharp blades of grass, and are frustrated by lack of vision of the way out of their rustling captivity. It is only when they hit on the unlikely idea of *collaboration* that the dwarf stands on the giant's shoulders and catches a vision of the way ahead and out of their painful situation.

Fine words are not enough, hopes are not enough. If the problem is *urgent* and *important* we must have confidence in our ability to find solutions and seek national and international commitments to make them work.

The first commitment, I suggest, is to strengthening and enabling of national tuberculosis control programmes (Commitment 1). Much has been spoken at this meeting and written about this but let us remember Dixie Snider's warning 'If you do what you always did, you'll get what you always got.' There are still countries without TB control programmes and although there must be flexibility to

- **Finding smear-positive cases**
- **Affordable treatment**
- **Compliance**
- **Management structures**
- **Adequate finance**

Commitment 1 National TB control programmes

accommodate differences in management in different countries, the principles of tuberculosis control are well established and they have been shown to work. Identifying infectious tuberculosis cases who have bacteria in their sputum smears is the top priority. These infectious cases then require adequate, affordable drug treatment which is sustainable for the necessary duration, demanding compliance from patients but also from the health delivery system. In order to sustain these practical goals, there has to be a well organized management structure, fitting in with the national health care model and adequate finance to sustain the planned programme.

Before allowing science fiction to carry us to the future, let me reaffirm the importance of continued support and evaluation of existing diagnostic services (Commitment 2).

Case finding	**Active/passive**
Education	**National/local targeted**
Sputum smear	**Supplies**
Culture	**Quality control**
	Sentinel laboratories
Chest X-ray	
Trial of treatment	
Polymerase chain reaction	
	Colour
	Single tube
	Decrease contamination
Phage	**Luminescence**
Drug resistance markers	
	Probes/PCR

Commitment 2 Faster diagnosis

Passive case finding of symptomatic patients at health centres is dependent on trained health workers but active case finding through community surveys should detect TB cases with chronic cough even earlier. Health education about tuberculosis and lung disease can be targeted at different populations to assist with earlier diagnosis. Sputum smear is the most widely used diagnostic test but it demands skilled and very patient technicians, supplies of slides and stains, a microscope and adequate sputum samples. Culture facilities for *Mycobacterium tuberculosis* are a greatly underrated resource in most countries. Many countries only have one sentinel laboratory but how important this is as a reference centre! There needs to be a commitment to maintaining it, providing quality control, perhaps organized *regionally* or *internationally*.

In affluent countries chest X-rays are a helpful diagnostic facility and often the first screening test undertaken. In the AIDS era, non-typical X-ray appearances of tuberculosis are frequent. Often a trial of treatment first with a broad-spectrum antibiotic and then with anti-TB therapy is a standard diagnostic procedure for management of suspected cases, particularly children.

Molecular methods of diagnosis are exciting new developments, already in research practice in affluent countries. We must be committed to developing appropriate technology for the less affluent countries to reduce bacterial identification from 8 weeks and antibacterial sensitivity tests from 12 plus weeks to a few days. Let us not be defeated by worries of contamination but develop foolproof, simplified and affordable diagnostic tests, using these exciting new technologies. You will recall that diagnostic serology for infectious diseases using ELISA technology was developed 30 years ago but it took the HIV epidemic to make ELISA-based tests available everywhere in the world. There is every reason why we should demand new molecular methods be made appropriate, affordable and available just as widely in the future, perhaps using the same optical readouts as ELISA assays. Making new assays work in the laboratory is only the start of the challenge. The tests have to be made into kits, commercialized, manufactured, distributed and popularized in the Third World. This process is expensive and will require special financial support, since commercial organizations are unlikely to make money on the product.

Increasing patient compliance is perhaps the most pressing challenge to those who wish to control TB (Commitment 3). Supervised or directly observed therapy is the ideal but optimal intermittent regimens using long-acting drugs, perhaps given once a week, would help improve compliance. Different incentives for patients must be tested and are clearly dependent on the finance, social structure and culture of each community. In some situations travel costs are reimbursed, drugs are free and even salary is given to patients on treatment. In other countries effective programmes have demanded payment from those requiring anti-TB therapy, which may be reimbursed, with interest on successful completion of chemotherapy. We have heard about alternative distribution systems and the debate about using existing primary health care structures. Encouraging and *empowering*

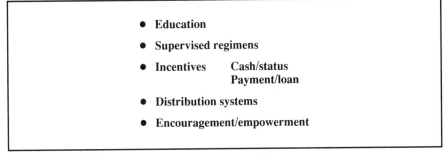

Commitment 3   Increasing patient compliance

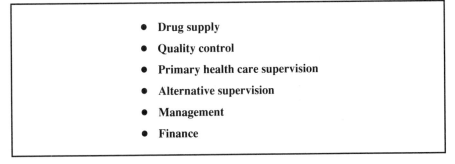

Commitment 4   Increasing programme compliance

patients and communities to take on these important responsibilities must be the ideal way forward. Let us commit ourselves to testing and implementing ways to optimize patient compliance.

Failure to take medication is often not the fault of the patient but of the TB programme (Commitment 4). Drugs are either not available or of dubious quality. The demanding national issues of selecting an essential drug list, procurement of antituberculous drugs at optimal prices and distribution of drugs to health centres requires skilled logistics management, as we heard from Diana Weil and Richard Laing. Supervision of local health services demands a robust management structure and adequate finance to support these services. Since poor compliance leads to multiple drug resistance there must be a commitment to ensuring that drugs are available. The philosophy urged by Philip Hopewell is worth repeating 'that successful completion of therapy is the responsibility of the provider and the programme.'

Education underlies all our efforts at TB control (Commitment 5). Although national education programmes via the media can help, targeted education towards highly influential groups needs to be a priority. Politicians, medical and paramedical workers, traditional healers, shopkeepers and pharmacists, teachers

- **Targeted (highly influential) groups**
  Politicians
  Medical and paramedical workers
  Traditional healers
  Shopkeepers/pharmacists
  Teachers/pastors

- **Targeted (high risk activity) groups**
  Sex workers
  Police/armed forces
  Driver
  Businesses

Commitment 5   Education

and pastors are all important as they can then act as teachers themselves. In the tropics and in poor socio-economic situations, those who are HIV-positive today are at risk of tuberculosis tomorrow: so education targeted at early detection or perhaps TB chemoprophylaxis in those who are at high risk of HIV is indicated.

The HIV epidemic has taught us many lessons in public health education and particularly that the most effective messages are relayed by individuals who are talking to and identifying with their own peer group.

The commitment to new drugs (Commitment 6) is a challenge to the pharmaceutical industry but also to governments who encourage research and can

- **Pharmaceutical/commercial interest**
- **National priority**
  Research
  Partnership with industry
- **Change formulation**
  Screen old compounds
  Combinations
- **Drug resistance**
- **New strategies**
- **TB genome project**
- **Animal models**

Commitment 6   New drugs

enhance commercial involvement, perhaps using incentive schemes in partnership with academic institutions and industry. New formulations to give longer bioavailability of existing or new compounds are urgently needed. New strategies are required to develop antimycobacterial agents which kill multiple-drug-resistant organisms and drugs which penetrate both the intracellular compartment and the areas of caseous necrosis. The TB genome project will help towards this goal but animal models are also needed for *in vivo* screening of potentially useful drugs. If we are not careful we can lull ourselves into a false sense of security, that we already have all the drugs we need. Not only must we keep ahead of drug-resistant mutants but I am not convinced that we yet have an effective sterilizing drug which kills persisters or dormant bacilli and which penetrates the areas of caseous necrosis.

Francis Bacon wrote in 1620 'He that will not apply new remedies must expect new evils, for time is the greatest innovator.'

- **Education**
- **Prevent transmission:**   **Sexually transmitted diseases**
  Condoms
  Screen blood supply
  Drug abuse
- **Slow down progression**   *Pneumocystis*
  Reduce cofactors   **Tuberculosis**

  (Antivirals)

Commitment 7   Appropriate intervention for HIV disease

In the affluent countries of the world huge resources are being spent on treating those who are HIV-positive (Commitment 7). Life expectancy after seroconversion is, on average, 11 or more years, and the most effective interventions to date have been prophylaxis of the major opportunistic infections particularly against *Pneumocystis*. So far, antivirals have prolonged life expectancy by only about a year.

At the present time, in developing countries interventions have been limited to: education about HIV transmission, some use of condoms and screening of blood supplies.

Figure 1 shows CD4 count on the vertical axis and years after seroconversion on the horizontal axis. In affluent countries the CD4 count slowly falls leading to AIDS by a mean of 11 years, and antivirals, when given at a low CD4 count below 400, prolongs life by up to a year. In the tropics the data are not so clear but it appears that the natural history of HIV disease is faster with the loss of CD4 cells perhaps speeded up by recurrent infections and especially tuberculosis. Giving antivirals is not going to help this situation much and a more relevant intervention is to prevent the endemic infections which stimulate CD4 cell

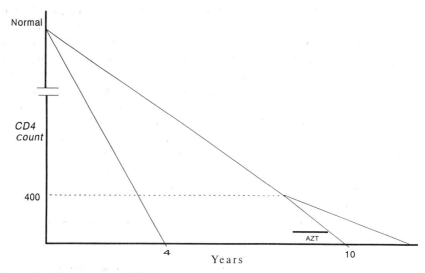

Figure 1   The evolution of HIV disease

proliferation and viral replication.

Many studies in the developing world are still documenting seroprevalence in different groups, rather than measuring the impact of interventions.

The HIV epidemic is like a fire burning on the living room carpet. We are observing the speed at which it spreads, the noxious fumes and particulate content in the smoke. We must intervene to help put out the fire.

Tuberculosis is the most obvious infection to try and prevent and several studies are currently in progress to look at the efficacy of different chemoprophylactic regimens. Although there is some evidence of efficacy in preventing reactivation of TB and slowing progression to AIDS, it would be a mistake to implement this intervention until compelling evidence is available—not only for efficacy but for feasibility of implementation and cost-effectiveness of the intervention. It seems unlikely that chemoprophylaxis will ever be feasible for HIV-positives on a national scale but more likely targeted to special groups such as occupational groups. However, there is a compelling logic to offer chemoprophylaxis to those who test HIV-positive in TB endemic areas as an incentive for voluntary HIV testing. In some countries, like Zambia, the person in the Ministry of Health who is responsible for TB control (Roland Msiska) is now also in charge of the AIDS programme. These linkages provide new opportunities for linked initiatives.

No longer can we watch the epidemic spread and expect the growing numbers of HIV positives to remain silent. Their increasing clamour for intervention demands our attention. Answers are needed urgently about the efficacy and feasibility of using TB chemoprophylaxis in this group.

Hypersensitivity skin reactions to sulphur containing drugs, cotrimoxazole and

- **TB genome project**
- **Defining protective immunity**
- **Protective vaccine**
- **Therapeutic vaccine**
- **Polyvaccine**

Commitment 8   A new vaccine

thiacetazone are now well documented in about 20% of HIV-positives and challenge us to provide guidelines for treating HIV-positive TB patients in situations where thiacetazone is still part of the standard tuberculosis therapy.

The TB genome project allows us to predict confidently a great increase in understanding of *M. tuberculosis* proteins, antigens, cell wall components and potential drug targets. Despite 50 years of BCG we still cannot define protective immunity to tuberculosis. Let us commit ourselves to a better vaccine than BCG with protective and perhaps also therapeutic potential (Commitment 8). The ability to transfer DNA into and out of mycobacteria allows for the realization of the exciting dream of a multivalent vaccine, carrying immunogenic determinants against several different pathogens, potentially being carried inside a fast growing mycobacteria, which has such a good inbuilt adjuvant activity.

Finally, unless we can convince presidents and politicians that tuberculosis is a national priority, the epidemic of TB will continue to increase alarmingly, particularly in Africa, Asia and Central and South America. TB is a disease of poverty but, with the HIV epidemic, its potential to spread to and from immunodeficient individuals makes it an urgent priority. We have the tools to contain the epidemic. The biotechnology revolution is giving us new and improved tools but unless there is a political will to support TB control, many will die unnecessarily. It seems likely to me that the Dean of the London School of Hygiene and Tropical Medicine Richard Feachem's prediction will soon be true that the

- **National priority**
  Health
  Education
  Finance
- **Special interest groups**
- **Community care**

Commitment 9   Commitment to political partnership

DALY, the disability adjusted life year, will become part of the everyday language of those who have to make the decisions about funding priorities. There will be great interest in the underlying assumptions taken to arrive at morbidity effects in the World Bank's *World Development Report* on health published in July 1993 and in the report on the *Global Burden of Disease*. However, the conclusions about cost-effective interventions are likely to be highly influential in guiding resource allocation. The 3–6 fold increase suggested for TB control programmes provides a valuable mandate for effective advocacy for support of the TB effort.

Political pressure can be generated by *national and international special interest groups, by the press* and by *those working in the community* (Commitment 9). There are many of those people here today. Let us challenge each other not to accept defeat but to foster a partnership with politicians to fight this highly emotive and dangerous but curable and preventable disease.

- **National TB control programmes**
- **Faster diagnosis**
- **Patient compliance**
- **Programme compliance**
- **Education**
- **Affordable new drugs**
- **HIV interactions**
- **New vaccine**
- **Political partnership**

Figure 2   Commitments for the future

Figure 2 might look like a tablet of stone containing the 10 commitments but the numerate amongst you will notice only 9 are listed. The final commitment is to fight *Poverty* and that demands a much wider commitment internationally to reducing the economic inequalities which allow tuberculosis to remain such a preventable scourge all over the world.

Rather than be divided about our goals let us reassert our commitment to controlling this disease. Biomedical, clinical and social sciences all have an important part to play in the battle against TB and this meeting has reminded us how valuable it is to share aspirations with those who are developing and managing control programmes. What we need to find now are the resources and people to allow the dreams of controlling tuberculosis effectively to become a reality.

Index

Index compiled by A.C. Purton